HOOKED

Explorations in Bioethics and the Medical Humanities

Series Editor: James Lindemann Nelson

This series aims to include the most theoretically sophisticated, challenging, and original work being produced in the areas of bioethics, literature and medicine, law and medicine, philosophy of medicine, and history of medicine. *Explorations in Bioethics and the Medical Humanities* also features authoritative contributions to educational contexts and to public discourse on the meaning of health and health care in contemporary culture and on the difficult questions concerning the best directions for biomedicine to take in the future.

Dubious Equalities and Embodied Differences: Cultural Studies on Cosmetic Surgery
  by Kathy Davis

Hippocrates' Maze: Ethical Explorations of the Medical Labyrinth
  by James Lindemann Nelson

Healing the Self: Ethical Issues in Chronic Illness, Rehabilitation, and Palliative Care
  by Bruce Jennings

Mass Hysteria: Medicine, Culture, and Mothers' Bodies
  by Rebecca Kukla

Hooked: Ethics, the Medical Profession, and the Pharmaceutical Industry
  by Howard Brody

HOOKED

Ethics, the Medical Profession, and the Pharmaceutical Industry

Howard Brody

ROWMAN & LITTLEFIELD PUBLISHERS, INC.
Lanham • Boulder • New York • Toronto • Plymouth, UK

ROWMAN & LITTLEFIELD PUBLISHERS, INC.

Published in the United States of America
by Rowman & Littlefield Publishers, Inc.
A wholly owned subsidiary of The Rowman & Littlefield Publishing Group, Inc.
4501 Forbes Boulevard, Suite 200, Lanham, Maryland 20706
www.rowmanlittlefield.com

Estover Road
Plymouth PL6 7PY
United Kingdom

British Library Cataloguing in Publication Information Available

Library of Congress Cataloging-in-Publication Data

Brody, Howard.
  Hooked : ethics, the medical profession, and the pharmaceutical industry / Howard Brody.
    p. ; cm. — (Explorations in bioethics and the medical humanities)
  Includes index.
  ISBN-13: 978-0-7425-5218-0 (cloth : alk. paper)
  ISBN-10: 0-7425-5218-7 (cloth : alk. paper)
  1. Medical ethics. 2. Pharmaceutical industry—Moral and ethical aspects. 3. Physicians—Professional ethics. I. Title. II. Series.
  [DNLM: 1. Ethics, Medical—United States. 2. Conflict of Interest—United States. 3. Drug Industry—United States. 4. Physicians—United States. 5. Public Policy—United States. W 50 B8643h 2007]
  R724.B76 2007
  174.2'951—dc22   2006018423

Printed in the United States of America

∞™ The paper used in this publication meets the minimum requirements of American National Standard for Information Sciences—Permanence of Paper for Printed Library Materials, ANSI/NISO Z39.48-1992.

If we put horse manure in a capsule, we could sell it to 95 percent of these doctors.

—Harry Loynd, president of Parke,
Davis and Company, 1951–1967

CONTENTS

ACKNOWLEDGMENTS

A great many people have assisted me in the research and writing of this volume. I have tried to note all of them in specific endnotes, and apologize to anyone I have missed.

I turned at various times to Bob Goodman, Joel Lexchin, Peter Mansfield, Mike Wilkes, Jeanne Lenzer, and John Abramson for advice and assistance. I especially value the support and counsel of Rick Bukata and Jerry Hoffman. My involvement with their "Primary Care Medical Abstracts" courses aided me in identifying literature and shaped my views on the deleterious impact of pharmaceutical funding on physician education. Many colleagues in the Department of Family Practice and in the Center for Ethics and Humanities in the Life Sciences, Michigan State University, supported and encouraged my research.

Anders Kelto served as my student research assistant and assisted me with the initial stages of accumulating a computerized bibliography. Anders joined me and my faculty colleagues John Goddeeris and Andy Hogan in a research study of the financial aspects of the medicine-pharmaceutical interface. While this project did not lead to the hoped-for publication, I have made use of our findings at several places in this volume.

Neill Bogan, Carl Elliott, and Jim Nelson read the manuscript and made helpful suggestions.

My thanks to the Rowman and Littlefield staff: acquisitions editor Chris Anzalone, production editor Marian E. Haggard, and copyeditor Gary J. Hamel.

A final note: The pharmaceutical industry and the medical profession represent a moving target. Readers who are aware of the most recent breaking news often wonder how to interpret what a book author says about a topic, not knowing how long before the passage they are reading was actually written. So, for the record, I would like to note that I largely completed work on this manuscript in July 2005. I continued to make small revisions into the early months of 2006; most of those later revisions are so identified in the endnotes.

ABBREVIATIONS

AAFP	American Academy of Family Physicians
AARP	American Association of Retired Persons
ACCME	Accreditation Council for Continuing Medical Education
ACT UP	AIDS Coalition to Unleash Power
AG	Attorney General
AIDS	Acquired Immunodeficiency Syndrome
AMA	American Medical Association
AWP	average wholesale price
BAM	Business for Affordable Medicine
CAUT	Canadian Association of University Teachers
CCOHTA	Canadian Coordinating Office for Health Technology Assessment
CDC	Centers for Disease Control [currently, Centers for Disease Control and Prevention]
CEO	Chief Executive Officer
CLASS	Celecoxib Long-Term Arthritis Safety Study
CMD	Current Medical Directions
CME	continuing medical education
CML	chronic myelogenous leukemia
COX-2	cyclo-oxygenase-2 inhibitor drug
CRO	contract-research organization
DHEW	Department of Health, Education, and Welfare [currently, DHHS]
DHHS	Department of Health and Human Services
DM	district manager
DSM	*Diagnostic and Statistical Manual of Mental Disorders*
DTC	direct-to-consumer
DTCA	direct-to-consumer advertising

EKG	electrocardiogram
FDA	Food and Drug Administration
FTC	Federal Trade Commission
GIST	gastrointestinal stromal tumor
GP	general practitioner
HCFA	Health Care Financing Administration [currently, Centers for Medicare and Medicaid Services (CMS)]
HHS	[U.S. Department of] Health and Human Services
HIPAA	Health Insurance Portability and Accountability Act
HIV	human immunodeficiency virus
HMO	health maintenance organization
HRG	[Public Citizen] Health Research Group
IBS	irritable bowel syndrome
ICU	intensive care unit
IND	investigational new drug
MADD	Mothers Against Drunk Drivers
MECC	medical education and communications company
MIT	Massachusetts Institute of Technology
NCI	National Cancer Institute
NHLBI	National Heart, Lung, and Blood Institute
NIH	National Institutes of Health
NIPD	National Institute of Pharmaceutical Development [hypothetical]
NSAID	nonsteroidal anti-inflammatory drug
OIG	Office of the Inspector General
PBM	pharmacy benefit manager
PDA	personal digital assistant
PDUFA	Prescription Drug User Fee Act
PhRMA	Pharmaceutical Research and Manufacturers of America
R&D	research and development
SLAPP	strategic lawsuit against public participation
SMO	site-management organization
SSRI	selective serotonin re-uptake inhibitors
TRIPS	trade-related intellectual property agreement
UCLA	University of California at Los Angeles
UCSF	University of California at San Francisco
USDA	United States Department of Agriculture
VA	Veterans Administration
VIGOR	Vioxx Gastrointestinal Outcomes Research
WHO	World Health Organization
WTO	World Trade Organization

Introduction

THE TIPPING POINT

Tom and Ray Magliozzi, the *Car Talk* guys on National Public Radio, couldn't stop laughing as they described the poetic justice that once befell one of their acquaintances. The fellow was driving home from work during the wee hours of the morning when he passed an unguarded construction site. Right next to the street stood a pile of brand-new, four-by-eight-foot sheets of half-inch plywood—exactly what he needed for a home remodeling project. He decided upon what the old Army veterans used to call a "midnight requisition," and piled a dozen sheets of plywood on the top of his car. This being a spur-of-the-moment larceny, he had no rope to tie down the load. But he reasoned that if he drove slowly—he was only a few blocks from his house—nothing would happen. Hardly any other cars were on the road that late. The pile of wood seemed to weigh a ton; it wouldn't be going anywhere.

All went well until the one other car on the road at that hour cut suddenly in front of him at an intersection. He touched the brakes as gently as he could. As the Magliozzi brothers described it between guffaws, he then saw events occurring through his windshield as if in special-effects slow motion. Each sheet of plywood slid forward, one at a time, and landed in the street in front of his car. As each sheet slid forward, it took with it some portion of the automobile—the grill, the headlights, the front fenders, the hood. Finally he contemplated a pile of plywood and most of the front end of his car lying in the middle of the intersection.[1]

The plywood had reached what Malcolm Gladwell calls "the tipping point."[2] The tipping point is a common feature of social change. Before one reaches the tipping point, it appears that the social system is firmly stuck where it is. Perhaps people have for years tried to reform or alter it, but its inertia has frustrated all their efforts. Suddenly, once the tipping point is reached, the very inertia that previously frustrated change now pushes the change forward more rapidly, and more powerfully, than anyone could have guessed.

Another feature of the tipping point is that it appears at first glance to be an event of little consequence—no different than all the other tiny shoves that people have been applying to the stuck system for a long time without visible result. It follows that at the moment it occurs, one would hardly ever be correct in claiming that the tipping point had been reached. (Any more than the Magliozzi brothers' acquaintance could have been able to guess in advance what exactly was going to happen when he put his foot on the brake.) Only in hindsight would one as a rule be confident in identifying the tipping point.

What does all this have to do with the medical profession and the pharmaceutical industry?

A tipping point of sorts may have occurred in the spring of 2004. The event that later history might pick out from all that happened was a legal action filed by the attorney general (AG) of the state of New York, Eliot L. Spitzer, on June 2. The AG accused the giant drug firm GlaxoSmithKline of fraud. Many lawsuits had been filed in the previous several years by states' attorneys general against major drug firms, all claiming fraud. Those suits were mostly based on the allegation that the firms were overcharging the state Medicaid systems for their drugs by manipulating the pricing structure. The firms were supposed to charge Medicaid the lowest price they charged any customer, but companies had found a variety of ways to hide the fact that they had charged some favored buyers less than they were charging Medicaid.

But the New York fraud charges were quite different. Spitzer alleged that GlaxoSmithKline had deliberately concealed the results of four research studies of the antidepressant drug Paxil when used in children and adolescents. These four studies all showed that the drug either did not work well or that it caused harm. By contrast, a fifth study was interpreted to show that Paxil was helpful in treating childhood depression.[3] The firm rapidly published and then gave considerable publicity to the fifth study, while doing its best to conceal from the medical community the contrary results of the other four studies.

In 2003, British government regulators ruled that Paxil should not be used in the treatment of depression in children and adolescents because cases of suicide were more frequent among younger patients using that and a few similar drugs. On October 27, 2003, the U.S. Food and Drug Administration (FDA) also issued an advisory to that effect.[4]

The Wall Street Journal, whose editorial page tends to be a strong defender of the pharmaceutical industry, took Spitzer to task for filing this lawsuit. The Journal claimed that this was solely a matter of grandstanding and publicity seeking, since it was the FDA, not the state government of New York, that properly had jurisdiction over the regulation of drugs in the United States. But the Journal's editorial missed part of the point. By filing a more or less unprecedented action on behalf of the state, Spitzer was effectively making a claim about the FDA. He was accusing the FDA of having been sufficiently captured by the pharmaceutical industry so as no longer to be capable of protecting the citizens from potentially ineffective or unsafe drugs. He was claiming that the citizens of New York had no recourse other than to take matters into their own hands.

At about the same time that Spitzer filed his lawsuit, journalist Shannon Brown-lee wrote an article for the *Washington Monthly* with the subtitle, "Why You Can't Trust Medical Journals Anymore." Her target was less the pharmaceutical industry that financed studies like the Paxil trials than the physician-investigators who con-ducted the studies and then willingly did the bidding of the industry in the way that they reported, or failed to report, the results. Brownlee's choice of a subtitle carried with it an important message. In previous years, a vocal minority of physi-cians and scientists had warned ominously (though to little practical effect) that the medical literature was becoming seriously biased as a result of manipulation by the industry. Brownlee may have been one of the first laypeople to grasp fully what this meant for the public health—to fully understand the implications of the pub-lic water hole of scientific information becoming polluted.[5]

Brownlee also chose to frame her dismay in terms of *trust*. As a journalist, she was familiar with the idea of professional ethics. If she wrote an article praising a drug and did not disclose either to the editor or to the readers that she was in the pay of the drug company, she expected certain consequences to follow that would be deleterious to her future career. She could not understand how respected aca-demic physicians could participate in what appeared to be the same sort of behav-ior, yet be allowed to go on about their business as if nothing had happened. You physicians, she seemed to be saying, were supposed to have taken an oath to pro-tect our health. We trusted you. And now you have betrayed our trust.

In the wake of the New York lawsuit, a number of events occurred. Many major U.S. newspapers wrote editorials strongly condemnatory of the pharmaceutical industry, and calling for new legislation to require the publishing of research re-sults in a centralized registry.[6] At the time, most observers knew that a federal clinical trials registry existed—under the tutelage of the National Library of Medi-cine—but assumed that the industry posted its clinical trials in that registry only on a voluntary basis. Later it was revealed, to the surprise even of medical journal editors, that the law required industry compliance. The FDA had issued in 2002 some guidelines to govern industry registration of their clinical trials, but had ap-parently been either unable or unwilling to police the compliance.[7]

GlaxoSmithKline announced soon after that it would immediately begin making public information about all its ongoing clinical trials.[8] Merck and Eli Lilly quickly followed suit.[9] The industry apparently smelled a public relations disaster looming. By comparison, in 2001, Warner-Lambert had been accused by an investigative re-porter for the *Los Angeles Times* of working with compliant FDA officials to keep its diabetes drug, Rezulin, on the market despite mounting evidence that it was causing deaths from liver failure.[10] No public outcry followed that revelation and no state government filed suit against Warner-Lambert. The deaths of middle-aged people with diabetes apparently did not have a strong grip on the public psyche. The allega-tion that children and teenagers might commit suicide as a result of taking an antide-pressant medication was a different matter altogether. It seemed all too reminiscent of the thalidomide scare of the early 1960s. A drug that caused babies to be born without arms or legs got one's attention. The realization of how close that drug came to being sold in the United States caused sufficient public concern to move passage in Congress of tough legislation tightening regulation of the drug industry.

On June 30, 2004, the main spokesperson for the industry, the Pharmaceutical Research and Manufacturers of America (PhRMA), announced with some fanfare that it was reissuing and revising its code of ethics for research, calling for the complete and prompt publication of all results, positive or negative. The *New York Times* dismissed this as being purely voluntary and therefore lacking any enforcement teeth.[11] In September, a consortium of international medical journal editors stated that beginning in July 2005, they would refuse to accept for publication any clinical trials that were not registered at a publicly accessible trials registry.[12] This statement carried considerable weight because it seemed unlikely that drug companies would willingly forgo the potential publicity and prestige value of having their clinical trials published in such widely respected journals as the *New England Journal of Medicine* and *JAMA*.

At the end of September, Merck announced that it was voluntarily withdrawing its blockbuster drug, Vioxx, after it was linked to evidence of heart disease and stroke. For the rest of 2004 and into 2005, the media were full of stories about the safety of commonly used drugs, and the relative failure of the FDA to protect the public from these risks.

Perhaps, ten years from now, things will be pretty much as they are today. The industry will still fund the vast majority of clinical drug trials. The physicians who conduct the trials will be eager to maintain their funding and so will report, or fail to report, trial results in ways that favor the outcome that the industry wishes. The medical journals will continue to publish the resulting papers, perhaps duly disclosing the various financial conflicts of interest of the papers' authors, perhaps not. A small number of do-gooders will grumble about it, and the world will go on its way.

Or perhaps, in a decade, things will have changed. Perhaps the national clinical trials registry will have teeth in it. Journal editors will check submitted papers against the data posted in the registry to ensure that their readers are getting the full story. Perhaps the funding of clinical trials will have been taken in part or in whole out of the hands of the drug firms, so that physician-investigators who want research money will no longer feel beholden to individual companies for their support. Perhaps with more public funding of research, studies will be conducted that provide answers that physicians need to know to better treat patients, rather than solely the answers the companies want to know to better market their products. Perhaps physicians themselves will have a higher sense of professional integrity and will routinely refuse to participate in practices that they now just as routinely accept.

If change does occur, perhaps people will look back at the New York lawsuit against GlaxoSmithKline as a turning point in history. Or perhaps, in retrospect, a different event will seem more important. As I write this, it is too soon to tell.

ABOUT THIS BOOK

This book aims to:

- describe the present relationship between the medical profession and the pharmaceutical industry

- assess that relationship from the standpoint of ethics and policy
- where problems are identified, suggest positive changes

Medicine is "hooked" in two ways. In one sense, medicine's relation to the pharmaceutical industry, and the gifts and rewards that it dispenses, has been likened to an addiction. Addiction has been called the "disease of denial," and we will see that denial characterizes many aspects of medicine's assessment of this relationship.

Yet medicine and the pharmaceutical industry are also "hooked" in quite a different way. Remove the industry and its products, and a considerable portion of scientific medicine's power to help the patient vanishes. Once upon a time, physicians could wander out into the woods, gather a basketful of herbs and roots, and proceed to treat patients according to the best scientific standards of the day. Today, medicine and the pharmaceutical industry must find ways to thrive together if patients are to be well served.

My focus in this volume is on the relationship between the medical profession and the pharmaceutical industry—not the industry as a whole, and not on its relationship with the entire society.[13] For example, much of the public debate over pharmaceuticals in 2003–2004 has focused on one issue—the high prices charged for drugs in the United States. There is some connection between drug prices and the industry-profession relationship. Some behaviors of physicians work to drive up drug prices. If drugs cost too much for patients to afford, that affects the physician's professional responsibility to provide care for the patient. Still, I would argue that the high cost of drugs is a general social issue much more than an issue that *directly* arises at the profession-industry interface. Accordingly, I will say relatively little about drug prices and will not make any suggestions in the end that are *specifically* aimed at lowering drug prices.[14]

One might naturally wonder why I have chosen to focus narrowly in this fashion. There are a number of reasons. One is purely practical—it's probably impossible to write a single volume that addresses every aspect of the pharmaceutical industry in today's society. Another reason is a matter of choice—I am a physician, and I worry about the ethics and the integrity of my profession. Yet other reasons have to do with the general public interest. I would contend that it's no accident that medicine is configured as a "profession" in society. The idea of being a professional includes among other features that one is supposed to act in a *trustworthy* way. A profession is not just a way of making money; it's a form of public trust.

A big part of my argument is that medicine has for many decades now been betraying this public trust in the way that it has accepted various benefits from the pharmaceutical industry. Medicine and the industry together have been very creative in thinking up rationalizations to make it seem as if all this behavior really serves the interests of the public after all. And medicine has also managed to convince itself that its world is divided into an on-stage and a backstage portion. Patients, we imagine, see us on stage but cannot peek behind the curtains and see us backstage. So long as some of the embarrassing exchanges between medicine and industry occur backstage, we think that no one will notice and public trust in the profession will not be compromised.

But this on-stage–backstage thinking is wrong in two ways. First of all, the public is now peeking behind the curtain. Shannon Brownlee looked behind the curtain into medical research funding and did not like what she saw. Second, the professional goal is not merely to retain the trust of the public. A good con man, after all, is very good at getting people to trust him. The goal of a profession ought to be *to act in a trustworthy manner, to deserve the trust that people place in it*. Acting in a trustworthy manner often requires us to act *as if* we were on stage even when people cannot see us.

With these goals in mind, here's what comes next. First I will tell the stories of two drugs, Gleevec and Claritin. The Gleevec story is an ideal story from the industry's point of view—a new type of treatment for cancer that as of today appears to be wildly successful. The Claritin story might be the poster child for everything that is wrong with the industry. This poses a major question—what could we do to increase the number of Gleevec stories and to decrease the number of Claritin stories?

Next, because a lot of this book is about ethics and integrity, I need to explain in more detail what those terms mean in this context. I will develop an ethical framework by which we can judge the behavior of both the profession and the industry. This chapter is one big reason why a book like this is needed. Many volumes have been written in recent years about the pharmaceutical industry. But very few explicitly address ethics, and few look specifically at the industry-profession interface.

Much of this book will seem like industry bashing. So I also need to be as fair as I can be. I will next include a chapter in which I try my best to give the industry's point of view on all the issues that this book will address. I'll let the industry "side" present its "case" first. A good part of the remainder of the book will then be devoted to testing the plausibility of the industry's "case."

The large middle portion of the book is organized to illustrate the next big reason why I think this book is needed. The many books and the considerably greater number of articles I was able to identify on this topic generally address one level of the profession-industry interface. Some look at individual physicians accepting gifts from pharmaceutical company sales representatives ("reps"). Some look at universities accepting large research grants from the industry. Some look at how the FDA polices the industry. Some look at the industry's role in continuing medical education programs.

One of my central claims in this book is that *we won't understand the problem, and we won't be able to propose helpful solutions, unless we see how all these levels of activity are interconnected*. Accordingly, in each chapter in this large central portion of the book I will take up one of the levels of concern. In each chapter I will keep two questions in mind:

1. How is this level of activity connected to all the other levels?
2. How does what goes on at this level of activity inform us about the plausibility of the pharmaceutical industry's presentation of its case?

The chapters fall roughly into three groups: pharmaceutical research; activities claimed by the industry to constitute education; and the industry's relationship with its primary regulator, the FDA.

Normally in a book of this length one is doing pretty well simply to talk about the problems that exist today. There generally would not be sufficient space to go into a detailed history of all the parties to the present controversies. I will nevertheless, in some portions of the discussion, take the time to present some historical background. I will argue that with that background some of the difficulties we confront today suddenly start to make a lot more sense. This is especially true with regard to the relationship between physicians and drug reps, and the role of the FDA in regulating the industry.

The final section of the book is concerned with possible solutions. I talk generally about strategies for solutions and then talk in turn about two distinct sorts of solutions. One sort directly addresses physician professionalism. It assumes that unless physicians change how they behave and how they look at each others' behavior, certain things will never improve. We can pass laws and enact regulations, but ultimately a profession has to take responsibility for its own integrity. The second sort of solution does involve laws and regulations, because unless certain things change in the environment, the profession and its individual professionals will be swimming against too strong a current if they try to change their behavior in the needed ways. I argue in this book that unless we address *both* professional integrity and responsibility *and* external laws and regulations, we will not address the issue in its entirety.

I will finally look at two general strategies for solutions—the Management Strategy and the Divestment Strategy. The Management Strategy has been the most popular choice of professional organizations writing guidelines and codes of ethics. It assumes that the relationship between the medical profession and the pharmaceutical industry needs to be a very close one, and so the only viable option for reform is managing its problematic features better. I will argue in favor of the minority view to date, the Divestment Strategy.[15] Reliance on the Management Strategy is one big reason why things have steadily changed for the worse, despite the fact that thoughtful physicians began writing about these problems back in the 1960s and 1970s. I will go so far as to claim that the Management Strategy is in itself a part of the set of rationalizations, mutually constructed by the profession and the industry, constructed to retain the status quo. As radical as the Divestment Strategy sounds, it is the only reasonable way to solve the very serious problems that our analysis will uncover. (As Shannon Brownlee says, when you can no longer trust the "science" that you read in prestigious medical journals, then the problem is serious.) And in fact a careful look at the Divestment Strategy will show that it is not as radical as it is at first made out to be. Ultimately, the medical profession, the pharmaceutical industry, and the larger society will all benefit from a more hands-off sort of relation between medicine and the drug companies.

Finally, in an epilogue, I will discuss a bit of emerging evidence that a time for change may be at hand—that in fact, we have reached a useful tipping point in renegotiating the relationship between the medical profession and the pharmaceutical industry.

NOTES

1. This anecdote was broadcast as part of the National Public Radio program *Car Talk*, broadcast #0323, June 7, 2003.

2. The example I have used involves a "tipping point" that occurs due to laws of Newtonian physics. Gladwell instead has in mind a process of social change that follows the mathematical laws of epidemics; M. Gladwell, *The Tipping Point: How Little Things Can Make a Big Difference* (Boston: Little, Brown, 2000). I prefer my analogy because social change, once it occurs, hardly ever disappears to return to the previous status quo; whereas the "epidemic curve" describes an event that first waxes and then just as surely wanes.

3. I say "interpreted" here because there is some question as to whether the fifth study was actually positive. A memo prepared by physician-investigators within the firm initially considered that study also to be negative. W. Kondro and B. Sibbald, "Drug Company Experts Advised Staff to Withhold Data about SSRI Use in Children," *CMAJ* 2004; 170:783. By the time it was published, the results had apparently been recast in such a way as to make the results appear favorable for Paxil. M. B. Keller, N. D. Ryan, M. Strober, et al., "Efficacy of Paroxetine in the Treatment of Adolescent Major Depression: A Randomized, Controlled Trial," *J Am Acad Child Adolesc Psychiatry* 2001; 40:762–72. See also S. Boseley, "Company 'Held Back' Data on Drug for Children: Antidepressant Had No Effect, Leak Reveals," *The Guardian* (London), February 3, 2004. The leaked memo can be viewed at Alliance for Human Research Protection, "GlaxoSmithKline CEO: 'We had to absorb a number of hits,'" Alliance for Human Research Protection, 2004, www.ahrp.org/infomail/04/02/16.html. See chapter 7 for the means that might be used to distort or "spin" scientific research to reach a conclusion more favorable to the industrial sponsor.

4. FDA Public Health Advisory: Reports of Suicidality in Pediatric Patients Being Treated with Antidepressant Medications for Major Depressive Disorder (MDD) (Washington, DC: FDA Center for Drug Evaluation and Research, Oct. 27, 2003); www.fda.gov/cder/drug/advisory/mdd.htm (accessed August 10, 2004).

5. An earlier article to raise many of the same concerns was M. Kauffman and A. Julien, "Industry Cash a Potent Habit; Medical Research: Can We Trust It?" *Hartford Courant*, April 11, 2000:A1.

6. See for example: "For Truth in Drug Trial Reporting" [editorial], *New York Times*, June 20, 2004:12; "Missing Drug Data" [editorial], *Washington Post*, June 30, 2004:A20.

7. S. Vedantam, "Drugmakers Prefer Silence on Test Data," *Washington Post*, July 6, 2004:A1.

8. B. Meier, "Glaxo Plans Public Listing of Drug Trials on Web Site," *New York Times*, June 19, 2004:C2.

9. B. Meier, "Merck Backs U.S. Database to Track Drug Trials," *New York Times*, June 18, 2004: C1; L. Abboud, "Lilly Plans Broad Access to Results on Its Drug Trials," *Wall Street Journal*, August 3, 2004:B1.

10. D. Willman, "Risk Was Known as FDA OK'd Fatal Drug Study: New Documents Show Warner-Lambert Trivialized Liver Toxicity of Diabetes Pill Rezulin While Seeking Federal Approval," *Los Angeles Times*, March 11, 2001:A1.

11. "For Honest Reports of Drug Trials" [editorial], *New York Times*, September 11, 2004:A14.

12. C. De Angelis, J. M. Drazen, F. A. Fizelle, et al., "Clinical Trial Registration: A statement from the International Committee of Medical Journal Editors" [editorial], *N Engl J Med* 2004; 351:1250–51.

13. Sergio Sismondo, introducing a special issue of the journal *Social Studies of Science* on the pharmaceutical industry, writes, "Physicians' decision-making is the most common

locus of discussion in medical ethics. The papers in this special issue suggest that that is to take a narrow view of the ethical issues, a view that appears to come about because it privileges the position of physicians, both epistemically and ethically"; S. Sismondo, "Pharmaceutical Maneuvers," *Soc Stud Sci* 2004; 34:149–59. I agree that in the grand scheme of things, a physician-centric view of the matter is too narrow to be ideal, but Sigmondo's statement seems to presuppose that the issue has already been exhaustively discussed from the "narrow" viewpoint. My argument in this volume is that the issue has instead been neglected within the "narrow" confines of medical ethics. I would be happy to see this "narrow" study later provide raw material for an appropriately "broad" study of the topic that appropriately relates the medical profession to the larger social context.

14. One argument the industry uses to defend its high U.S. prices is that these profits are needed to fund research. I will directly address the way the industry conducts its research, because those practices lie at the interface between the industry and the medical profession. In the process I will explain, as many others have, why the industry argument about profits and research funding is not convincing.

15. At the time this book was being completed (roughly, before July 2005), the Divestment Strategy appeared to be a distinct minority view. This changed somewhat in January 2006 with a paper in a major medical journal by a number of prominent academic physicians, taking a stance mostly consistent with that strategy; T. A. Brennan, D. J. Rothman, L. Blank, et al., "Health Industry Practices That Create Conflicts of Interest: A Policy Proposal for Academic Medical Centers," *JAMA* 2006; 295:429–33. This paper in turn cited an earlier recommendation for divestment, upon which I have relied in chapter 16; A. Schafer, "Biomedical Conflicts of Interest: A Defence of the Sequestration Thesis—Learning from the Cases of Nancy Olivieri and David Healy," *J Med Ethics* 2004; 30:8–24. In one way, the otherwise excellent discussion by Brennan et al. fell significantly short of my own proposals. They continue to defend direct payment of research grants and contracts from drug companies to universities and hospitals, so long as the grant goes to the institution and not an individual physician-investigator. I call rather for channeling all such research funds through a neutral government agency (chapter 18). I do not have the same level of confidence implied by Brennan et al. that academic institutions can avoid their own conflicts of interest if they depend directly on individual firms for research support.

I

OVERVIEW

1

THE GOOD, THE BAD, AND THE UGLY: A STORY OF TWO MEDICATIONS

Gleevec did not come out of the blue. There is a whole culture at Novartis that puts a focus on the discovery arena. We have been concentrating our efforts for some time on high-risk research, on truly innovative science where the chances of success may be low but a certain investment is still required. Our goal is to benefit the human race in a unique way; we want to be true innovators, bringing new, important drugs to our patients, drugs that cure and prevent diseases, drugs that improve the quality of life.

—Dr. Daniel Vasella, CEO of Novartis[1]

Over a two-month period in the spring of 2001, the American news media carried two stories about the pharmaceutical industry and pharmaceutical research. One story dealt with a new drug, the other with a well-known drug on the market for some time. One story was widely circulated; the other was probably missed by most Americans. Between them the two stories display the different sides of the pharmaceutical industry and its power and highlight the concerns I want to address in this book.

THE GLEEVEC STORY

The first story involves Gleevec (generic name: imatinib), a drug that fits almost anyone's definition of a "medical breakthrough." Accordingly, it received quite favorable press attention. Gleevec is a member of a new class of anticancer drugs. Standard cancer chemotherapy, while in some cases life-saving, is beset with problems. Most chemotherapy drugs are not capable of telling the difference between cancer cells and normal cells in a very sophisticated way. As a rule, they kill cells that divide rapidly. Cancer cells divide rapidly, but so do many normal body cells, such as the cells in the bone marrow, hair roots, and the intestinal lining. This means that any drug that kills cancer cells will also cause severe side effects—suppressing the bone marrow so that the body cannot make vital red and white blood cells, causing hair loss and intestinal symptoms, and often making the patient feel extremely ill for several days or even weeks. Scientists have long been trying to find drugs that are more highly selective for cancer cells, killing only the bad cells while sparing the good ones. That has meant first finding a chemical process or other cell function that goes on only in cancer cells, and then using that insight to design a specific drug to shut down that process.

Around 1985, Drs. David Baltimore and Owen Witte, working in university and academic research labs, identified a basic mechanism that explains one type of leukemia, chronic myelogenous leukemia (CML), which usually strikes older adults. They found that because of an odd form of one chromosome, called the "Philadelphia chromosome," the CML cell possesses a defective signaling system. It has lost the ability to shut itself off after dividing and making new cells. The result is abnormal cells that keep dividing incessantly—the hallmark of cancer. Baltimore and Witte clarified the specific gene that made the Philadelphia chromosome into a cancer-causing agent and identified the specific enzyme made by this gene as one of a class called tyrosine kinases.

For the drug industry, the Philadelphia chromosome discovery was both good and bad news. The good news was that enough was now known about the basic molecular structure of one type of cancer cell to guide potential drug development to block a key cancer-causing process. The bad news was that the particular form of cancer appeared to be a financial loser. About six to seven thousand Americans are diagnosed with CML every year, compared to around two hundred thousand with either breast or prostate cancer. As Dr. Daniel Vasella, CEO of the giant drug firm Novartis, points out in his book on Gleevec, these figures would ordinarily cool any industry enthusiasm to launch a major research effort.[2] The costs to find the magic compound that turned off the erroneous cancer signal in the cell could be huge, but the market for the new drug might be too small to recoup the investment unless the drug were priced very high.

Alex Matter, a physician-researcher at the pharmaceutical firm Ciba-Geigy in Basel, Switzerland, was undeterred by these economic concerns. He had become a believer in the idea of "designer drugs" to fight cancer. As he saw it, the task was intimidating but not impossible. The hard part was that tyrosine kinase, beside causing the abnormal signal in CML cells, is part of chemical reactions in many types of normal cells. But Dr. Matter was sure that with perseverance and a bit of luck he could design a molecule that blocked only the bad type of tyrosine kinase while leaving all the others alone. He assembled a team: Nick Lydon to manage the actual laboratory work; Jürg Zimmerman, a chemist, to make the new compounds; and Elisabeth Buchdunger, a biologist, to test the compounds for their effects on human cells. They also established collaboration with Dr. Brian Druker at the Dana-Farber Cancer Institute in Boston, who could do further human-cell testing on promising compounds.

In early 1993, the team achieved promising results in their lab with one new compound Zimmerman had made called STI571. It seemed a far leap from the lab to testing in humans with cancer, and most of the industry scientists they talked to were cool to the project. Brian Druker, however, who had moved from Dana-Farber to the Oregon Health Science University in Portland, was enthusiastic about his own results with STI571 in human cells grown in tissue culture. Some animal studies were done, showing that STI571 appeared not to have any serious toxicity. But still no one in the company was pushing for human studies, and Druker grew impatient.

In 1996, Ciba-Geigy merged with another large Swiss company, Sandoz, to form the giant firm Novartis. Dr. Vasella, who had been leading Sandoz, was tapped to become CEO of Novartis. He met with Alex Matter, and could at that time have called a halt to all work on STI571 as a long shot and probable money loser. But he found Matter's enthusiasm and logic infectious and gave him the green light to proceed. Dr. Druker was promised some of the compound to begin human trials in the fall of 1996, but then another setback arose when some of the animals receiving the drug started to get sick. More animal studies were done at different doses, and finally it appeared that it would be safe to start studies in humans. Dr. Druker, still impatient, finally was given the go-ahead in the summer of 1998.[3]

Human studies of new drugs typically consist of three phases. Phase I is usually carried out in healthy volunteers, but with cancer drugs, because of their dangers, advanced cancer patients are often used instead. Phase I studies are very small and are intended to decide the safe dose. Subjects enrolling in Phase I trials are told explicitly that they would probably get no benefit themselves from the research— later patients will be better off if the drug works, so their volunteering for the research is a contribution to fighting the disease for the benefit of others. Then, in Phase II trials, a small number of patients with the actual disease are given the drug at the decided-upon dose to see if it shows any therapeutic activity. If the drug passes the Phase II trials, larger-scale studies (Phase III) are conducted on more patients suffering from the disease. The FDA ordinarily demands results from all three phases before considering approval of a drug for general medical use.

Dr. Druker and his colleagues started their Phase I trials on patients with CML who had failed to respond to interferon, the best available drug for the disease. At low doses of the new drug, which they were now calling Glivic, not much happened. But as new patients were enrolled and the dose was increased, the investigators were astonished to see some dramatic responses. The high white blood cell counts that are characteristic of out-of-control leukemia started to fall, and the abnormal bone marrow cells with the Philadelphia chromosome started to disappear. Perhaps best of all, few patients had serious side effects. A bit of fluid retention and some limb weakness were as much as most of the research subjects complained of. Compared to typical anticancer drugs, this was an astoundingly low side-effect profile.

The Matter-Druker team was meanwhile casting about for other cancers where Glivic might have activity. If Matter's theory was correct, these would be few in number, if any existed at all. The abnormal cancer-causing signals might be different for each type of cancer—indeed, common cancers like breast cancer might in the end turn out to consist of many subtypes, each with its own signal abnormality. The whole concept of "designer drugs" for cancer argued that each type of cancer would need its own individual drug. Still, it would be a plus for Novartis (and its bottom line) if Glivic turned out to be effective for some other forms of cancer, even if only in combination with other drugs. The best candidate to emerge was (sadly for the marketers) even more rare than CML—a type of intestinal cancer called gastrointestinal stromal tumor (GIST). Phase I studies were undertaken with GIST patients, and again extremely positive results with low levels of side effects were seen fairly early on.

Two articles by these research teams were eventually published in the *New England Journal of Medicine*. In a total of 454 subjects with late-stage CML, 95 percent had normal blood counts and 60 percent achieved the disappearance of the Philadelphia chromosome from their bone marrow. After being followed for an average of eighteen months, 95 percent of the subjects were alive, and 89 percent remained in the chronic phase, instead of progressing on to the final (blast) stage of the disease.[4] In 147 GIST subjects considered to be in the advanced stages of disease, 54 percent had a partial response and 28 percent appeared to have had their disease stabilized.[5] These results were notably better than those achieved with any other existing treatment for these cancers.

By late 1999, it seemed clear to the scientists doing the studies and to the staff of Novartis that they had a very promising drug, which cancer patients would be clamoring to get. The next big hurdle was whether they could get regulatory approval to move the drug onto the market, based on the promising but limited data they were accumulating in Phase I and Phase II trials. The entry of Glivic could be delayed for years if the FDA, for instance, demanded that the drug pass all the hurdles traditionally required and go through the more extensive Phase III trials. And there were reasons for worry. No matter how promising the trial results so far, the scientists could not know if Glivic could actually cure anyone, or how long the positive response to Glivic might last. Patients with CML and GIST might someday be able to go off the drug and do just fine for an indefinite period—a true cure. Or the patients might need to take the drugs for the rest of their lives to keep their diseases under control, but could do so fairly easily due to the low side-effect profile of the drug. Or, in the worst case scenario, Glivic would turn out to produce much more severe side effects when taken in the long term, or would work to suppress the cancer only for a few years, or both. The studies done so far simply could not tell.

But the Novartis people found the FDA fully sympathetic. The agency granted the company fast-track status due to the genuinely innovative nature of the drug. The FDA staff began to work in tandem with the Novartis group to be sure that the review process was expedited. On May 10, 2001, FDA approval of the drug was announced by the secretary of Health and Human Services (HHS), Tommy Thompson, in a rare news conference (FDA approval of a drug is hardly ever the occasion for a full press conference). Thompson noted that the FDA had set a new record, approving the drug in only two-and-a-half months from the date that Novartis submitted its final application. In the end, the worst damage that the FDA did to the company interests was to demand a minor name change. "Glivic," the FDA thought, was too close to the names of two other drugs and might cause confusion. The company responded by renaming the drug "Gleevec" for use in the United States, retaining the name "Glivic" for the rest of the world market.

The next challenge for Dr. Vasella and his Novartis team was to gear up to produce the quantities of Gleevec that would be demanded once word of the drug's success got out. To adhere to Dr. Vasella's vision, Novartis had to be prepared, first, to expand the size of their research trials to enroll as many sufferers of CML and GIST as possible, and later, to supply free drugs to many patients who could not otherwise afford Gleevec.

The result of this commitment was that Novartis's usual method of manufacturing drugs would not work here. The company was used to producing small batches of the chemical in a Swiss plant during the trial phase, in the meantime getting all the bugs out of the methods for large-scale industrial production, which would eventually occur at the company's large plant in Ringaskiddy, Ireland. The demands for Gleevec required that the Ringaskiddy plant get on line very quickly and master the twelve-step process required to make the complex Gleevec molecule. The Irish workers, excited to be part of this major pharmaceutical development, put in overtime to get their plant ready. As a result, Novartis set its own speed record, getting the first batches of the drug to wholesalers within a day after official FDA approval.

One challenge still remained—Novartis had to decide upon a price for its new wonder drug. The company eventually chose the price range of $2,000–$2,400 per month for the dose needed by CML patients in the chronic phase of the disease. Dr. Vasella commented, "We agree with those who say that the price we have set for Gleevec is high. But given all the factors, we believe it is a fair price."[6] The factors include the significantly improved quality of life as well as the medical benefits Gleevec provides, coupled with the fact that the few competing treatments for CML also have to be taken every day or every week for long periods of time, and cost just about the same as Gleevec does without performing as well. The high-end treatment for CML is bone marrow transplantation, which costs nearly $200,000 and has a very high complication and failure rate. Novartis also began a reduced-price and free-drug program for patients who could not afford the drug in the usual way. Dr. Vasella concluded:

> We at Novartis know we have been fair when determining our drug prices. But critics make it harder for society to believe that we are sincere in what we say—and in what we do. We hope that our behavior with regard to Gleevec, taking a huge investment risk despite a small patient population; accelerating our manufacturing process; creating a patient assistance program for the drug, will demonstrate that we truly care about patients. We can do so as long as we are successful, satisfying the interests of the shareholders by providing a return on investment. We would hope that once the general public learns that we are not simply heartless, faceless, and greedy industrialists, but people who care and want to help the patient population, then perhaps the same public will have a greater tolerance for drug prices and a willingness to listen to our arguments of why we must be allowed to make a profit.[7]

As one might imagine, the Gleevec story is not without its bumps in the road. The *New York Times* reported in mid-2003 that the worldwide charitable program to provide Gleevec for those unable to afford the cost had turned out to be equal parts charity and lobbying, with patients being urged to become protestors to demand that governmental programs in cash-strapped nations cover the full costs of the drug.[8] Nonetheless, Gleevec has continued to be an impressive drug for the small group of patients at whom it is targeted and represents a genuine innovation. Even in the worst-case scenario, if the drug stops working for CML and GIST after a few years, it will still have shown the way for scientists to work on a new generation of "designer drugs" aimed at blocking the specific chemical reactions that make cancer what it is. Dr. David Parkinson of Novartis told Nicholas Wade of the *New York Times* that Gleevec "emerged from 40 years of hard labor and is a validation that the approach will work if the science is right."[9] Nor has Novartis suffered financially; in 2003, the company reported that Gleevec had hit the one-billion-dollar mark in annual sales necessary for a drug to be classed as a "blockbuster."[10]

THE CLARITIN STORY

Two months before Gleevec hit the media, Stephen S. Hall wrote an article for the *New York Times Magazine* titled "Prescription for Profit."[11] Hall's concerns that led him to write the story were very mundane compared to the life-or-death story of patients with advanced cancer. Hall suffered from the drippy nose and red, itchy eyes of hay fever and other seasonal allergies—hardly a life-threatening problem, yet in its own way a major concern of American medicine, based simply on how many people suffer from these symptoms—an estimated thirty-five million. For years Hall had treated himself with the over-the-counter pill, Chlor-Trimeton, an old standby antihistamine. It worked great for his symptoms, but it also made him very sleepy. When Hall finally complained about this problem to a new allergist he was seeing, the allergist rummaged through his sample supply and handed Hall a week's worth of Claritin, manufactured by Schering-Plough (which, incidentally, also makes Chlor-Trimeton). Claritin was an antihistamine like Chlor-Trimeton, but of a new chemical family, which was supposed to be nonsedating. Hall was impressed: "I had seen the ads on TV—who hadn't? I figured I'd give it a try."[12]

Hall continued his tale: "So I went home and tried it. The little white pill was easy to swallow and had to be taken only once a day. There was just one problem: it didn't work. It didn't relieve my runny nose and red-rimmed, gunked-up eyes. When I told my allergist, he didn't seem particularly surprised. Only about 30 to 40 percent of his patients, he said, found the drug helpful."[13]

Hall was puzzled. He knew that Claritin was the most profitable antihistamine of all time, with annual sales of more than two billion dollars. As he noted, everyone had seen the TV ads for Claritin; it was one of the most aggressively marketed drugs of that day. Beside the usual advertising and providing of free samples to physicians, Schering-Plough has relied very heavily on direct-to-consumer advertising. The advertising pays off for the company in part because Claritin is so expensive—costing (in 2001) about eighty to eighty-five dollars for a month's supply compared to less than ten dollars for Chlor-Trimeton. Knowing all these facts, Hall assumed that the drug would work for the symptoms he complained of. So why was his allergist telling him that more than half of his patients failed to get any benefit from Claritin?

Hall started looking into the Claritin story. There are many twists and turns in the story, which goes back to the mid-1980s when Schering first started doing human research on its new antihistamine, loratadine (the generic name for Claritin), and submitting its data to the FDA to get approval to sell the drug. But for our purposes we need to focus on only one of Hall's findings about Claritin.

Going back to the 1987 meetings between FDA staff and Schering representatives, Hall highlighted the research approach that Schering used to get FDA approval for Claritin. Schering presented the FDA with research data to show that when loratadine was compared against placebo pills in randomized, double-blinded trials (research studies in which neither the physician nor the patient knows who is getting the "real" drug and who is getting the placebo or "dummy" drug), loratadine was nonsedating and was effective as an antihistamine. But the size of its effect was very small. It was only about 10 percent better than the placebo in relieving allergy symptoms—a much smaller effect than would be seen with older antihistamines like Chlor-Trimeton. The reason for this lack of effectiveness seemed obvious to the FDA staffers—Schering had tested only one dose of loratadine, ten milligrams. Claritin was then widely available as an over-the-counter drug in Europe (where it cost only ten to fifteen dollars for a month's supply instead of the eighty to eighty-five the prescription Claritin cost in the United States), and many Europeans took thirty or forty milligrams per day. They found that at that higher dose the drug works better, about as well as Chlor-Trimeton. But at that higher dose, the drug also causes drowsiness among an increasing number of those taking it. Schering avoided submitting any data to the FDA for doses greater than ten milligrams because they knew that if they could show more antihistamine effect, they would also have to admit that the drug caused sedation. But they were especially anxious to keep the label "nonsedating" because that was how they wished to market the drug for maximum profits.

Schering-Plough heavily marketed their drug to both physicians and John Q. Public based on the twin claims that it was an effective antihistamine and that it was nonsedating. They presented those claims in such a way that the reasonable person would conclude that the combination of effective antihistamine and nonsedation was a peculiar feature of the chemical nature of the drug loratadine. But the company knew, from the data that it had presented to the FDA in 1987, that loratadine was not a very effective antihistamine if it was given in a nonsedating dose, and that when you made it more effective as an antihistamine by increasing the dose, you also got a lot more sedation. Despite knowing all this, Schering-Plough deliberately and consistently maintained that their drug was both highly effective and special. Small wonder that Hall was shocked when his allergist told him how ineffective the drug really was in general use, and when Hall found out that if Claritin were to be prescribed at a dose where it was truly effective, it would also be just about as sedating as his old Chlor-Trimeton, which costs about one-tenth as much.

With its highly successful marketing campaign, Schering-Plough had created the proverbial goose that lays the golden egg, and they were anxious to ensure that nobody killed the goose. Hall wrote that the original patent on Claritin was soon to expire. When a drug firm develops a new drug, they receive a patent giving them an exclusive right to sell it under their brand name for twenty years. After that period, other drug manufacturers can market that drug as a generic medicine, usually driving down the cost considerably. Several generic manufacturers had begun to gear up to produce loratadine and to begin selling it after Schering's patent was up. Schering's response was to sue those manufacturers, claiming that in one way or another, the generic drug companies' applications to the FDA violated Schering's exclusive patents. From the generic companies' point of view (and Hall's), these lawsuits had no legal merit. Rather, they were an economic ploy. A large drug firm with its own in-house legal staff figures that a lawsuit of this sort will cost it approximately five million dollars. If the result of the lawsuit was to delay for *one day* the appearance of a generic version of loratadine, Schering would make back its money, assuming that Claritin sales continued at the then-current rate of two billion dollars annually. So these lawsuits were a rather bald delaying tactic aimed at securing an extended period during which Schering could reap the rewards of its highly effective marketing campaigns.

Hall noted one particular irony of the Claritin story. Based on all the Claritin marketing hoopla, one might assume that allergy sufferers have only two choices—take a medicine like Claritin at the ten-milligram dose, which is not very effective at relieving symptoms but at least won't put you to sleep, or else take the old standby medicines, which are very effective but which will knock you out. Because of the smoke screen this marketing campaign has laid down, two basic facts are unknown to many allergy patients. The first fact is that Chlor-Trimeton and the older, cheap antihistamines don't make *everyone* sleepy. In fact, as many as half of those taking them will have little or no sedation. To rush right to Claritin without at least giving a medicine like Chlor-Trimeton a trial first is really a waste of money—even if Claritin were as effective as it claims to be, which, as we have seen, it isn't. The second fact is that there is a totally different set of medications one can turn to for much more reliable relief of allergy symptoms without any risk of sedation—the corticosteroid nasal sprays. They are often cheaper than Claritin, are extremely effective in relieving allergy symptoms, are nonsedating, and for the vast majority of patients have no side effects at all. In fact, Schering-Plough itself manufactures one highly effective corticosteroid nasal spray. But millions of patients have seen the TV ads and rushed to their physicians demanding Claritin, and many physicians (sadly) don't have the time or the energy to teach patients these basic facts and to try to talk them out of it.

Hall mentioned yet another irony. Consider the fact that loratadine turns out to be not very effective as an antihistamine, and it is nonsedating simply because it is given in a low enough dose. Chlor-Trimeton is a much more potent antihistamine and even at its full dose, only about half of those who take it have significant sedation. Suppose we tried using lower doses of Chlor-Trimeton? With a bit of research, could we find an *ideal* dose, which caused a lot less sedation but which still relieved most people's allergy symptoms? Given how many millions of people suffer from allergies, this new research project would seem to have real value, even if allergy treatment hardly saves lives. But Hall's informants in the medical research and pharmaceutical areas told him that this study will probably never be conducted. Given the more pressing public health concerns, government agencies will not fund such a study. And the money to be made from selling the generic preparations of the older antihistamines over the counter are far too low to make it profitable for any drug company to sponsor that research by itself. So, despite the billions of dollars we spend on medical research every year, the answer to this simple question of the ideal dose of the older antihistamines will probably never be known.

THE BIG PICTURE

We've now reviewed two stories. The Gleevec story is shaping up as the classical medical success story. The Claritin story seems an exposé of all that could go wrong when powerful, profit-driven firms take over the world of medicines.

If there were a lot of Gleevec stories and only a few Claritin stories, I would not be writing this book. No system is foolproof. If most of the new drugs introduced were real medical breakthroughs as Gleevec seems to be, and were marketed honestly, we could tolerate the occasional excess of greed and arrogance such as that displayed by Schering-Plough.

But that's not the world of the drug industry over the past forty to fifty years in the United States. There have been only a few Gleevec stories and a great many Claritin stories. As I will document in later chapters, Schering-Plough does not deserve to be singled out; the way that firm behaves is simply par for the course.

Each year about fifteen or twenty new prescription drugs appear on the market. If we are lucky, one of them might be a Gleevec-type drug—a real improvement in medicine's ability to treat some serious disease. All the rest will be what doctors call "me-too" drugs—not substantially better than drugs already on the market, or better only at the cost of causing worse side effects. The drug firms put out these me-too drugs in hopes that through some marketing spin, they can convince physicians or the consumer or both that this drug is in some way special or superior and thereby grab a chunk of the market. Claritin was just one example of this marketing strategy.

It is, however, one thing to tell stories, and quite another to do a careful ethical analysis. Is there anything *ethically* wrong with an industry that behaves typically in Claritin-type ways? The next chapter will provide an ethical framework that will allow us to approach this question.

NOTES

1. D. Vasella with R. Slater, *Magic Cancer Bullet: How a Tiny Orange Pill Is Rewriting Medical History* (New York: HarperBusiness, 2003), 94.
2. Vasella, *Magic Cancer Bullet.*
3. For a somewhat different version of events from those recounted by Dr. Vasella, see M. Goozner, *The $800 Million Pill: The Truth Behind the Cost of New Drugs* (Berkeley: University of California Press, 2004), 199. In Goozner's account, based on interviews with some of the principals, Owen Witte initially tried to interest several drug firms in tyrosine kinase blocking molecules but got nowhere. After Bruce Druker got excited about the potential of STI571, he lobbied Ciba-Geigy relentlessly for many years before any further development

occurred. While Druker knew that Nick Lydon at Ciba-Geigy shared his enthusiasm, no one farther up the chain of command took a positive outlook, and Druker is convinced that only his lobbying efforts kept the drug program alive at that point. Goozner claims that Dr. Vasella became a strong advocate of developing the drug only after Novartis received massive mailings from cancer sufferers who had heard about Gleevec's first promising clinical results.

4. H. Kantarjian, C. Sawyers, A. Hochhaus, et al., "Hematologic and Cytogenetic Responses to Imatinib Mesylate in Chronic Myelogenous Leukemia," *N Engl J Med* 2002; 346:645–52.

5. G. D. Demetri, M. von Mehren, C. D. Blanke, et al., "Efficacy and Safety of Imatinib Mesylate in Advanced Gastrointestinal Stromal Tumors," *N Engl J Med* 2002; 347:472–80.

6. Vasella, *Magic Cancer Bullet*, 180.

7. Vasella, *Magic Cancer Bullet*, 172. Typical of industry spokespersons, Vasella claims that Novartis took huge financial risks in investing in Gleevec research and that the price of the drug was only fair in terms of the need to recoup these costs, but he provides no estimate of what it actually cost Novartis to do the research. Vasella reportedly told science writer Nicholas Wade that Novartis had invested between $600 million and $800 million in the research and development of Gleevec; N. Wade, "Swift Approval for a New Kind of Cancer Drug," *New York Times*, May 11, 2001:1.

8. S. Strom and M. Fleischer-Black, "Drug Maker's Vow to Donate Cancer Medicine Falls Short," *New York Times*, June 5, 2003:A1.

9. N. Wade, "Powerful Anti-Cancer Drug Emerges from Basic Biology," *New York Times*, May 8, 2001:1.

10. F. Fleck, "A Healthy Novartis Increases Stake in a Rival," *New York Times*, January 23, 2004:W1.

11. S. S. Hall, "Prescription for Profit," *New York Times Magazine*, March 11, 2001:40–45 ff.

12. Hall, "Prescription for Profit," 40.

13. Hall, "Prescription for Profit," 40.

2

AN ETHICAL FRAMEWORK

The louder he talked of his honour, the faster we counted our spoons.

—Ralph Waldo Emerson[1]

There is another difficulty in trusting to the honor and conscience of a doctor. Doctors are just like other Englishmen: most of them have no honor and no conscience: what they commonly mistake for these is sentimentality and an intense dread of doing anything that everybody else does not do, or omitting to do anything that everybody else does.

—George Bernard Shaw, *The Doctor's Dilemma* (1911)[2]

To better understand the relationship between the medical profession and the pharmaceutical industry, we must accumulate pertinent facts and assess our findings in light of some sort of basic ethical framework. The purpose of this chapter is to lay out a framework that we can refer back to as we proceed.

I will discuss why trust matters in the physician-patient relationship and what makes a physician (or the entire profession) trustworthy. I will address the moral status of the activities of the pharmaceutical industry and then explore the nature of conflicts of interest, examining whether any exist between the profession and the industry. I will also address some ethical issues relating to relative power. Finally, I will ask whether existing codes of ethics from professional organizations provide us with an adequate set of ethical principles.[3]

BASIC ETHICAL DUTIES OF PHYSICIANS

Most believe that becoming and practicing as a physician is a somewhat different matter, morally, from simply setting oneself up in business. Business people are expected to be ethical—for instance, not to shortchange their customers or to deliver an inferior product when the customer has paid for top quality. But an ethical businessperson is supposed to put aside her own self-interest, with the goal of serving the customer, only to a limited extent. The customer is assumed to know best what is in his own interest and act accordingly. Physicians, by contrast, are expected to put aside many of their own personal interests and to devote themselves instead to promoting the interests of their patients.[4]

To put the matter in a different way, we are willing to assume that businesses will provide us with the best products and services precisely when businesses can make the maximum profit off doing so. But we are not, as a rule, prepared to make the same assumption about medicine—that the unalloyed profit motive will ensure that our physicians give us the best medical care possible. This point of view was probably most famously expressed by George Bernard Shaw: "That any sane nation, having observed that you could provide for the supply of bread by giving bakers a pecuniary interest in baking for you, should go on to give a surgeon a pecuniary interest in cutting off your leg, is enough to make one despair of political humanity."[5]

This conclusion is less controversial than the argument that leads to it. Some thoughtful writers believe that the ethical "code" of conduct that requires the physician to lay aside self-interest and to serve the needs of the patient is simply the same ethical set of rules and principles that govern all of us in our society. Medical ethics, that is, is just a special case of the larger morality of the community.[6] Others argue that medicine has what might be termed an *internal* morality, distinct from the common, societal morality but rather limited in scope. Physicians are not excused from following the common moral code of the community; the internal morality of medicine is an extra obligation they undertake as part of the practice of medicine. The internal morality is the substance of the claim that medicine is not *merely* a business.

The physician first trains in and then participates in a historical tradition that can be termed a *practice*.[7] A practice is a complex human activity that usually can be mastered only with some difficulty after a prolonged period of training. A practice is characterized by some inherent standards that define what it means to be *good* at it; and in the case of some practices, the notion of "good" that defines the standards of the practice is a moral sense of "good" and includes ethical content. The moral content of such a practice may include both a statement of goals the practice is supposed to seek and also of the means that will be acceptable or unacceptable in reaching those goals.[8]

Medicine has as its goals a number of activities that relate to human health and illness. Physicians try to cure diseases when they can. They try to give patients advice about keeping healthy and avoiding disease. They manage the effects of chronic diseases that cannot be cured. They reassure people who feel badly but who have no diagnosable disease. And they relieve the suffering and provide compassionate care to the irreversibly ill and the dying.

Edmund Pellegrino, a physician-philosopher, argued that these goals of medicine lead to an understanding of medicine's basic internal morality via what he termed the "fact of illness" and the "act of profession." The *fact of illness* is that there is usually a serious gap in power and capability between the physician and the patient. In most medical settings, the patient and the physician are hardly on equal terms. The physician typically knows much more about health and illness than the patient does, and the patient usually feels much more vulnerable and at risk. The fact of illness would seem on its face to rule out a marketplace ethic as a suitable ethic for medicine. The idea of equals coming together freely to negotiate a mutually beneficial contract characterizes very poorly the brute facts of the encounter between physician and patient.

The physician's ethical response to the "fact of illness," Pellegrino continues, is the "act of profession." Pellegrino is concerned not with the noun *profession*—describing a corporate body of individuals, as when we speak of the "medical profession"—but rather the verb *to profess*. To profess is to speak out in public and to make a promise to which one is willing later to be held accountable.

"Professing" medicine, according to Pellegrino, entails making a promise to try your best to serve the patient who comes to seek your help and never to take advantage of the patient's vulnerability. It is to proclaim among other things that how much money the physician makes should be subordinated to a commitment to the patients' well-being.[9] This is, more or less, the enduring moral core of the ancient Hippocratic Oath. The importance of this act of promising is recognized by most medical schools, which still have graduates take some form of oath, even if the precise Hippocratic wording has in some cases been supplanted by modern substitutes.

Why the focus on the *public* promise making implied by "professing"? Illness often strikes in ways that do not permit us to seek out only physicians we personally know or whose credentials we have personally validated. At any time we might suffer a sudden crisis and be brought to a hospital emergency department or similar facility. If a person walks up to us and says, "I'm Dr. Jones," our social and cultural customs allow us to make many assumptions about Dr. Jones and what we can count on her to know and to do. For example, we don't have to quiz Dr. Jones as to whether she once took a course in human anatomy; her status as a physician entitles me to assume she has a working knowledge of that subject. Moreover, we can assume that information we tell Dr. Jones will be treated as confidential—we don't have to negotiate a specific agreement as to whether or not to keep information private.[10] In short we can *trust* Dr. Jones to take care of me. When we speak of "professing" medicine, we speak of making a promise to the entire community. Without such a promise, it would not make sense for individual patients to trust previously unknown physicians in times of crisis.

The basic concept of "trust" turns out to be an extremely complicated idea. To mention just two wrinkles, I might trust my friend George without question if it came to taking care of my dog for two weeks while I was on vacation, but I might not trust George for a minute if it came to paying back a hundred-dollar loan. So to say, "I trust George," is an incomplete sentence; we would have to add, *to do what*? We would also want to discern whether my trust in anyone, to do anything, is *justified*. I might, for instance, as a patient, be fully justified in trusting my physician to know what drugs are generally best for high blood pressure. I would be completely unjustified if I were to trust my physician never to make a mistake.[11]

Fortunately, for our purposes in this book, we need not delve into most of these finer points about trust. We can arrive at our destination if we agree simply that, in general, (1) patients trust physicians to dedicate themselves to the patients' well-being and health, and (2) patients are, or ought to be, justified in trusting physicians to act in this manner.

Both physicians and patients easily forget the importance of trust, simply because we take it so much for granted and could hardly begin to imagine what it would be like to try to practice medicine without it. Trust obviously makes physicians' work much easier, but that in turn means that patients generally get much better care most of the time because this level of trust exists. Patients can trust too much, and, for instance, not ask some hard questions that might lead physicians to realize that a serious error is about to be made. But in general, trust is the grease that keeps the wheels of medical practice turning smoothly for the benefit of physician and patient alike. Anything that would compromise the general sense of trust between physicians and patients counts as a serious threat to both parties as well as to the society as a whole.

The basic trust in medicine must, however, be a two-way street. What if patients trusted physicians blindly and physicians secretly acted in ways that would make patients distrust them if only they knew? This is not the sort of ethical physician-patient relationship we have in mind when we praise the "trust" inherent in the relationship. It is not enough for patients to trust physicians; in addition, physicians ought to be *trustworthy* individuals. They must genuinely strive to be the sorts of professionals whom it would be reasonable for patients generally to trust.

Pellegrino's "fact of illness" and "act of profession" help us to fill out the list of the *means* that physicians may use to achieve the various goals of the practice of medicine. It is important that physicians not employ simply any means at all; there must be a commitment to the sorts of means that make physicians trustworthy in the eyes of the community. We have seen that this includes fidelity (faithful commitment) to the interests of the patient. The list of means also includes doing things in accord with a standard of scientific knowledge and skill, avoiding doing any harm to the patient unless the harm brings about a compensating benefit, and being honest in how one describes and portrays medical practice.

Table 2.1 summarizes this account of the internal morality of medicine.

Table 2.1. List of Goals and Ethical Means to Achieve Them

Goals of Medicine[1]	Ethically Appropriate Means
Prevention of disease and injury	Competence in medical knowledge and skills
Promotion and maintenance of health	Avoiding harm without compensatory
Relief of pain and suffering caused by illness	benefit
Cure of disease where possible	Honest portrayal of medical knowledge and
Care of chronic disease that cannot be cured	skills
Avoidance of premature death	Fidelity to therapeutic relationship
Care toward a peaceful death	

[1] This particular list of goals is modified slightly from a report of an international consensus panel; D. Callahan, "The Goals of Medicine: Setting New Priorities," *Hastings Cen Rep* 1996; 26(6): S1–S26.

The rhetoric and the reality of the "profession" of medicine's internal morality require some clarification. When physicians are waxing fulsome, they often speak as if serving the interests of patients *always and completely* dominates the "good" physician's attention. This leads to justified criticism of disingenuousness. A few physicians seem willing to accept careers in which their lives are given almost entirely to service, in a saintly devotion to the well-being of their patients; these physicians appear happy to forgo most of their personal interests. But sainthood is not expected of the average physician, either by his professional peers or by the general public. There must be some *reasonable* balance between the physician's self-interest and the commitment to serve the patient, and just how to draw the line of "reasonableness" is highly contentious. But some general conclusions seem uncontroversial. What if a physician has saved $50,000 toward the college education of her children and one of her long-standing patients needs a liver transplant and lacks $50,000 to pay the full cost of the potentially life-saving surgery? We would expect that the physician would perhaps write several letters and make several phone calls to try to find other sources of payment for this surgery. But I would not claim that "professing" medicine means that this physician is obligated herself to pay the $50,000 out of her child's college fund. On the other side of the line, the physician who has a waiting room full of patients and who leaves at 5:00 P.M. just because he doesn't wish to work any longer that day has clearly failed to live up to his "profession."

ETHICAL STATUS OF THE PHARMACEUTICAL INDUSTRY

We have seen so far that the physician is obligated to place the interests of the patient ahead of his own interests at least to some degree, and also that the peculiar circumstances of medicine and illness require that the trust of the patient and society be maintained and that physicians behave in trustworthy ways. We now need to put the pharmaceutical industry into the equation.

There are at least three ways in which the pharmaceutical industry plays a morally good role in our society and deserves full credit for its praiseworthy behavior. First, at a purely business level, the industry employs a large number of people and earns substantial profits for its shareholders. As businesses, the major pharmaceutical firms are usually held to be exemplary. I wish to make clear that I am adopting an ethical stance of general agreement with the values of a capitalist society. As long as one commits no crime or fraud and violates no important principles of business ethics, it is a good thing to make money by producing something that people wish to buy. The fact that the pharmaceutical industry makes a profit is not something that should be viewed as ethically questionable; and even the fact that it makes a *large* profit is not by itself ethically suspect. We cannot eliminate "profiting off the misfortunes of others" unless we are prepared to radically restructure large segments of our society. My basic argument requires none of that restructuring.[12]

Everything I have just said about the ethical goodness of running a profitable business presumes fair and ethical means. It has been charged by a number of experts that the pharmaceutical industry all too often does *not* use fair and ethical means—that the industry is rife with corporate crime, and that it acts to manipulate the market rather than to compete fairly.[13] When we encounter such charges we should assess them soberly and ask what ethical and policy implications follow if they can be substantiated. What we should not do is condemn an entire industry simply because it is profitable and powerful.

The next way in which the industry plays a morally good role is that it does not make a profit making just any old product—as the common phrase has it, it is not in the business of making widgets. Rather its business is making medicines that promote human health and that occasionally save lives. To the extent that health is a more important human good than the mere satisfaction of desires and appetites, making medicine is ethically a more exemplary line of work than making, say, video games—and by the same reasoning, a considerably more exemplary line of work than making tobacco products or junk foods. Those who work for the pharmaceutical industry can go home at night feeling a bit prouder of what they do than those who work for many other industries.

Leonard Weber, in his analysis of business ethics in health care, emphasizes that this morally good role imposes a moral obligation on the industry.[14] Having staked out this ethical claim—having in effect "professed" to a sort of moral high ground within the business world—the industry must impose on itself the corresponding level of moral obligation; it cannot enjoy the benefits without shouldering the burdens. This can be seen most clearly in instances such as the anthrax bioterrorism scare in the United States in late 2001. The firm that manufactures ciprofloxacin, which was thought to be the drug of choice to combat anthrax, ethically ought not (as the Bayer company did for a time) concern itself primarily with profits and exclusive rights to market the drug. The firm should attend first and foremost to the public health need for adequate and prompt supplies of the drug, even if its profits are thereby lessened.[15]

Attending to the needs of public health may be morally required for the industry. By contrast, the third morally good role the industry might play in society goes beyond what is morally required and enters the realm that ethical theory designates as "supererogatory," similar to the saintly physician who cheerfully accepts poverty just so that she can more effectively serve the neediest patients. One episode that seems to fit the supererogatory category is Merck's decision not only to manufacture Ivermectin, a drug effective in treating river blindness in parts of Africa, but also to make the drug available for that purpose for free.[16] In an industry known often for abandoning or for failing to develop drugs for third-world diseases in favor of less essential but more lucrative drugs for sale in the developed world, simply having decided to proceed with the manufacture of Ivermectin might have been praiseworthy. Bayer may have had a public health obligation to make ciprofloxacin readily available at lower cost, but no one would argue they had an obligation to give it away for free. A similar act by most drug companies today is maintaining a charitable program whereby individual, needy patients can apply for and receive free supplies of expensive medications. Doing charitable works that go beyond the bounds of moral obligation is as praiseworthy when performed by the pharmaceutical industry as it would be if done by anyone else.

CONFLICTS OF INTEREST

We have seen that practicing medicine involves professing a moral commitment to one's patients and that in a number of ways the pharmaceutical industry fulfills an ethically good role in our society. To some, the conjunction of those two conclusions resolves any potential moral concern. Here we have two ethically good groups of folks serving the end of promoting human health, so everything is just fine, thank you. If it were so simple, this book would not now be before you.

Let us imagine a patient whose cholesterol levels are above normal. The levels are near but not yet quite as high as the levels listed by various standard guidelines for beginning drug therapy to try to prevent heart disease and stroke. The patient has made some attempt—for how long and exactly how whole-heartedly might be questioned—to lower the cholesterol levels through dietary modification and exercise, but so far without success. The patient, let us say, has relatives who have suffered from heart disease, but otherwise has no major risk factors besides the high cholesterol (such as smoking, hypertension, or diabetes).

We could imagine in this case a physician concerned to apply the best current scientific knowledge to the specific circumstances of this patient and to make a recommendation that she regards as being in the patient's best interests. Included in the interests of this patient are reducing long-term cardiovascular disease risk and avoiding the side effects, inconvenience, and cost of medications. On balance we could imagine this physician concluding that the patient should be advised to work just a bit harder at diet and exercise modification and recheck the cholesterol in six months. The decision to administer lipid-lowering drugs would be deferred to the future.

Is this advice, arguably in the best interests of the patient, also in the best interest of a drug company that manufactures a statin drug for lowering cholesterol? It would appear not. The company has an interest in recruiting this patient to join the throng currently consuming these relatively expensive and also often effective drugs.

Let us now imagine a second physician, who is also asked to advise this patient. This second physician has been conditioned by the pharmaceutical industry over time to see his personal interests as closely allied with those of the industry. It may be that this physician has received monetary rewards or substantial gifts for prescribing a high volume of drugs manufactured by one or more companies. Or it may simply be that this physician frequently visits with drug company sales representatives ("drug reps") or reads the drug company ads in medical journals and has come to believe the message that these sources convey. This second physician, we would imagine, would be relatively more likely to advise our patient to start immediately on a statin drug. (He might also, in addition, recommend a particular statin based not on scientific evidence but rather on his personal relationship with a particular rep or his liking for a certain ad. But we should note that a "tilt" in favor of the industry might be manifested not only as a predilection for one drug or manufacturer, but also more subtly as a predilection for drug management of medical problems over other modes of treatment and prevention.)

If the general public is privy to the contrary advice given by these two physicians, what would the reaction be? To the rational observer, two things would appear to be true. First, there is a conflict of interest between the medical profession
and the industry in regard to this particular patient. Second, that conflict of interest creates a potential conflict of loyalty for the physician. It is likely that the second physician has strayed from the ethical duty to which he has "professed." He is
now serving a set of interests different from the patient's. In the eyes of a discerning, rational public, the second physician has shown himself to be less *trustworthy*
than the first. The patient cannot have the same confidence in the second case that
the physician is looking out primarily for what is best for the patient. And that is
true whether the conflict of interest has arisen because the physician's personal
interest (in getting money or freebies) has inserted itself or whether the physician
is personally disinterested but has unwittingly been influenced by the industry.

When we try to define precisely what we mean by "conflict of interest," we discover that the issue is far thornier than it first appeared. Edmund L. Erde, a philosopher, has explained that the complexity arises because "conflict of interest" is used to
cover so many different sorts of cases in different practical contexts. He argues that
these differences make any simple, clear definition of "conflict of interest" largely
pointless, since the definition is bound to leave out some considerations of moral
concern. He suggests instead that we investigate what we might call the lay of the
land, a survey of the territory where conflicts of interest occur. Erde proposes that
we could view the territory in the manner summarized in the diagram in figure 2.1.

"Conflicts of Interest"			
Descriptive		Performative	
Personal motives	Social arrangements	Warnings	Accusations of breach of obligation

Figure 2.1. Schematic Diagram: Senses of "Conflicts of Interest"

Most uses of the term "conflict of interest" have both a descriptive and a performative intent. We try to tell our listeners how the world is arranged and also to
prompt them to take some action based on our moral assessment of the world.
(Erde argues that there is not much point in seeking a *solely* descriptive account of
"conflict of interest," since, as a practical matter, we only use the term when we
intend to express some degree of moral unease if not actual disapproval.)

Looking for a moment solely at the descriptive element of language, we might
mean to point out that an individual physician (for example) is motivated to act in a
way that might compromise one or more of her professional duties because of the
existence of a competing interest. Alternatively, we might mean to point out the
existence of social arrangements that create a risk or probability that physicians will
be tempted to act contrary to professional obligations, even if any individual physician is highly motivated to remain true to the duties owed to the patient. That is,
one but not the other of the two descriptive intents "accuses" the physician of "bad
motives."

The performative aspect of our utterance might also differ on different occasions.

We might in some cases wish to warn the individual physician, or other stakeholders, to beware of the risks of a breach of professional duty down the road. In other instances we might judge that the breach of professional duty has already occurred and we seek to hold individuals accountable for that behavior.

For those who still insist on a short definition, Erde offers this summary statement: "[T]o have a [conflict of interest] is to be in a situation in which one might plausibly be thought to do something immoral due to a motivation that might tempt most role holders (or this individual). The implication is that many persons of typical moral fiber would be likely to neglect the duties of their roles for the sake of [the temptation or motivation identified]."[17]

Erde adds two further observations. First, he proposes a basic link between conflict-of-interest language and the underlying concept of *trust in a social role* (including professional roles). Erde doubts that we would ever have come to talk about conflicts of interest were it not for the existence of social roles that have designated duties attached to them, where other people are more or less forced to trust the person occupying the role to carry out those duties efficiently and responsibly. (It is neither possible nor desirable to have the person occupying the social role watched every minute by an oversight panel; and even if this could be done, we'd have to decide whether we could trust the panel.) Conflicts of interest are therefore morally important because they address the trust *or trustworthiness* attached to social and professional role behavior. Thus, Erde's notion of conflict of interest meshes well with our previous analysis of the internal morality of medicine and of trust and trustworthiness.

Second, Erde suggests that the distinctions suggested by the often-heard phrases, "*potential* conflict of interest" or "*apparent* conflict of interest" are bogus and misleading. The distinctions he has already proposed handle the need to make any such qualifications. For instance, the difference between a warning and an accusation tells us whether we think a breach of professional obligation is merely possible or has actually occurred. In actual usage, the qualifiers "apparent" or "potential" seem to be employed as a way to soften the term "conflict of interest," making it more palatable. We wish both to point out conflicts of interest and also to reassure the involved parties that we are not accusing them of ethical lapses.[18]

This desire to have it both ways comes at a cost. It is quite true that to accuse somebody of a breach of duty, when a warning is more appropriate, is morally wrong. But it also appears to send the erroneous message that people should not be blamed for becoming involved in systemic arrangements that reasonably ought to give rise to warnings.

Some conflicts of interest are, for all practical purposes, unavoidable. One patient each day is going to be the last patient the physician sees. The physician is usually going to feel somewhat torn between getting home and giving this last patient all the care and attention that optimal standards require. We cannot imagine any realistic arrangement that would completely eliminate this problem.

But as we'll see in considerably more detail below, other arrangements—including many that typify today's relationships between medicine and the pharmaceutical industry—are not necessary or inevitable. They are "practically" impossible to eliminate only on a set of assumptions that could in turn be open to question.

If one voluntarily occupies a position that exposes one to a system of pressures that increase risk of a later breach of professional obligation, and if one's social role involves trust and trustworthiness as a central feature, then one could reasonably be held morally accountable for one's willingness to place oneself within the scope of that conflict of interest. To use a very crude analogy, if I allow a two-year-old child to play in the yard right next to a busy street, I increase the risk of that child's being injured or killed. If someone holds me morally blameworthy for my actions in allowing the child to play there, it misses the point for me to object, "You have no right to criticize me. First, the child was not, in fact, actually harmed. Second, it is not as if I personally ran over the child with a car myself." Admittedly, using poor judgment about where to allow the child to play is not as bad a moral breach as directly hurting the child, but my innocence of the larger crime cannot excuse me from culpability for the lesser offense.

The reason why my behavior is morally blameworthy is made more obvious if we imagine my using these excuses when berated by the child's mother. She is likely to respond, "But I *trusted* you to take good care of him while I was out shopping." Two separate goods are at stake here—first, the good of the child's safety, and second, the mother's ability to go about her business with a reasonable sense of trust in her child's well-being while she is absent. To the extent to which I occupy a role in which I expect others to trust me, I am obligated to hold myself to a higher standard of behavior. I can be morally blamed for engaging in actions that would lead reasonable persons to withhold their trust. If I am a member of a profession and occupy a professional (collective) role, I have done even more harm if my behavior might prompt other members of the public to refuse to trust other members of my profession in the future because of the way that I personally behaved. All of this goes to show that in some cases I *can* reasonably be blamed for conflicts of interest, even when I have displayed no bad motives (but have merely participated in certain social arrangements) and even when no one can accuse me of actually having violated a professional duty.

The distinctions Erde has proposed also help us understand why the presence or absence of *felt conflict* may have little to do with whether a conflict of interest exists. If the only descriptive sense of conflict of interest involved personal motives, then I might object, when warned or accused, that the onlooker is in no position to know what my true motives are. But conflict of interest, descriptively, can apply equally well to social arrangements that are visible to all. In such cases, where reasonable people would conclude that a social arrangement creates serious temptations to deviate from professional duty, the physician who voluntarily elects to become involved in those arrangements can be held morally accountable, even if he knows that he has no bad motives and even if he feels and perceives no moral conflict. Indeed, in such cases, the moral accountability could be adjudged to be more serious because of the *lack* of perception of a conflict—the physician, in effect, has confessed to a level of moral obtuseness that seems unacceptable in a *trustworthy* professional.

Erde's definition includes the word "plausibly." The account we have given of conflict of interest implies a "reasonable person" type of standard. The onlooker could be *wrong* about a purported conflict of interest if, on reflection, we conclude that the arrangement pointed out is not at all likely to affect the person's loyalty or judgment in a negative fashion. To take one example, top scientists at the National Institutes of Health (NIH) were accused of having numerous conflicts of interest that the previous leadership had permitted. Pressure was placed by Congress on the new director, Dr. Elias Zerhouni, to crack down on these abuses. Some critics therefore charged that the new, much stricter conflict-of-interest rules proposed for the NIH early in 2005 swung the pendulum too far in the opposite direction. For instance, some NIH scientists lost no time in complaining that the new guidelines forbade even their secretaries from owning any stock in a company that manufactured a product within their general area of research.[19] Now, leaving aside the larger question of whether stricter guidelines were in fact called for, one might argue that no one could *plausibly* assert that a secretary's owning stock in a certain company could have any inappropriate influence over the way NIH scientists conduct their research. In this case, one could easily refute the assertion of a morally serious conflict of interest.

On the other hand, let us look at an example, also from the NIH, in which it is rather more plausible to ascribe conflicts of interest. In July 2004, an expert panel convened by the National Cholesterol Education Project of the NIH's National Heart, Lung, and Blood Institute (NHLBI) issued revisions to existing guidelines on treating elevated cholesterol levels.[20] The overall impact of the revisions was to lower the threshold for treating patients with statins and to increase the dosages of these drugs that some patients would require. Critics immediately pointed out that the majority of the panelists had financial ties to the companies that manufacture statins, and that these ties had not been disclosed in the original journal article.[21] A group of physicians, organized by the Center for Science in the Public Interest, sent a petition to the directors of NIH and NHLBI objecting both to the scientific basis for the cholesterol recommendations and also to the conflicts of interest of the panelists.[22] The petition received a response from Dr. Barbara Alving, acting director of NHLBI, in which she stated, "The members of expert panels charged with developing guidelines are selected for their scientific and medical expertise, their stature and track record in the field, and their integrity."[23]

Dr. Alving's reply prompted a British signatory to the petition, Dr. Malcolm Kendrick, to recall a quip of P. G. Wodehouse's, "When an Englishman says 'trust me' it's time to start counting the spoons."[24] To back up a couple of steps, what could the NHLBI mean in claiming that the panelists were "selected for their integrity"?

1. The panelists were involved in no social arrangements that would lead reasonable people to question their judgment about the wider use of statins.
2. The panelists were screened with some other objective instrument, a sort of "integrity scale," prior to appointment.
3. In the subjective opinion of whoever appointed the panel the panelists were persons of integrity.

We know that #1 could not have been the criterion because the panelists were in fact involved in those sorts of social arrangements. It is very doubtful that #2 was the criterion, since we have heard of no such instrument or its use among NIH panelists. That leaves #3.

The reason to have a notion of "conflict of interest" in the first place is that we realize that our subjective judgments about certain matters may be flawed. When we can make more money by deviating from our strict professional obligations, we have a very strong tendency to judge our own motives in the kindest possible light and to imagine the deleterious consequences of our actions to be minor or nonexistent.

Therefore, when the NHLBI finds it necessary to proclaim that expert panelists subject to obvious financial conflicts of interest are persons of "integrity," the proclamation is morally suspect on several levels. "Conflict of interest" in this situation means reasonable people, knowing what they know about the relationship that follows from receiving financial rewards, have reason to doubt these scientists' ability to assess the evidence regarding statins in a fair-minded way. To insist that these scientists are people of integrity is to urge reasonable people to put aside these reasonable thoughts and to trust instead the subjective judgment of the people doing the insisting. But people who ignore plausible evidence of a systemic conflict of interest are people whose subjective judgments about integrity have quite reasonably been called into question. These parties' judgments about integrity are further called into question when they seem blind to the disconnect between, on the one hand, admitting that the panelists take money from drug manufacturers, and on the other hand, insisting that these are nevertheless people of integrity.

One final comment on the term "conflict of interest" is in order here. Another philosopher, Arthur Schafer, begins his analysis of the concept by quoting from a frequently cited paper by Dennis Thompson, who defines conflict of interest as "a set of conditions in which professional judgment concerning a primary interest (such as a patient's welfare or the validity of research) tends to be unduly influenced by a secondary interest (such as financial gain)."[25] Schafer disagrees and offers an alternative formulation: "A person is in a conflict of interest situation if she is in a relationship with another in which she has a moral obligation to exercise her judgment in that other's service and, at the same time, she has an interest tending to interfere with the proper exercise of judgment in that relationship."[26] One of the reasons Schafer dislikes Thompson's initial formulation is the misleading nature of the term "interests." It is not merely the case that the patient has an *interest* in being well cared for, or that the physician has an *interest* in caring well for the patient. The physician has a *professional duty* to care for the patient at a level of reasonable competence and fiduciary commitment. By contrast, the physician has no *duty* to make more money. The phrase "conflict of *interest*" could suggest that the two competing forces tempting the physician in different directions are of *equal* moral weight. Such a mistaken view, which fails to appreciate that serious professional duties are being threatened by *mere* "interests," might fuel the objections of those who attack conflict-of-interest concerns as representing a nitpicking, holier-than-thou mentality.

TRUST AND TRUSTWORTHINESS IN RESEARCH

So far we have been attending primarily to the relationship between the physician and patient in the medical treatment or therapeutic setting. What happens to concepts such as "trust," "trustworthiness," and "conflict of interest" when we shift to the research setting, better described as an investigator-subject relationship rather than as a physician-patient relationship?[27]

Some would argue that nothing fundamentally changes when this shift occurs. The physician is still a physician and still should be viewed as a fiduciary, entrusted to give the patient-subject the *best available* medical care. I believe that this is incorrect. The investigator-subject relationship in the research setting is a fundamentally different form of relationship and requires a different ethical analysis. This is because the goal of the research setting is not to provide therapeutic benefits for individual patients; rather it is to acquire new knowledge that can aid in the medical care of future patients.[28] Saying that the research setting is ethically different from therapy is *not* to say that the research subject deserves any *less* ethical protection than the patient. It is rather to say that the ethical dangers come from a different direction, and new ethical defenses are required to meet the challenge.

The principal ethical duty of the investigator is to protect research subjects from exploitation. A major (but not the only) tool to prevent exploitation is to insist upon each subject's adequately informed consent.[29]

We will later review evidence that a good deal of the clinical research activity funded by the pharmaceutical industry is more an extension of the industry's marketing effort than a true contribution to medical science. The major goal of some research is the increase in sales of the company's product—even if the means to achieve that result is to spin or tweak the research data to make differences sound more impressive than they are, or even to suppress unfavorable data outright.

Human subjects participating in research trials may do so for basically selfish reasons—because they believe that trial participation will give them the best chance of cure. But the informed consent process, if it works as it is supposed to work, ought to help such subjects to realize that any benefit they might receive from a trial is uncertain at best. One would hope that most appropriately informed subjects wish to participate in research at least in part for altruistic reasons. They wish to see medical science advance and to make that knowledge available for the treatment of future patients.

For these reasons there is a serious problem of trust and trustworthiness in at least some industry-sponsored clinical research. It is unjustly exploitive of human subjects to allow them to imagine that they are contributing to the advance of science if in fact the design of the study has been manipulated specifically to obtain data that the company will use to its marketing advantage, rather than to answer any scientific question of real interest or importance. (This would be the case, for instance, if a low dose of the company's antidepressant drug is compared to a high dose of a competitor's drug as a way to "prove" that the company's drug has fewer side effects.[30]) If such "research" trials are allowed to go forward at all, it would seem to be essential that the process of informed consent acknowledge the frankly commercial nature of the activity. If research subjects are going to experience the risk and inconvenience of taking a study medication and being tested for various outcomes, they should know the exact purposes for which the final results will be used. Moreover, it would seem a specific violation of the rights of human subjects for a pharmaceutical firm ever to suppress or conceal the results of clinical trials, as happened with the studies of SSRI-class antidepressants in children and adolescents.[31]

Subjects deciding whether to enter into a research trial would also reasonably wish to know about any financial incentives and financial conflicts of interest that involve the investigator and the physician (often their personal physician) who recruits them for the trial. When physicians may be paid between one thousand and five thousand dollars for recruiting a patient for a company-sponsored study, this might reasonably be disclosed as part of a mandatory informed-consent process.[32] At the very least, the subjects might then be able to demand their fair share of the "take."

ETHICAL AND PRUDENTIAL CONSIDERATIONS

Defenders of cozy relationships between the industry and the profession have generally objected at this point that it is highly insulting to accuse physicians of being "bought" by the industry in the manner we have just described. Returning to the case of the physician treating the patient with a high cholesterol level, one could come up with a fully satisfactory scientific rationale for beginning drug therapy in this patient. Data could be brought forth to show that this patient will experience a better medical risk-benefit ratio by starting on statins now.[33] The lesson (it is alleged) is therefore that physicians are careful, scientific professionals who make thoughtful judgments, always keeping the patient's interests foremost. All the drug industry does, through its promotional and advertising activities, is keep these professionals aware of new developments in pharmaceuticals. Thus, for example, Dr. Bert Spilker, PhRMA's senior vice president of scientific and regulatory affairs, accused two critics who would "ban all contact between drug industry sales representatives and physicians" as "fear[ing] that physicians are so weak and lacking in integrity that they would 'sell their souls' for a pack of M&M candies and a few sandwiches and doughnuts. . . . As a physician, I find it hard to imagine that any of my colleagues would compromise professional concern for their patients. Certainly the vast majority of physicians are able to resist this temptation and make decisions solely based on the best medical interests of their patients."[34]

Later we will examine the evidence to support this assertion of noninfluence. For now, the point to explore is simply how much of the discussion is an ethical one and how much might better be classed as prudential. That is, is it a question of what is morally right, or is it a question of what is simply a smart thing to do?

Let us return to the point about public trust and trustworthiness. The average rational spectator, seeing the two physicians give different advice to the patient with high cholesterol, would conclude that the second physician (influenced by industry promotion) is less trustworthy as a patient advocate or fiduciary. That conclusion follows in fairly straightforward fashion merely from noting the existence of a conflict of interest. It might be that the second physician was not consciously aware of any bias toward any particular drug or toward drug versus nondrug therapy. One could probably locate a third physician who would have recommended immediate statins for the patient but who never talked with drug reps or read drug ads. Still, a judgment has been made about the trustworthiness of a group of physicians—in today's environment, the vast majority of physicians—and as we previously argued, that judgment is at least in part an ethical judgment.

To portray the matter solely as an *ethical* one, however, may lead to important misperceptions. Physicians understandably react in indignation when someone seems to be challenging their professional ethics on the basis of accepting one drug company pen or coffee mug or eating a sandwich at a "free" drug lunch. Doesn't making such mundane transactions between profession and industry a matter for *ethical* scrutiny suggest an unrealistic level of perfectionism—if not, less charitably, an attitude of smug self-righteousness among the critics?[35]

There are several possible rejoinders to this line of critique. We will ask later whether it is justifiable to consider "just one" sandwich or pen rather than the long-term pattern of relationship signified by those exchanges. For now, it's important to relocate the debate to the realm of ethics and prudence rather than "pure" ethics.[36]

Prudence enters into the matter because most physicians readily claim to be very busy people, making what they choose to do with their time a pressing concern. It is also an *ethical* concern to the extent that spending one's time doing certain things might make one less available to perform patient care functions and so less dedicated to the care of one's patients. There is therefore some overlap between the realms of ethics and prudence.

How is time management relevant to the ethical question of avoiding actual conflicts of interest as a professional while remaining in an ongoing relationship with industry? We have seen that the rational spectator might conclude that the physician is acting in a less trustworthy fashion because that physician has been observed to engage in certain sorts of relationships and transactions with industry. The rational spectator knows that in the world of business promotion, such interactions can be expected to lead to biases in the direction of the interests of the promoter. There is a general tendency in that direction even though any particular bit of information exchanged may be unbiased. Moreover, the drug industry pays a lot for the ads, drug reps, and free drug samples—amounting to more than twenty billion dollars annually in the United States.[37] If the result is *not* physician behavior that coincides better with the companies' interests, the industry is wasting a tremendous amount of money.[38]

The ethical judgment of trustworthiness, we now realize, is made only in the context of a judgment about the physician's time management. Imagine two physicians who both went to the "free" drug lunch, ate the sandwich, and listened to the sales pitch. One proceeds to go into the office and to start writing prescriptions. The other, however, is worried about the potential bias of the company's marketing message, and so before she goes back to work, she spends an hour on the computer or in the medical library cross-checking the accuracy of what the company rep said.

Our first question is: which of these two physicians is more trustworthy? Presumably our rational spectator would bestow that accolade on the second physician. But let us take this judgment a bit farther. The first physician, we now realize, has an ethics-trustworthiness problem. He has exposed himself to potential bias and has done nothing to correct it, even though he should realize that the bias might interfere with his fiduciary duty to his patients.[39] What, then, do we say about the second physician? From a mere trustworthiness viewpoint she is exemplary, but she would seem to have a serious time-management problem. Why spend all that time cross-checking the biased information received from the company source? In less time she could have simply learned the unbiased information about what drug to prescribe by reading any number of independent professional and scientific sources.[40]

The vast majority of physicians who expose themselves to the commercially biased messages of the industry do not spend the time needed to check out the accuracy of what they have heard or read. In that setting, their protestations of being dedicated, scientific prescribers, who cannot be swayed by a pen or a donut, ring rather hollow, especially in the face of empirical evidence of the frequency of inaccurate information in company pitches and presentations.[41] If the truth be known, the physicians who eagerly attend the "free" lunches for the drug company do so not so they will later have to spend extra time, but rather because most think that listening to the sales pitch *substitutes for* more strenuous and time-consuming research. But if that is the case, the second physician who actually does spend the extra time seems to have painted herself into an ethical corner as well. She has indeed established herself as a more scientific and trustworthy patient advocate, but only at the cost of proclaiming herself to have a good deal of time on her hands. If she has so much extra time and is dedicated to patient service, why not see a couple more patients rather than scarf down free sandwiches? (We assume that the average physician enjoys a sufficient income not to *need* the freebies supplied by the drug companies).

A further consideration is that the term "freebie" is relative. In actuality, patients pay for the sandwiches, pens, coffee mugs, and so forth, in the form of higher drug prices. Our second physician, who is willing to spend extra time to be an unbiased prescriber, nevertheless is willing in effect to charge her patients extra just so she can have that sandwich at lunch. Admittedly, her single personal act of refusal to consume that sandwich will not decrease the price of drugs for any of her patients. But she bears some responsibility for participating in a pattern of behavior that, multiplied across all physicians, has real and arguably deleterious consequences for patients.

In sum, the conflicts of interest between the individual practicing physician and the pharmaceutical industry are a matter of some ethical as well as prudential concern. Historically, the relationship has not been seen as ethically problematic, and so when the ethical concerns are spotlighted, practitioners commonly respond with anger, outrage, and various rationalizations, all of which can be complicated to disentangle. To see why this is so, it will be necessary later to explore in some detail the history of this relationship during the twentieth century.

ETHICS AND POWER

The individual physician, however, is not the only level at which we must explore the ethical implications of the relationship with industry. When we begin to explore the various levels and their interconnections, it may be helpful to consider links between ethics and *power*.

During the formative years of today's bioethics, the term "power" was seldom alluded to explicitly. "Doing something because it is the right thing to do" and "doing something because you have the power to get away with it, or because others with more power make you do it" seemed to be completely antithetical concepts. This ignoring of power was unfortunate, because a central ethical question in medicine is "How can physicians use their power wisely and responsibly?"[42]

It is relatively easy to see the power implications of the relationship between the individual physician and the patient. As we argued before, this is basically an unequal relationship in which the average patient is relatively vulnerable and so lacking in power. Patients nevertheless *can* exercise considerable power in the relationship. For example, many experts decry the widespread misuse and overuse of antibiotics in U.S. medical practice, with antibiotics being prescribed routinely for viral illnesses that cannot benefit from such treatment, causing a public health threat of bacteria developing resistance to commonly used drugs. Physicians who prescribe antibiotics in such circumstances commonly say that the patient expects these drugs, that it would take too long to try to talk the patient out of wanting the drug, and that the patient will simply go shopping until he finds a physician willing to prescribe it. It would appear that in the matter of antibiotic prescribing, many physicians have somehow handed the power over to the patient. So a simple formula of "physician is powerful, patient is powerless" won't do. If we are to explore all the ethical ramifications of this relationship to the bottom, we will have to assess in a very finely grained fashion exactly who has power over what and in what circumstances. We can then ask what would count as responsible and irresponsible uses of power.

Then we could expand this exercise to the corporate level and talk about the network of power relationships among all players in our system. Recall in our two cholesterol examples that we have depicted two very different levels at which the profession-industry relationship might occur. In one case we saw the possibility that an individual physician might prescribe for an individual patient in a biased fashion. In the other case we saw the possibility that nationally respected scientists might be biased in the process of writing consensus guidelines that could conceivably be used as a tool by thousands of physicians in writing future prescriptions for their patients. Obviously the power implications, as well as the possible remedies to prevent future abuses, are quite different at these two levels—even though, as I will argue in this book, it would be mistaken to view these two "cases" as somehow having nothing to do with each other.

As we proceed, we will address all of the following levels of interaction between the profession and the industry:

- the individual physician receiving gifts, information, and free samples from drug reps
- groups of physicians attending formal continuing medical education courses funded in part by the industry
- industry support of medical professional organizations

- industry support of "grass roots" patient advocacy groups
- industry advertising aimed directly at consumers
- industry support of medical journals
- industry support of research, and consulting and speakers' fees paid to individual investigators and "opinion leaders"
- industry's role in lobbying government for favorable laws and regulations
- the role of the FDA in regulating the industry

THE STORY OF A CANADIAN LAWSUIT

A case study may illustrate further what it means to view some of these relationships in terms of power. The Canadian Coordinating Office for Health Technology Assessment (CCOHTA) is funded by Canadian federal, provincial, and territorial government units to help make informed health policy. One of its jobs is to advise on the cost-effectiveness of drugs. Because of the price controls imposed in Canada by the provincial health plans, CCOHTA's decision that two drugs provide equivalent benefits can have profound economic consequences for a manufacturer. The Canadian health system will typically then agree to pay for the lower-priced drug and the more expensive drug may lose a major share of the market.

In 1997, CCOHTA did a scientific review of statin drugs for lowering cholesterol. The agency followed its usual procedures, notifying the involved drug companies of its report, sharing a preliminary draft, and meeting with company representatives. CCOHTA then prepared to issue a report that more or less treated statins as a single class of drugs with largely equivalent effects—a conclusion that would surprise hardly anyone familiar with the scientific literature or with daily clinical practice. The senior vice president for science of the American Heart Association agreed that CCOHTA's conclusions were reasonable.

Bristol-Myers Squibb, however, took exception to the implication that its statin drug, pravastatin (Pravachol), was not necessarily superior to other statins. The company filed suit claiming that CCOHTA was guilty of "negligent misstatements" and demanding that the report not be issued. The lower court in Ontario denied the motion and the company then appealed.

The appeals court ruled against the company in June 1998. The judge, in denying the company's demand for an injunction, noted that ruling for Bristol-Myers Squibb would essentially render CCOHTA useless, since it would declare open season, inviting any other drug firm immediately to sue if it did not like the recommendations.

The legal defense that led to CCOHTA's "winning" its case cost the agency a total of $230,000 Canadian. That sum was 13 percent of CCOHTA's annual budget. By contrast, if we were to assume that the case also cost the company the same amount in legal fees, the total expense amounted to one single day of sales revenues for Pravachol in Canada.[43]

At just about the same time that CCOHTA was conducting its statin study, the province of Ontario commissioned a study of proton pump inhibitor drugs for treating ulcers and acid reflux. Anne Holbrook, a physician and pharmacist at McMaster

University, led the panel, which concluded in 1999 that all the proton pump inhibitors worked about the same. AstraZeneca was manufacturer of Prilosec (or Losec as it was known in Canada), one of the more expensive drugs. Dr. Holbrook received a letter from a Toronto law firm threatening to "take appropriate steps, including the commencement of appropriate legal proceedings," if the guidelines proposed by the panel were distributed.

Dr. Holbrook wisely referred the lawyers for AstraZeneca to the province of Ontario as the sponsor of the study. The company never sued, so the province of Ontario never faced the large legal fees that CCOHTA had to pay. Apparently the firm was content with the fear factor alone, warning academic physicians what sort of hornet's nest they would be putting their heads into if they acted against the interest of big drug companies.[44]

The CCOHTA lawsuit is analogous to what has been called a "SLAPP," for "strategic lawsuits against public participation." Such a lawsuit is brought without any hope of prevailing in the courts. The goal is either to delay an outcome for a sufficient time so that a large profit can be made, or else to exert a chilling effect on others through the threat that they will be sued in the future and will have to spend vast amounts of time and money to defend themselves against baseless charges. A SLAPP can be effectively brought only by a party who has a disproportionate share of financial resources. In ethical terms, the lawsuit is an abuse of power. The legal system in Canada seemed incapable in this instance of rectifying the power imbalance and leveling the playing field; the adage that "every person has a right to his day in court" here worked to protect the powerful against the relatively powerless. So at present, ethical condemnation (or more effective government regulation) may be the only tools at our disposal to try to prevent such abuse.[45]

We can, in general, describe our foray into the profession-industry relationship as this sort of assessment of the relative power of the interacting parties at all levels and in all relevant circumstances, and the identification of "hot spots" where serious power imbalances appear to lead to abuses. We can then proceed to ask what interventions might in the future better restore some balance of power. Other things being equal, we wish to empower patients and ordinary citizens, even if this to some extent threatens the self-interest of the industry or the profession.

A further case study that illustrates the difficulties in making these sorts of power assessments is provided by direct-to-consumer (DTC) advertising of prescription drugs, a practice that has escalated in the United States since 1997. Consider the following arguments relevant to this practice:

- Physicians commonly complain about DTC ads because they already feel significant time pressure in the average patient visit, and this is increased if patients come in asking questions about DTC ads for specific medications, requiring long explanations about why the medication may not be appropriate for the patient.[46]
- The industry defends DTC ads as contributing to public education. People may learn what as-yet-undiagnosed diseases they might suffer from, and also what medications might be available to treat the disease.[47]

- Critics of the industry note that the tendency in DTC ads is to "medicalize" problems of everyday living and to try to convince the public that they need medication for these problems.[48]
- Those concerned about prescription costs note that physicians often prescribe brand-name drugs when requested specifically by patients, even when cheaper alternatives are available, so that DTC ads seem to drive up the costs of medical care.[49]

Several conclusions are possible. One is that DTC ads empower patients, while physicians, jealous of their prerogatives, respond negatively to this power shift and their own perceived loss of power. On this analysis, if the ads make patients come to see the physician with a variety of searching questions that require careful answers, that is precisely what medical care is supposed to be all about. Another possible conclusion is that the drug industry is using its money and influence to manipulate patients, who then use their relative power within the system to manipulate physicians in a manner that ends up serving the financial interests of the industry. It is possible that both patient empowerment and patient manipulation are occurring simultaneously, and careful empirical research would be needed to determine the precise contribution of each. At any rate, a full ethical and policy analysis demands an assessment of how each party to the transaction uses his power and what impact this has on the other parties.

In a capitalist society, it appears to run against the grain to claim that there is something unethical going on just because a company or an industry has grown large and wealthy. Wealth is supposed to be the reward for doing the right things. But the example of SLAPP, and questions we will address later about the lobbying power of the pharmaceutical industry, remind us that too much concentration of wealth and power in the hands of a single interest group can create unfortunate social consequences. We will, as we go through this book, periodically encounter analogies to the times a hundred years ago, when the novel *The Jungle* set the stage for the creation of the FDA, and when President Theodore Roosevelt had to do battle with the "trusts." Some think that we are overdue for another time of trust-busting, that we have forgotten the lessons of the beginning of the twentieth century. An ethical analysis that is open to considering issues of power will aid us in determining whether that prescription has merit.

ORGANIZATIONAL CODES OF ETHICS

It might seem odd that I have proceeded this far with a discussion of the ethical basis for judging interactions between the medical profession and the pharmaceutical industry without having made any explicit mention of the codes of ethics of various medical-professional groups. One might imagine that these codes would provide the most direct and informative statements of professional ethics.

There are, however, serious problems with and challenges to professional-organizational codes. What if a certain behavior is unethical but the vast majority of physicians currently engage in it? An organization that depends at least in part on members' dues for its survival may be reluctant to brand the larger portion of its membership with the label "unethical." On the other hand, it may be tempting to take the high road in writing, knowing full well that few medical organizations have the necessary staff or resources to police compliance with ethical codes. Everyone wins, it may appear—the organization gets credit for its uncompromising ethical stance, and members may go about their business with impunity.

The American Medical Association's (AMA) recent role in professional ethics may illustrate some of these problems. The AMA issued guidelines on accepting gifts from the pharmaceutical industry in 1991 and updated them in 2002.[50] Both dates coincided with upswings in governmental interest in physicians receiving drug-company gifts. The 1991 guidelines followed hard on Senate committee hearings chaired by Senator Edward Kennedy, and the 2002 update came during a time when numerous government agencies were reviewing the problem and when individual states were considering mandatory reporting laws.[51] Nonetheless, AMA staff insisted that the organization's ethical reflections preceded rather than followed the threat of government intervention or regulation.[52]

The 1991 guidelines begin:

Many gifts that are given to physicians by companies in the pharmaceutical, device, and medical equipment industries serve an important and socially beneficial function. For example, companies have long provided funds for educational seminars and conferences. However, there has been growing concern about certain gifts from industry to physicians. Some gifts that reflect customary practices of industry may not be consistent with the principles of medical ethics. To avoid the acceptance of inappropriate gifts, physicians should observe the following guidelines.[53]

Several things appear evident. First, the statement begins by praising the industry for providing socially beneficial gifts, almost as if the framers feared to be seen as ungrateful for past largesse. Second, there is mention that practices routine in business might not be consistent with medical ethics, but there is no clear statement of the medical-ethical principles that *ought to* guide the gift relationship. It may be implicit, if one takes the AMA's *Principles of Medical Ethics* as a whole, that "physicians continue to hold the welfare of their individual patients as their primary ethical responsibility. . . . Second to patient welfare is the acknowledgment that the public's trust in the medical profession must be safeguarded."[54] But this clear statement of foundational ethical principles does not appear within the gift guideline itself. Finally, the focus is completely on gifts received by individual physicians; no mention is made of any ethical concerns about professional organizations receiving gifts or grants from the industry.

The lack of mention of the professional-organization level of gift giving might have something to do with the AMA's own history during this period. In 1997, the leadership of the AMA found it necessary to backtrack in the face of heavily negative publicity after it announced a multimillion-dollar deal to allow Sunbeam Corporation to use the AMA's name on health-related products.[55] Several highly placed AMA officials were forced to resign in the ensuing scandal.[56] Some critics saw more of the same in the AMA's decision, following the updating of its ethical guidelines on pharmaceutical gifts, to accept drug company grants to support an educational program to promulgate the new guidelines.[57]

What of the substance of the AMA ethical guidelines? Generally, physicians are allowed to accept company gifts if: (1) no strings are attached, (2) the gift is somehow linked to or useful to patient care, and (3) the gift is of minimal or nominal value. These apparently reasonable provisions are nonetheless open to criticism. It is not clear that the monetary value of a gift determines the degree of influence it may have over the physicians' prescribing. Ten gifts of low value that constantly remind the physician of the drug's brand name, for instance—like pens or notepads—may be more influential than a single, larger gift. And gifts exert influence not by themselves, but as part of, and as tokens of, human relationships. Most of us were taught as children to feel obligated to those who give us gifts, regardless of value, and the industry has proven adept over the years at milking this early acculturation for all it is worth.[58]

One can also quibble over the notion of "no strings attached." There is no explicit tie between a pen or a free lunch and any specific promise from the physician to prescribe a certain quantity of the drug being pushed. But as we will see later when we discuss drug reps, no physician would have to talk to too many colleagues before she learned that the higher prescribers for any drug are usually rewarded with more gifts of higher value. It may be difficult or impossible to eliminate the implicit sense of the tie between getting gifts and doing what the industry wants the physician to do.

Finally, we must ask what the results were of the 1991 and 2002 AMA pronouncements. Again, those within the organization saw great success. A reporter for the AMA's journal claimed that the practice of inviting physicians for a free dinner plus a hundred-dollar honorarium to hear a company pitch, which had involved an estimated one hundred seventy-five thousand physicians annually during the late 1980s, would become completely defunct in the wake of the 1991 guidelines.[59] Commenting on the need to revisit the guidelines in 2002, AMA staff wrote, "The initial impact of these [1991] guidelines was a marked abatement of the excesses. . . . However, with a new generation of physicians and a dramatic expansion in the industry's sales force, awareness of and adherence to these guidelines have waned over time."[60]

I have, however, been unable to locate any credible information from non-AMA sources that either the 1991 or the 2002 guidelines have had any discernible influence whatsoever. The available anecdotal evidence strongly suggests that it was business as usual after both guidelines were issued.[61] If anything, promotional events such as dinners-with-honoraria steadily increased between 1991 and 2002.[62]

Other organizations have tried to provide different sorts of ethical guidance. The American College of Physicians adopted a somewhat more forthright and critical set of statements in 1990, with more extensive ethical rationale and argument.[63] Instead of a quasi-objective standard based on value of gift, relevance to patient care, and so on, they proposed a subjective standard: "A useful criterion in determining acceptable activities and relationships is: Would you be willing to have these arrangements generally known?"[64] This publicity criterion has generally been viewed with approval by commentators. But it is also open to criticism.

An overly sensitive physician might be ashamed of an arrangement that actually violated no ethical rules. A particularly thick-skinned physician would not mind if his patients knew all about his most egregious conflicts of interest. In a perverse way this ethical guideline might even appear to reward ethical obtuseness.[65]

Jerome Kassirer, in his recent book, is generally dismissive of all efforts to deal with the ethical problems of drug company interactions via voluntary codes of ethics promulgated by professional organizations. He compares physicians to lawyers and other professionals and notes the unique lack of enforcement mechanisms in the way physicians' organizations deal with conflict of interest. In his view, the lack of any real teeth in the guidelines sends a stronger "ethical" message than anything within the guidelines themselves. He concludes, "That physicians are not held to the standards of journalists, attorneys and other professionals is one of the great scandals of our time."[66]

The basic ethical framework developed in this chapter allows us to proceed to the details of the profession-industry relationship. The next step to give some structure to the inquiry is to ask how the world in which this relationship takes place looks to the pharmaceutical industry and its defenders. That, in turn, will lead to an analysis of what is meant by a "free market" in pharmaceuticals.

NOTES

1. R. W. Emerson, "The Conduct of Life: Worship" (1870), www.bartleby.com/66/5/21105.html (accessed March 16, 2005).

2. G. B. Shaw, *The Doctor's Dilemma* (New York: Penguin, 1980), 9–10.

3. It is one thing to baldly state an ethical rule, principle, or concept, and quite another to argue for and defend that rule sufficiently to persuade other thoughtful people to accept it if they are not inclined already to do so. This chapter will present an ethical position but will not engage in a rigorous defense of it. Nonetheless, I do not expect a great deal of dispute over the ethical positions I have taken here. In health care ethics there is a spectrum along which issues range themselves according to their relative degree of controversy. Compared to difficult issues such as abortion, human cloning, and physician-assisted suicide, I regard the ethical framework relevant to the pharmaceutical industry as lying well toward the noncontroversial end of the spectrum. The problem is not discerning the basic ethical rules and concepts that apply; it is deciding what actual behaviors and policies those rules require in the real world, and perhaps even more difficult, developing the political will to do what's required.

4. For a different theoretical foundation upon which to base an analysis of relationships with industry, see A. Wazana and F. Primeau, "Ethical Considerations in the Relationship between Physicians and the Pharmaceutical Industry," *Psychiatr Clin North Am* 2002; 25:647–63. These authors employ a Kantian framework but propose conclusions very similar to those argued for elsewhere in this book, and agree that conflict of interest is a key ethical issue.

5. Shaw, *Doctor's Dilemma*, 7.

6. T. Beauchamp, "Internal and External Standards of Medical Morality," *J Med Philos* 2001; 26:601–19; R. M. Veatch, "The Internal and External Sources of Morality for Medicine," in *The Healthcare Professional as Friend and Healer*, ed. D. Thomasma and J. L. Kissell, 75–86 (Washington, D.C.: Georgetown University Press, 2000); R. M. Veatch, "The Impossibility of a Morality Internal to Medicine," *J Med Philos* 2001; 26:621–42.

7. A. MacIntyre, *After Virtue* (South Bend, Ind.: Notre Dame University Press, 1981); see especially p. 175.

8. H. Brody and F. G. Miller, "The Internal Morality of Medicine: Explication and Application to Managed Care," *J Med Philos* 1998; 23:384–410; F. G. Miller and H. Brody, "The Internal Morality of Medicine: An Evolutionary Perspective," *J Med Philos* 2001; 26: 581–99.

9. E. D. Pellegrino, "Toward a Reconstruction of Medical Morality: The Primacy of the Act of Profession and the Fact of Illness," *J Med Philos* 1979; 4:32–56.

10. In the wake of HIPAA legislation, it might seem that the ability to rely on physician confidentiality is generated externally by federal law; but the physician's sense of obligation to maintain confidentiality long predated this particular bit of legislation.

11. I am grateful to Rodger Jackson, in an unpublished doctoral dissertation, for providing an especially finely grained analysis of trust. R. L. Jackson, "A Philosophical Exploration of Trust" (Ph.D. thesis, Department of Philosophy, Michigan State University, 1996). Jackson in turn relied on work by Annette Baier; see for instance A. Baier, "Trust and Antitrust," *Ethics* 1986; 96:231–60. I am also grateful to Robert Arnold for suggesting the need for a brief analysis of "trust" here.

12. Because of this ethical stance, I will later have a great deal of trouble with a commonly heard assertion—that the prices charged for many drugs today in the United States are "too high." At the end, some of the policy changes I will recommend would (one hopes) result in the lowering of some drug prices. But I remain very suspicious of any argument designed to show that one can decide what drugs "ought" to cost *purely on ethical grounds*. If a free-market, capitalist society means anything at all, I assume that it means that we should suspect any assertion of the "ethically correct" price of any good or service other than the price actually set by market conditions. If on the other hand we discover that a drug company is able to make a higher profit than it would under conditions of an ideally free market because it has used its economic or political clout to manipulate the market in its own favor, then we are entitled at least to point out that fact—especially if the company routinely responds with "free market" rhetoric when its activities are questioned.

13. J. Braithwaite, *Corporate Crime in the Pharmaceutical Industry* (Boston: Routledge & Kegan Paul, 1984); for a more recent update see J. Braithwaite, "Transnational Regulation of the Pharmaceutical Industry," *Annals of the American Academy of Political and Social Science* 1993; 525:12–30.

14. L. J. Weber, *Business Ethics in Healthcare: Beyond Compliance* (Bloomington: University of Indiana Press, 2001).

15. D. Socolar and A. Sager, "Windfall Profits Despite Discounted Price: Small Manufacturing Cost for Cipro Yields Estimated $70 Million Windfall," Health Reform Program, Boston University School of Public Health, 2002; http://dcc2.bumc.bu.edu/hs/Upload070102/ CIPRO%20windfall%20profits%20brief%20-%2028%20June%202002%20.pdf.

16. F. Hawthorne, *The Merck Druggernaut: The Inside Story of a Pharmaceutical Giant* (Hoboken, NJ: John Wiley & Sons, 2003), 15–17.

17. E. L. Erde, "Conflicts of Interest in Medicine: A Philosophical and Ethical Morphology," in *Conflicts of Interest in Clinical Practice and Research*, ed. R. G. Speece, D. S. Shimm, and A. E. Buchanan, 12–41, quote p. 30 (New York: Oxford University Press, 1996).

18. Erde, "Conflicts of Interest in Medicine." For a more legally-oriented analysis of conflicts of interest in research particularly, see P. N. Ossorio, "Pills, Bills and Shills: Physician-Researcher's Conflicts of Interest," *Widener Law Symposium J* 2001; 8:75–103.

19. I am grateful to Robert Arnold for suggesting the need for this qualification. Whether the new NIH conflict-of-interest guidelines proposed early in 2005 were a long overdue corrective, a politically-driven overreaction, or some of each, is a matter beyond the scope

of our discussion. On some of the initial objections, see R. Alonso-Zaldivar, "NIH Employees Object to New Ethics Rules: A Senior Agency Official Says the Restrictions on Drug Industry Consulting Payments to Staff Researchers Are Necessary," *Los Angeles Times*, February 24, 2005:A14.

20. S. M. Grundy, J. I. Cleeman, C. N. Merz, et al., "Implications of Recent Clinical Trials for the National Cholesterol Education Program Adult Treatment Panel III Guidelines," *Circulation* 2004; 110:227–39.

21. D. Ricks and R. Rabin, "Panel's Ties to Drugmakers Not Cited in New Cholesterol Guidelines," *Long Island Newsday*, July 15, 2004:A6; J. P. Kassirer, "Why Should We Swallow What These Studies Say?" *Washington Post*, August 1, 2004:B3. For a more dismissive view of the controversy see A. Zuger, "How Tightly Do Ties between Doctor and Drug Company Bind?" *New York Times*, July 27, 2004:F1.

22. M. Goozner, "Petition to the National Institutes of Health Seeking an Independent Review Panel to Re-Evaluate the National Cholesterol Education Program Guidelines," September 23, 2004. http://cspinet.org/new/pdf/finalnihltr.pdf (accessed November 12, 2004).

23. B. Alving, Letter to Merrill Goozner, undated, [October 2004]:8.

24. M. Kendrick, "Conflict of Interest—Time to Count the Spoons?" *Red Flags Weekly Newsletter*, August 11, 2004; www.redflagsweekly.com (accessed November 21, 2004).

25. D. F. Thompson, "Understanding Financial Conflicts of Interest," *N Engl J Med* 1993; 329:573–76.

26. A. Schafer, "Biomedical Conflicts of Interest: A Defence of the Sequestration Thesis—Learning from the Cases of Nancy Olivieri and David Healy," *J Med Ethics* 2004; 30:8–24; quote p. 19.

27. L. R. Churchill, "Physician-Investigator/Patient-Subject: Exploring the Logic and the Tension," *J Med Philos* 1980; 5:215–24.

28. F. G. Miller, and H. Brody, "A Critique of Clinical Equipoise: Therapeutic Misconception in the Ethics of Clinical Trials," *Hastings Cen Rep* 2003; 33(3): 19–28; H. Brody and F. G. Miller, "The Clinician-Investigator: Unavoidable but Manageable Tension," *Kennedy Institute of Ethics J* 2003; 13: 329–46.

29. E. J. Emanuel, D. Wendler, and C. Grady, "What Makes Clinical Research Ethical?" *JAMA* 2000; 283:2701–11.

30. D. J. Safer, "Design and Reporting Modifications in Industry-Sponsored Comparative Psychopharmacology Trials," *J Nerv Ment Dis* 2002; 190:583–92.

31. Psychiatrist David Healy has perhaps been most outspoken on the way that the commercialization of clinical trials threatens the rights of human subjects; D. Healy, *Let Them Eat Prozac* (Toronto: James Lorimer and Company, 2003), 374. Healy quotes Jonathan Quick of WHO: "If clinical trials become a commercial venture in which self-interest overrules public interest and desire overrules science, then the social contract which allows research on human subjects in return for medical advances is broken." J. Quick, "Maintaining the Integrity of the Clinical Evidence Base," *Bull World Health Organ* 2001; 79:1093. See also J. La Puma, C. B. Stocking, W. D. Rhoades, et al., "Financial Ties as Part of Informed Consent to Postmarketing Research: Attitudes of American Doctors and Patients," *BMJ* 1995; 310:1660–63; S. Garattini, V. Bertele, and L. Li Bassi, "How Can Research Ethics Committees Protect Patients Better?" *BMJ* 2003; 326:1199–201; T. Lemmens, "Piercing the Veil of Corporate Secrecy about Clinical Trials," *Hastings Cen Rep* 2004; 34(5): 14–18; B. M. Psaty and C. D. Furberg, "COX-2 Inhibitors—Lessons in Drug Safety," *N Engl J Med* 2005; 352:1133–35.

32. M. Munro, "Bounty-Hunting Doctors Recruit Human Guinea Pigs: Doctors Earn Thousands by Talking Their Patients into Being Subjects in Drug Trials," *Ottawa Citizen*, February 23, 2004:A1.

33. This, at any rate, is what is argued by the authors of commonly cited clinical guidelines. For a summary of the evidence against the use of statins in patients who have not already shown signs of coronary disease, see J. Abramson, *Overdosed America: The Broken Promise of American Medicine* (New York: HarperCollins, 2004), 129–48; and "Do Statins Have a Role in Primary Prevention?" *Therapeutics Letter* (University of British Columbia) #48, April–June 2003, www.ti.ubc.ca/PDF/48.pdf (accessed November, 23, 2004).

34. B. Spilker, "The Benefits and Risks of a Pack of M&Ms: A Pharmaceutical Spokesman Answers His Industry's Critics," *Health Aff (Millwood)* 2002; 21:243–44; quote p. 243.

35. "At best, [the] comments [of an earlier writer recommending less contact with the industry] appear naive; at worst, they smack of a holier-than-thou moralism that harks back to a bygone era." S. Verma, "'A Matter of Influence': Graduate Medical Education and Commercial Sponsorship" [letter], *N Engl J Med* 1988; 318:52. One may find similar sentiments expressed in numerous letters to the editors in medical journals.

36. H. Brody, "The Company We Keep: Why Physicians Should Refuse to See Pharmaceutical Representatives," *Ann Fam Med* 2005; 3:82–85.

37. PhRMA, "Pharmaceutical Marketing and Promotion: Tough Questions, Straight Answers," Washington, D.C.: PhRMA, 2004; www.phrma.org/publications/policy//2004-11-10.1095.pdf (accessed November 23, 2004). PhRMA's figures show total promotional costs in excess of $25 billion in 2003. Of this, direct-to-consumer advertising uses up about $3.3 billion; the remainder is marketing aimed primarily at physicians. Marcia Angell argues that PhRMA's promotional figures understate the true expenditures; M. Angell, *The Truth about the Drug Companies: How They Deceive Us and What to Do about It* (New York: Random House, 2004). The figures are sufficiently immense in either case.

38. The classic statement of this observation is, "No drug company gives away its shareholders' money in an act of disinterested generosity." M. D. Rawlins, "Doctors and the Drug Makers," *Lancet* 1984; 2:814.

39. M. G. Ziegler, P. Lew, and B. C. Singer, "The Accuracy of Drug Information from Pharmaceutical Sales Representatives," *JAMA* 1995; 273:1296–98.

40. D. Griffith, "Reasons for Not Seeing Drug Representatives" [editorial], *BMJ* 1999; 319:69–70.

41. Ziegler et al., "The Accuracy of Drug Information," M. A. Bowman, "The Impact of Drug Company Funding on the Content of Continuing Medical Education," *Mobius* 1986; 6:66–69; D. Bardelay, "French Doctors Report Sales Representatives' Visits," *Essential Drugs Monitor* 1994; 17:21.

42. J. Ladd, "Medical Ethics: Who Knows Best?" *Lancet* 1980; 2:1127–29; H. Brody, *The Healer's Power* (New Haven: Yale University Press, 1992).

43. A. A. Skolnick, "Drug Firm Suit Fails to Halt Publication of Canadian Health Technology Report," *JAMA* 1998; 280:683–84.

44. M. Shuchman, "Consequences of Blowing the Whistle in Medical Research," *Ann Intern Med* 2000; 132:1013–15; D. Hailey, "Scientific Harassment by Pharmaceutical Companies: Time to Stop," *CMAJ* 2000; 162:212–13.

45. G. W. Pring and P. Canan, *SLAPPs: Getting Sued for Speaking Out* (Philadelphia: Temple University Press, 1996). The lawsuits that gave rise to the "SLAPP" designation were, as a rule, filed against citizens' groups opposing land development by the development companies. The intent of the lawsuits was to discourage citizens from exercising their rights to petition the government, such as local zoning boards. In ruling against the merits of such suits and favoring rules or legislation to limit them, courts commonly relied heavily upon the basic constitutional right of peaceable petition. By contrast, a "SLAPP" directed against a scientist, and designed to prevent scientists in the future from taking stands unfavorable to the pharmaceutical industry, does not interfere with that scientist's ability to petition any governmental

agency. It is therefore questionable whether the "SLAPP" designation properly applies to the latter class of lawsuits, even though the ethical problems of power imbalance are similar. Supporting a somewhat more expansive reading of SLAPP is K. Olson, "Restoring Anti-SLAPP's Backbone," *Recorder* (San Francisco), September 18, 2002:4.

46. Abramson, *Overdosed America*, 150–59; J. Frey, "Selling Drugs to the Public—Should the UK Follow the Example of the US?" *Br J Gen Pract* 2002; 52:170–71; M. B. Rosenthal, E. R. Berndt, J. M. Donohue, R. G. Frank, and A. M. Epstein, "Promotion of Prescription Drugs to Consumers," *N Engl J Med* 2002; 346:498–505.

47. A. F. Holmer, "Direct-to-Consumer Advertising—Strengthening our Health Care System," *N Engl J Med* 2002; 346:526–28; PhRMA, "Pharmaceutical Marketing and Promotion."

48. R. Moynihan, I. Heath, and D. Henry, "Selling Sickness: The Pharmaceutical Industry and Disease Mongering," *BMJ* 2002; 324:886–91.

49. B. Mintzes, M. L. Barer, R. L. Kravitz, et al., "How Does Direct-to-Consumer Advertising (DTCA) Affect Prescribing? A Survey in Primary Care Environments with and without Legal DTCA," *CMAJ* 2003; 169:405–12; M. Petersen, "Increased Spending on Drugs Is Linked to More Advertising," *New York Times*, November 12, 2001:C1; M. B. Rosenthal, E. R. Berndt, J. M. Donohue, A. M. Epstein, and R. G. Frank, "Demand Effects of Recent Changes in Prescription Drug Promotion," Kaiser Family Foundation Publication # 6085, 2003, www.kff.org.

50. AMA Council on Ethical and Judicial Affairs, "Gifts to Physicians from Industry" [editorial], *JAMA* 1991; 265:501; AMA, "Policy Finder: E-8.061 Gifts to Physicians from Industry," AMA, 2001, www.ama-assn.org/ama/pub/category/4001.html.

51. Senate Labor and Human Resources Committee, *Examining Practices of U.S. Pharmaceutical Companies and How Drug Prices and Prescriptions are Affected* (Washington, D.C.: U.S. Government Printing Office, 1991); W. Leary, "Doctors Given Millions by Drug Companies," *New York Times*, Dec. 12, 1990:B13; M. Petersen, "Vermont to Require Drug Makers to Disclose Payments to Doctors," *New York Times*, June 13, 2002:C1.

52. K. Morin and L. J. Morse, "The Ethics of Pharmaceutical Industry Gift-Giving: The Role of a Professional Association," *Am J Bioeth* 2003; 3(3): 54–55.

53. AMA Council, "Gifts to Physicians."

54. Morin and Morse, "The Ethics of Pharmaceutical Industry Gift-giving," 54.

55. J. P. Kassirer and M. Angell, "The High Price of Product Endorsement," *N Engl J Med* 1997; 337:700.

56. J. Kaiser, "Furor Over Company Deal Roils AMA," *Science* 1997; 278:26.

57. M. McCarthy, "Drug Firm Support of American Medical Association Ethics Effort Draws Fire," *Lancet* 2001; 358:821; S. Okie, "AMA Blasted for Letting Drug Firms Pay for Ethics Campaign," *Washington Post*, Aug. 30, 2001:A3.

58. The most extensive discussion of whether the monetary value of a gift from industry makes any ethical difference is D. Katz, A. L. Caplan, and J. F. Merz, "All Gifts Large and Small," *Am J Bioeth* 2003; 3(3): 39–46. The AMA representatives who commented on this paper took pleasure in pointing out that Katz et al. had also been supported by a grant from the pharmaceutical industry; Morin and Morse, "The Ethics of Pharmaceutical Industry Gift-Giving." On the culture and psychology of gifts, see also M. M. Chren, C. S. Landefeld, and T. H. Murray, "Doctors, Drug Companies, and Gifts," *JAMA* 1989; 262:3448–51; and J. Dana and G. Loewenstein, "A Social Science Perspective on Gifts to Physicians from Industry," *JAMA* 2003; 290:252–55.

59. T. Randall, "AMA, Pharmaceutical Association Form 'Solid Front' on Gift-Giving Guidelines," *JAMA* 1991; 265:2304–5.

60. Morin and Morse, "The Ethics of Pharmaceutical Industry Gift-Giving," 54.

61. See for example J. Sharfstein, "Pfizer Night at Boston Billiards," *N Engl J Med* 1997; 337:134; D. Grande and K. Volpp, "Cost and Quality of Industry-Sponsored Meals for Medical Residents," *JAMA* 2003; 290:1150–51.

62. Of many examples that could be cited, see C. Adams, "Doctors on the Run Can 'Dine 'n' Dash' in Style in New Orleans—Drug Companies Pick Up Tabs and Make Sales Pitches; Free Christmas Trees, Too," *Wall Street Journal*, May 14, 2001:A1.

63. American College of Physicians, "Physicians and the Pharmaceutical Industry," *Ann Intern Med* 1990; 112:624–26.

64. American College of Physicians, "Physicians and the Pharmaceutical Industry," *Ann Intern Med* 1990; 112:624–26; quote p. 624.

65. See for example Erde, "Conflicts of Interest in Medicine," especially pp. 25–27. Another critic of the guideline is J. P. Kassirer, *On the Take: How Medicine's Complicity with Big Business Can Endanger Your Health* (New York: Oxford University Press, 2005), 197. I would not, myself, be quite so negative about the ACP's guideline. I believe that at least one factor contributing to the sense of the "normal" most physicians have about their interactions with drug reps is a perceived distinction between on-stage and backstage medical activities. The waiting room and the exam rooms of one's office are on-stage. Reps are often received, and their freebies enjoyed, in the back rooms of the office, presumed to be out of sight to patients. The shock of awareness of how "backstage" activities would appear to patients if they could see them, has, I believe, been a useful ethical corrective for many (presumably well-motivated) physicians.

66. Kassirer, *On the Take*, 200.

II

SPECIFIC ISSUES AND PROBLEMS

3

THE PHARMACEUTICAL INDUSTRY AND THE FREE MARKET

The pharmaceutical industry earns nearly two-thirds of its profits in the United States since drug prices in the rest of the industrialized world are largely government controlled. Those profits rely almost entirely on laws that protect the industry from cheap imports, delay home-grown knockoffs, give away government medical discoveries, allow steep tax breaks for research expenditures and forbid government officials from demanding discounts while requiring them to buy certain drugs.

—Gardiner Harris in the *New York Times*[1]

You just don't get it. . . . We've got more money than God.

—Philip Morris executive[2]

HOW THE PHARMACEUTICAL INDUSTRY VIEWS THE WORLD

In 1997, 79 percent of the U.S. public thought that the pharmaceutical industry was doing a good job. In only seven years this had eroded to 44 percent (see figure 3.1).[3]

The industry, not surprisingly, believes that these public perceptions are based on misunderstandings. If we are going to assess the true relationship between medicine and the pharmaceutical industry, and suggest proposals that would improve that relationship, we must first try to understand how the industry itself sees the world it lives in. We may, in the end, find reason to disagree with this depiction, but for now let us suspend judgment and try to understand the industry's own sense of itself and its environment.[4]

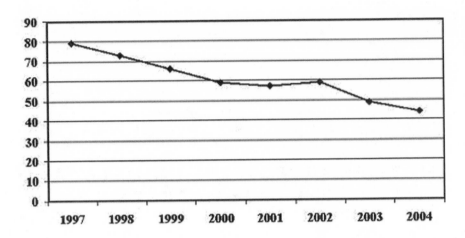

CHAPTER THREE

Figure 3.1. Percent of U.S. public judging the pharmaceutical industry to be doing a "good job," 1997–2004.

According to its world view, the industry makes high profits and is a very desirable stock for investors to purchase. It achieves this high market value by the very best of means, discovering and then producing new drugs to treat deadly diseases, and advancing the possibilities of medical science. It plows its profits back into more research and development, despite the inherent risks of those activities. This proves how well the free market works for pharmaceuticals.[5]

The industry regards patent protection as a critical element of the free market. The term "intellectual property" is commonly used in industry material to suggest that patent protection is an inalienable right and that taking it away or even limiting it amounts to simple thievery.[6]

Industry spokespersons have little patience with critics who ask how a free market can exist when the same pharmacy sells the same drug for five or ten widely different prices depending on the purchaser's insurance status.[7]

Pharmaceutical research is both risky and costly. To use an oil industry metaphor, the company must drill many dry holes before it hits a productive well. As Dr. Vasella noted in his story of Gleevec, the majority of employees in the research division of a pharmaceutical company may, over an entire career, never have the good luck to work on a successful drug.[8] They will have spent their whole lives in the essential but unromantic task of discovering what doesn't work. The Tufts University Center for the Study of Drug Development, funded by the pharmaceutical industry, estimates that in 2000 the cost of research on the average new drug was about $800 million.[9] Internal studies by industry consultants put actual research costs at about double the $800 million figure.[10]

Most other nations have a national health system and negotiate discounted drug prices, paying usually half or two-thirds what Americans typically pay (see figure 3.2).[11] According to spokespersons for the industry, Americans' willingness to pay top dollar for drugs is subsidizing the rest of the world's pharmaceutical research. If the United States ever became so misguided as to bring the cost of drugs down

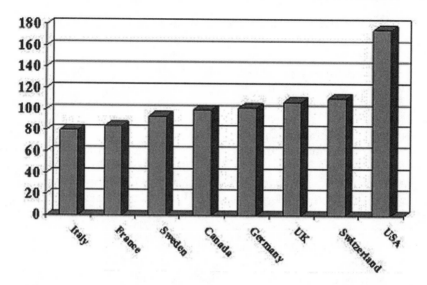

Figure. 3.2. Average price of prescription drugs in various countries, 2003.

to the average level in other developed countries, the bottom would fall out of re-search on new pharmaceuticals.[12] Sidney Taurel, CEO of Eli Lilly, wrote, "I sin-cerely believe that, by compromising these principles [a market-based system of pricing and patent protection], we could see the collapse of true innovation in bio-medicine, therefore vanquishing the hopes of making advances against devastating illnesses like Alzheimer's, cancer, heart disease, and diabetes."[13]

The industry's marketing is really a form of education, keeping physicians and the public up-to-date on the latest medical discoveries.[14] Physicians have every reason to believe that the education they receive from industry sources is trust-worthy. First, the drug companies care deeply about their scientific reputations. Second, market competition would quickly be the undoing of anyone making false claims; salespeople from rival companies would instantly pounce on and reveal the misinformation.

The industry manages to do these good works despite the pressure from its competitors—the generic drug makers, who can make money selling drugs de-spite having to pay only a tiny fraction of the cost of research and development—and from meddlesome regulators, notably the FDA.[15] Small wonder that the mes-sage the industry wishes to convey to the nation is "leave us alone." The industry is doing extremely well for itself, for its investors, for the public, and for the advance-ment of medical science, all at once. Any further regulation or restriction, like any other interference into the workings of the free market, would of necessity be harmful. "Hands off my industry," was the blunt headline selected to accompany the opinion piece by Sidney Taurel of Eli Lilly, in the *Wall Street Journal* in No-vember, 2003.[16]

Now that we have seen how the industry views the world, we must assess the accuracy and the implications of that view. The rest of the middle section of this book will address that task.

THE FREE MARKET: ETHICAL CONCERNS

Here and in the next several chapters we will address the industry's position on the profit margin that it needs to generate to fund research and the way those funds are spent. We have seen that the industry, in defending its high profits, makes extensive use of the rhetoric of the "free market" to shoot down proposals for reform or regulation.

The rhetoric therefore demands our ethical scrutiny. If we find that the reality does not match the rhetoric, the industry's objections to certain reform proposals lose their force. The industry cannot have it both ways, wrapping itself in the mantle of the free market when it serves its purposes and then deviating from free-market behavior when that is the easier way to make a buck. If the industry itself engages in anti-free-market behavior, it has no grounds to object when anti-free-market reforms are proposed to rein in its excesses.

While the price of drugs is not our primary concern in this book, physicians cannot remain indifferent to drug prices if they are to fulfill their roles as patient advocates. If drugs that could greatly ameliorate suffering are not available to some segment of the public, physicians should be concerned. If the industry charges very high prices for drugs, and if it then uses some of that money to reward physicians (via gifts or research grants or other benefits), the physicians who pocket those rewards become to some degree morally complicit. If lowering prices would have allowed more patients to benefit from these drugs, then the physicians who have accepted the industry largesse have participated in a system that has denied care to those patients.

Finally, we will encounter some cases in which the industry has gone over the line and committed fraud. One way to think about these fraudulent behaviors is to view them as aberrant. A few physicians are jailed every so often for Medicare or Medicaid fraud, and the vast majority of honest physicians hope that they will not be judged negatively because of the few bad apples. But another way to view the fraud is to see that everyday industry policy deliberately skates as close to the thin ice as possible. If a skater falls through the ice, it is not aberrant; it is a natural and indeed expected consequence of how business is done. John Braithwaite wrote in 1984, "To my amazement, two American executives I interviewed explained that they had held the position of 'vice-president responsible for going to jail' and I was told of this position existing in a third company."[17] He found that lines of authority in those pharmaceutical companies had been drawn deliberately so that this individual would be the fall guy in case of a serious legal problem. The vice president in question expected to be duly compensated for this service.

A FREE MARKET IN PHARMACEUTICALS?

The rhetoric often heard from PhRMA and its allies focuses on the notion that any change in the ground rules of how drugs are marketed or sold in the United States would be a violation of the sacred "free market." For example, PhRMA President

Alan Holmer told an audience at the University of Pennsylvania Leonard Davis Institute of Health Economics on January 24, 2003:

> The U.S. is the undisputed leader in bringing innovative medicines to market, and the center for research in the burgeoning field of biotechnology. The reason for U.S. leadership in this field is simple: we have the freest market for prescription medicines in the world. . . . If we adopt European-style price controls, we endanger not only medical advances but, also, economic leadership in this field.[18]

So there are two obvious questions to ask. First, *should* the market for pharmaceuticals be a "free" market? We have seen reasons to argue that because of the special nature and human need associated with pharmaceuticals, we should not treat them like any other consumer commodity. But a second important question is *whether* the market for pharmaceutical products in the United States *is* a free market, and if so, by what definition and by whose standards.

A so-called free market can be distorted by a disproportionate concentration of wealth in one segment of the market. We have noted the pharmaceutical companies' high profits, but it is worth taking a minute to grasp exactly how high those profits have been—at least before the recent industry downturn. Dr. Marcia Angell, in her attack on the industry, points out a telling fact. Ten of the largest U.S. pharmaceutical companies are on the list of *Fortune* 500 companies; a little math therefore demonstrates that the pharmaceutical industry makes up 2 percent of the total companies on that list. In 2002, these ten companies were responsible for *more* profits ($35.9 billion) than were *all the other 490 companies combined* (33.7 billion). Put another way, the pharmaceutical industry accounted for 2 percent of the *Fortune* 500 companies, but 52 percent of these companies' total profits.[19]

Princeton economist Uwe E. Reinhardt points out that the industry is a hybrid creature, half capitalist and half the result of government regulation. In the United States we have set up the industry as a for-profit venture instead of a nonprofit utility. But the industry could not exist in its present form were it not for two major deviations from the ideal "free" market—first, the exclusive monopoly rights granted by patents; and second, the ability to practice price discrimination because of the prohibition of drug resale (e.g., the rules that officially prohibit cheaper Canadian drugs from being re-imported back to the States). Partly because the industry has these two distinct faces, the American consumer gyrates between demanding that the companies produce new cures for cancer and sell them as cheaply as generic aspirin, and insisting that the pharmaceutical stocks owned by our retirement fund increase in value to the maximum possible extent. "Caught between these inconsistent standards of behavior is an industry that will naturally never get it quite right."[20]

Alan Sager and Deborah Socolar of the Health Reform Program of the Boston University School of Public Health summarize reasons why the pharmaceutical market is neither free nor competitive:

- The wide disparities in the prices different groups pay for drugs is by itself a strong signal of the lack of a free market. Under ideally competitive circumstances, prices tend to converge.

- Closely associated with the first reason are the high prices charged in the United States compared to other countries. In an ideally free market, prices not only converge, they converge in a way that tracks the marginal costs of additional production. But the costs of drugs in the United States are many times the cost of actually manufacturing the pills or capsules.
- While there may be a number of big drug firms, only a few firms sell major drugs in any one therapeutic class, such as antidepressants, antiulcer drugs, or cholesterol-lowering drugs. Within some of these categories, the top-selling three drugs account for between 70 and 90 percent of the total market. That means that within such classes there is very limited competition.
- As drug firms merge (as many have in the last decade), competition decreases further.
- The suppression of generic competitors by the brand-name drug companies, which we will discuss in the next chapter, is a further sign of monopoly or oligopoly rather than of a "free" market.[21]
- A "free" market cannot exist in the face of widespread fraud and criminal behavior. We have already seen that Braithwaite regarded the pharmaceutical industry as especially crime prone back in the 1980s.[22] Events such as the TAP-Lupron investigation, which we will look at below, hardly reassure us that the industry has changed its ways in the intervening years.

Katharine Greider provides another reason to question the "free market" rhetoric:

[T]he truth is, it's hard to tell exactly what everyone's paying [for prescription drugs]. Why? Because, incredibly, it's a *secret*. What's the actual price wholesalers pay for medication? Sorry, that's a secret. Proprietary information, the industry insists. And exactly what kind of price breaks and rebates are negotiated by the PBMs [pharmacy benefit managers] who administer benefits for 200 million people? Trade secret. In other words, what's paid for any given drug most of the time is entirely beyond public scrutiny.[23]

As Reinhardt noted, the modern U.S. drug industry departs most radically from any ideally free market with the patent protection of brand-name drugs. The industry tends to conflate the free market and patent protection ("intellectual property rights") in one breath as if to question either is un-American. And indeed patent protection has a long tradition within American society. But patents ultimately count as governmental interference with the free market. Patents represent a societal judgment that if left to its own devices, the free market will insufficiently reward invention and innovation. Government must therefore step in and disrupt the free market so as to bestow monetary rewards upon innovators. The innovators and the government make a bargain. The government grants the innovator exclusive rights to sell the invention for a period of time; in exchange the innovator publicly records the invention so that later anyone will be able to manufacture it. The system is supposed to ensure that future innovators will have sufficient financial incentive to improve existing products.

The bargain between government and innovators could go sour either way. If too short a period of patent protection is granted, the financial incentive is too low and future innovation stagnates. If the period is too long or if exclusive sales are protected in other ways, the public suffers by having to pay artificially high prices for many years. If the bargain needs to be renegotiated, it would seem that both the innovators and the government should have a say. By claiming patents as rights, the industry claims a privilege of dictating these matters to the government unilaterally. The industry might, at the present time, have the political and financial muscle to succeed in dictating in this fashion. But it cannot reasonably claim that it is thereby upholding the free market.

We find even more reasons to doubt the "free market" rhetoric when we look at the story of Xigris.

THE XIGRIS STORY

In a way it's a shame to pick on Xigris, which is, at least in concept, truly a breakthrough drug. Eli Lilly devoted two decades and reportedly hundreds of millions of dollars to the development of the drug, also known as activated protein C. It is a relative of a molecule produced by the human body to block inflammation and clotting. It's a complex protein, and figuring out how to manufacture it in bulk required a lot of research. The drug is supposed to be used in cases of septic shock—life-threatening shock caused by overwhelming infection. Lilly calculated that seven hundred fifty thousand people suffer from septic shock in American intensive care units each year and thought the drug's sales would reach one billion dollars.

Lilly priced Xigris at $6,800 per treatment. As the company told the *Wall Street Journal*, this price was based both on the high cost of developing and manufacturing the drug, as well as "on the benefit it gives patients."[24] This last phrase is a code within the industry that basically means, "If the drug does something people think is important, such as saving a life, we can charge a lot for it even if the actual cost of the drug is quite low." Critics charge that this phrase translates into "whatever the market will bear."

For all its promise, Xigris ran into trouble. A major clinical trial showed that 25 percent of patients getting Xigris died compared to 31 percent of patients getting standard treatment—in the minds of many physicians, not an overwhelming difference. The FDA advisory panel that reviewed Xigris split ten to ten on whether to approve the drug. Dr. H. Shaw Warren and his colleagues published a critical review in the *New England Journal of Medicine* in 2002, noting that the proposed mechanism for Xigris's effectiveness (preventing or destroying clots in tiny blood vessels) had never been proven and that a small number of patients in the clinical trials had developed severe bleeding complications. Warren and colleagues argued along with half the FDA advisory panel that more studies were needed before Xigris could be given a green light for general use.[25] Nevertheless, some intensive care experts were convinced that Xigris was a wonder drug and should become the standard of care for serious sepsis. These experts were soon receiving one-thousand-dollar-a-day speaker fees from Lilly to spread their message around the country.

In a time of skyrocketing drug costs, Xigris came with a huge price tag and questions about how well it worked. Many hospital intensive care units responded by limiting its use to the most severely septic patients—which, according to the trials, had been the subgroup of patients that did the best when given the drug. Lilly was disappointed to see its hoped-for blockbuster drug selling only $100 million dollars' worth in 2002.

Lilly tried to get Xigris back on track. The company found a powerful ally in Nevada state senator Sandra Tiffany. She was in a coma suffering from sepsis in a Burbank, California, hospital when she received Xigris, and recovered. The physician who treated Senator Tiffany was soon approached by a public relations firm hired by Lilly, and Senator Tiffany has since worked closely with the agency, giving numerous TV interviews. She also was a potent lobbyist when Lilly petitioned the U.S. Centers for Medicare and Medicaid Services to grant Xigris "new technology" status. The petition succeeded—meaning that the federal government will subsidize Xigris up to half the cost of treatment, or $3,400.

When even this federal subsidy did little to push new prescriptions for the drug, Lilly contracted with a new public relations firm to change its marketing strategy. The new slogan was that it constituted *unethical rationing at the bedside* of dying patients not to use the drug. The new approach put Lilly in touch with a group of physicians and bioethicists who were planning a study of rationing of treatment in intensive care units. Lilly gave this group a $1.8 million grant to study the ethics of rationing. (To nullify charges of conflicts of interest, the group set up a special oversight committee to ensure that Lilly did not influence the deliberations of the panels, and Xigris itself was excluded from the committee's reviews).[26]

As far as we know, nothing fraudulent occurred in the Xigris case. The same cannot be said for the activities of TAP Pharmaceuticals around their drug, Lupron.

THE TAP-LUPRON STORY[27]

Dr. Joseph Gerstein thought that his job with a Massachusetts managed-care organization involved deciding which drugs should be included in the HMO formulary. He did not imagine that it also involved becoming a whistle blower in a federal investigation.

The sudden change of job description occurred when Dr. Gerstein looked at two hormonal drugs for prostate cancer, Zoladex and Lupron. He found that the scientific evidence showed that both had equivalent actions and side effects. Zoladex was cheaper, so it seemed like a no-brainer—Zoladex went onto the formulary and Lupron came off. Soon Dr. Gerstein was approached by a representative from TAP Pharmaceuticals, offering a $20,000 "educational" grant to the HMO if he would reverse his decision and put Lupron back on formulary. When Gerstein, shocked at what seemed a blatant bribe, refused, TAP offered more and more inducements. After Gerstein reported this offer to federal investigators and continued to discuss the deal with TAP at their urging, the total amount offered to him rose to half a million dollars.

If the company was willing to pay such a huge inducement, why did they not simply lower the price of Lupron by the equivalent amount? Gerstein would have been happy to put Lupron back on formulary as long as it was priced as low as Zoladex. He had nothing against Lupron as a drug, and objected only to the high price. But if TAP lowered the price of Lupron, it faced trouble with Medicare. Medicare was paying a high price for Lupron based on the reported AWP, the "average wholesale price," or list price. If TAP started giving discounts to HMOs, Medicare would demand similar discounts.

The game that TAP was playing became evident after more investigation. Medicare pays for drugs that are administered intravenously in physician's offices and in hospitals, even as it (at the time) refused to cover outpatient medicines. The patient pays a copayment of 20 percent. The physician administers the drug and then collects the fees from Medicare and from the patient. According to the indictment eventually handed down by the federal grand jury, TAP representatives offered urologists treating prostate cancer an incredible array of goodies in exchange for administering Lupron—so-called "educational" grants that in actuality went for parties and bar tabs, trips to golf and ski resorts, and medical equipment. Basically, the physicians were getting Lupron at a discount, and then recouping the full list price from Medicare (and from the patient). In the most extreme cases, the physicians were getting free samples of Lupron from the company and then billing Medicare and the patient for the supposed costs of each dose, with the knowledge and the urging of company representatives.

The whole plan was based on keeping all these incentives secret from the Feds. TAP advised its sales force to instruct physicians to keep quiet: "Doctor, by discussing your costs of Lupron with other physicians, you run the risk of that information getting back to HCFA [Medicare's Health Care Financing Administration]. If HCFA then realized that AWP is not a true reflection of the price, the AWP could be affected, thus lowering the amount you may charge."[28]

While Gerstein was assisting the federal investigation from outside the company, another whistle blower was working from the inside. Doug Durand left Merck and became vice president for sales at TAP in 1995. At Merck he was used to having legal counsel watch over all promotional activities. He was surprised when he arrived at his new company and found they didn't even have any in-house legal counsel. Legal advice might interfere with sales, was the attitude of his new employers.[29]

Some months after joining TAP, he attended a meeting at which his staff were discussing paying urologists an up-front 2 percent "administration fee" if they agreed to prescribe Lupron. When one of the regional managers expressed his concerns about getting caught, another looked at Durand and joked, "How do you think Doug would look in stripes?" That led Durand to worry about more than his own integrity and reputation—he started to wonder whether, as Braithwaite had put it, he was the vice president in charge of going to jail. After trying unsuccessfully to change some of the worst company policies, he decided to share his notes with federal prosecutors.

Following the federal investigation, four urologists pleaded guilty to fraud and twelve company managers were indicted on multiple counts; the company eventually settled by paying fines of $875 million, then the largest fine ever paid in a health fraud case. Sources with knowledge of industry practices argued that the TAP case was more likely the tip of the iceberg than an aberration.

It is instructive to compare the Xigris story with the Lupron scandal. While there were questions about how much better Xigris is than other treatment, no one was saying that either Xigris or Lupron are bad drugs. If they were not being used more widely, it was due to one reason only—their high cost. That being the case, if there were a truly free market for pharmaceuticals, the consequences would have been easy to predict—the company would either lower the cost of the drug or sales would continue to fall. Both Lilly and TAP were willing to spend millions of dollars to push their respective drugs by doing everything imaginable *except* lowering their prices. Lilly has said that its goal is "to make sure that patients who meet the eligibility criteria for the use of Xigris receive the treatment." But they could easily achieve that goal by lowering the cost of the drug. It would appear that Lilly's true goal is rather to defend their "right" to charge whatever they wish for the drug. In other words, Lilly is interested in the opposite of a free market. The company wishes to use its economic power and influence to manipulate the market to its own advantage. As far as we know, it has till now (unlike TAP) used purely legal means.

MANAGED CARE AND PHARMACY BENEFIT MANAGEMENT

The pharmaceutical industry views the world as full of powerful and hostile forces, and surely one of the most powerful forces is the health insurance industry. For some years indemnity insurers such as Blue Cross-Blue Shield plans could simply pass any cost increases through to the employers who paid the bills for their workers. Few health insurance plans covered prescription drugs, except those taken inside the hospital. But at least since 1980, insurers have been pressured to limit cost increases, and it has become more common for prescription drugs to be at least partly covered. On the surface, this sets up a situation highly unfriendly to the pharmaceutical industry. A large insurance plan has great clout in the marketplace. If the insurer demands a deep discount, the drug company can either accept the lower price or give up a large block of business. This is true especially when several similar drugs are on the market in a given therapeutic category—what industry critics call "me-too" drugs. If all proton-pump inhibitors work roughly as well as each other in treating peptic ulcer disease and gastroesophageal reflux, the maker of one such drug has little bargaining power if the insurer can turn to another company and get an equally good drug at a lower cost. Any insurance plan can do exactly what Dr. Gerstein first decided to do when faced with the choice between Zolvadex and Lupron—choose the cheaper drug and demand that the other company match the discount if they wish their drug to be listed on the plan's approved formulary.

To at least some extent, the market forces work as described. Managed-care patients usually end up receiving drugs at a relative discount. As we have previously noted, however, the lack of transparency in the practices of the pharmacy benefit managers, the intermediate firms with which most managed-care organizations contract to negotiate with drug companies, makes it difficult to know who is getting a deal and who is being fleeced.[30]

Nevertheless, pharmaceutical companies have found many ways to manipulate this system to minimize the damage to their bottom lines. In April 2003, Bayer paid a fine of $257 million, the largest Medicaid fraud settlement on record. The company wanted to offer Kaiser Permanente managed-care plans a discount on its anti-biotic, Cipro, to undercut a challenge from Johnson & Johnson's rival drug, Floxin. To ensure that Medicaid never found out, Bayer arranged for the Cipro to show up in bottles without Bayer's national drug code number and labeled "distributed by Kaiser Foundation Hospitals." A Bayer executive who had been sent to an ethics training seminar (to the company's later regret, no doubt) blew the whistle on the deal.[31]

It might seem that I am deliberately blackening the industry's reputation by choosing to focus on criminal behavior. The problem is that often the industry conducts its business in secret. It may be only when a lawsuit is filed or a criminal prosecution is launched that internal company documents ever see the light of day. Those internal company documents, in turn, might be critical in revealing standard operating procedure inside the company.

Cutting deals with drug companies is a difficult and time-consuming business for managed-care plans. This has prompted most programs to outsource the task. Firms called pharmacy benefits managers (PBMs) began to proliferate. After a series of mergers, three giant companies eventually came to dominate the field—Medco, Caremark, and Express Scripts. Each PBM now had contracts with managed-care plans covering tens of millions of people, giving it huge muscle in the marketplace.

The pharmaceutical industry rose to the challenge in typical fashion. Large pharmaceutical firms bought the PBMs.

The specific case that has probably received the most publicity is the purchase of Medco by Merck. Eventually Merck decided that owning a PBM was more of a liability than a benefit and spun off Medco again as a supposedly independent company. But lawsuits continued to charge that Medco did Merck's bidding even after the divestment.[32]

The PBMs claimed that, whoever owns them, they provide excellent value. They bargain hard and negotiate significantly lower prices. Suppose, as often has happened, that the PBM negotiates a deal with a large drug company to place an expensive brand name drug at the top of a managed-care plan's formulary list. Cost-conscious physicians would demand to know why they are being forced to prescribe one of the most expensive drugs for the patient's condition when many cheaper medications are available. The PBM's answer is that appearances are deceiving. Maybe they are getting the brand name drug at a deeply discounted price, so that it is actually just as cheap as any competitor drug. Or maybe, in exchange for listing the brand-name drug on the formulary, the company has agreed to deep discounts on several other drugs they manufacture, so that the net savings to the insurance plan is large. Regardless of the details, the PBM insists, first, that members of the plan benefit from lower drug costs; and second, that the PBM passes almost all the savings on to those who pay for the insurance, keeping only a small percentage for themselves.

The only problem with believing these arguments put forth by the PBMs is that these firms resolutely refuse to open their books to any independent, outside scrutiny. They claim that their entire business hinges on how well they negotiate. If they open their books they are giving away all their vital trade secrets. The end result of this secrecy has been a spate of lawsuits. All the major PBMs are now involved in layers of legal challenges. So far, they have successfully fought off legislative as well as judicial attempts to force them to become more accountable.[33]

The question that remains largely unanswered today is how much PBMs have actually used the free market to drive down the prices of drugs, and how much the pharmaceutical industry has been able to capture PBMs so as to further manipulate the market to their own advantage. To whatever extent the "capture" scenario is the true one, we have even less reason to believe that anything resembling a free market in pharmaceuticals exists in the United States.[34]

When drug firms have considerable power to manipulate the market, it is bad enough when that power is used to increase the prices that U.S. consumers have to pay for prescription medicines. The outcome is much worse if a company dumps an unsafe drug on unsuspecting patients overseas, in exercise of its "free market" search for profits.[35] In the mid-1980s, Cutter Biological (a subsidiary of Bayer) developed a new, heat-treated version of its Factor VIII concentrate, the anticlotting material required by hemophiliacs. The new version of the drug effectively prevented the transmission of HIV, which had infected 74 percent of the users of the old concentrate. Cutter found itself with a large supply of the old concentrate on its shelves and proceeded to sell this product aggressively in markets in South America and Asia. All the while the company continued to insist that the old product was safe.

The story of Cutter's actions came out only when two New York Times reporters, Walt Bogdanich and Eric Koli, sorted through internal Cutter documents released as a result of domestic lawsuits, when American hemophilia patients who had become HIV-infected from the old concentrate sued. No high-priced lawyers were on hand to demand justice for victims in poor nations overseas. Ms. Li Wei-chun of Hong Kong, whose son died of AIDS at age twenty-three in 1996 after having used the nonheated concentrate in the 1980s, told the Times reporters, "They did not care about the lives in Asia. . . . It was racial discrimination."[36]

One final anecdote may convey the degree to which the pharmaceutical industry respects the free market. Eleven large U.S. corporations formed Business for Affordable Medicine (BAM) in the fall of 2001. The goal of this coalition was to support legislation that would plug loopholes in the 1984 Hatch-Waxman Act (which we will discuss in detail in the next chapter), in order to speed the entry of cheaper generic drugs into the market. These corporations were tired of seeing their health care costs for their employees escalate and eat into their profit margins. The corporate interests were joined by ten governors and a small group of labor leaders.

Early in 2002, people began to notice that some of the initially enthusiastic corporate members of the alliance had dropped out. Most of these companies, such as Marriott and Caterpillar, were somewhat tight-lipped about the precise reasons that they had withdrawn. No one wants to say out loud in public that they had succumbed to arm-twisting. But commentators noted that the large drug companies had launched a campaign to put pressure on their fellow corporate leaders to stay away from the coalition.

On their side, the drug industry was far from tight-lipped. Jackie Cottrell, a spokesperson for PhRMA, told Wall Street Journal reporters, "We think the BAM effort is misguided. . . . We have been and will continue to be very bold in asking BAM members to review issues and reconsider their membership."[37]

Many commentators therefore found it ironic when, in 2004, the drug giant Novartis was found to be singing a different tune. An internal memo was leaked to the press, showing the company urging its own employees to buy more generic, over-the-counter, and mail-order drugs so as to reduce the firms' employee health care expenses.[38]

We have seen that one form of interference in the free market is the patent system, and that many disputes about patents in the industry take place over the role of generic drugs. We'll explore that set of issues in more detail in the next chapter.

NOTES

1. G. Harris, "Drug Companies Seek to Mend Their Image," *New York Times*, July 8, 2004:C1.

2. Quoted in D. Kessler, *A Question of Intent: A Great American Battle with a Deadly Industry* (New York: Public Affairs, 2001), 127. A public relations consultant had suggested to the executive some ways to trim money from the budget of an advertising campaign, and received this reply.

3. Harris Interactive, "Reputations of Pharmaceutical and Health Insurance Companies Continue Their Downward Slide," *Harris Interactive Health Care News* June 22, 2004; 4(11), www.harrisinteractive.com/news/newsletters/healthnews/HI_HealthCareNews2004 Vol4_Iss11.pdf (accessed March 6, 2005). In March 2005, only 21 percent of respondents to a survey gave the pharmaceutical industry a "favorable" rating. In a Wall Street Journal/ NBC News poll, January 2005, only 3 percent thought the drug companies were "working for the public good," while 76 percent saw the industry as mostly concerned about profits; L. Abboud, "Stung by Public Distrust, Drug Makers Seek to Heal Image," *Wall Street Journal*, August 26, 2005:B1.

4. One of the best general resources for understanding the industry's self-image is the PhRMA website, www.phrma.org.

5. PhRMA proclaims on its website: "The U.S. free market is working—not only to encourage pharmaceutical innovation, but also to help contain health-care costs. . . . The best way for governments to control health-care expenditures—and to provide quality care for patients—is to rely to the maximum extent feasible on the delivery of health care through market-based private plans that promote consumer choice and compete on the basis of quality and total costs." www.phrma.org/issues/drugcosts/market.cfm (accessed March 6, 2005).

6. For example, "intellectual property protection" was the rallying cry of the U.S. industry when it fought strenuously to prevent South Africa from making generic versions of protease inhibitors, when that nation could not afford to pay Western prices for those drugs to fight its massive AIDS epidemic. P. Bond, "Globalization, Pharmaceutical Pricing, and South African Health Policy: Managing Confrontation with U.S. Firms and Politicians," *Int J Health Serv* 1999; 29:765–92; D. Barnard, "In the High Court of South Africa, Case No. 4138/98: The Gobal Politics of Access to Low-Cost AIDS Drugs in Poor Countries," *Kennedy Inst Ethics J* 2002; 12:159–74.

7. To give just one example of widely varying prices for the same drug, generic ranitidine (an antacid), General Motors would pay $181.22 for ninety tablets by mail order from the pharmacy benefit manager, Medco (including the customer's $5 copay); a GM employee at a retail pharmacy would pay $62.88; an uninsured person at the same store would pay $78.62; someone ordering on line from the discount firm Costco would pay $22 for one hundred pills; and another benefit manager, Caremark, on its mail order site, charges U.S.

government customers $105.42. The official, so-called "average wholesale price" or AWP of ninety generic ranitidine is $264. B. Martinez, "Generic Drugs by Mail Can Be a Raw Deal," *Wall Street Journal*, February 15, 2005:B1.

8. D. Vasella with R. Slater, *Magic Cancer Bullet: How a Tiny Orange Pill Is Rewriting Medical History* (New York: HarperBusiness, 2003).

9. J. A. DiMasi, R. W. Hansen, and H. G. Grabowski, "The Price of Innovation: New Estimates of Drug Development Costs," *J Health Econ* 2003; 22:151–85.

10. For discussion on both sides of this issue, see Public Citizen, "Rebuttals to PhRMA Responses to the Public Citizen Report, 'Rx R&D Myths: The Case against The Drug Industry's R&D "Scare Card,"'" *Public Citizen*, November 28, 2001, www.citizen.org/print_article.cfm?ID=6514 (accessed March 6, 2005); M. Goozner, *The $800 Million Pill: The Truth behind the Cost of New Drugs* (Berkeley: University of California Press, 2004).

11. A. Sager and D. Socolar, "2003 U.S. Prescription Drug Prices 81 Percent Higher Than in Other Wealthy Nations," Health Reform Program, Boston University School of Public Health (Data Brief #7), October 28, 2004; http://dcc2.bumc.bu.edu/hs/US-foreignrxpricegap 28Oct04.doc (accessed March 6, 2005).

12. The research funded by the industry (it is claimed) meets not only the highest scientific standards, but also the highest ethical standards. In 2002, PhRMA issued a set of guidelines for research integrity; PhRMA, "Principles on Conduct of Clinical Trials and Communication of Clinical Trial Results," November 20, 2002; www.phrmaorg/publications/policy//2003-11-20.871.pdf (accessed January 14, 2004). Among other things the guidelines require assiduous care to protect human research subjects, and require appropriate and timely publication of research results with the role of all involved investigators and authors stated honestly.

13. S. Taurel, "Hands Off My Industry," *Wall Street Journal*, November 3, 2003:A14.

14. Richard Levy, PhD of the National Pharmaceutical Council in Reston, Virginia, presented physicians with an especially spirited defense of pharmaceutical marketing as education. He wrote: "The high marketing expenses incurred by the pharmaceutical industry reflect the intensity of the effort required to communicate this important information. The communicators require thorough training and an extensive support infrastructure." He continued: "The medical literature is extensive, but access to it in the real world of medical practice is difficult. The pharmaceutical sales force represents an extremely efficient and effective means of obtaining information. By investing 5 or 10 minutes, and without traveling to a medical library, physicians who have little time to read can obtain the information they need. Sales calls are expensive for the company but are a valued service to physicians." R. Levy, "The Role and Value of Pharmaceutical Marketing," *Arch Fam Med* 1994; 3:327–32, quote p. 329. According to the industry's own figures, more is spent on research than on promotion; according to the calculations of other observers, considerably more is spent on promotion than on research and development, by a factor of at least two. See, for example, U. E. Reinhardt, "Perspectives on the Pharmaceutical Industry," *Health Aff (Millwood)* 2001; 20:136–49.

15. Fran Hawthorne, for her book about the FDA, interviewed a number of pharmaceutical industry executives and discovered that to them, the FDA "is the all-powerful, arbitrary, nitpicky naysayer that keeps their desperately needed medicines off the market until they run a zillion unnecessary tests to prove things they already proved. The agency is unreliable, one week saying it wants to help manufacturers get their products out to patients quickly; then the next week panicking after too many reports of dangerous side effects. It is mysterious; there is no way of knowing just what a company must do to move its product past the regulatory box-checkers. At best, the FDA is a bunch of bureaucrats who mean well but are scared to be the first to approve something new. Most of all, the agency must be

obeyed." F. Hawthorne, *Inside the FDA: The Business and Politics behind the Drugs We Take and the Food We Eat* (Hoboken, NJ: John Wiley and Sons, 2005), x.

16. Taurel, "Hands Off My Industry."

17. After the *Park* case before the U.S. Supreme Court, which held the company's chief executive mostly liable for corporate wrongdoing, this behavior presumably ceased; J. Braithwaite, *Corporate Crime in the Pharmaceutical Industry* (Boston: Routledge & Kegan Paul, 1984), 308.

18. A. F. Holmer, "How Can We Not Afford Prescription Drugs in America? The Value of New Medicines for Patients," www.phrma.org/publications/publications/24.01.2003.678.cfm; accessed September 14, 2003.

19. M. Angell, *The Truth about the Drug Companies: How They Deceive Us and What to Do about It* (New York: Random House, 2004), 11.

20. Reinhardt, "Perspectives," 137.

21. A. Sager and D. Socolar, "Lower U.S. Prescription Drug Prices Are Vital to Both Patients and Drug Makers—but Instead, U.S. Prices Have Been Rising Rapidly Relative to Those in Other Wealthy Nations," Health Reform Program, Boston University School of Public Health, July 24, 2003; www.bumc.bu.edu/www/sph/hs/images/Health_Reform/Lower_drug_prices_protect_patients.pdf (accessed January 26, 2005).

22. Braithwaite, *Corporate Crime*.

23. Katherine Greider, *The Big Fix: How the Pharmaceutical Industry Rips Off American Consumers* (New York: PublicAffairs, 2003), 9–10. The staff of the Senate Select Committee on Aging learned in the early 1990s that drug firms often make large purchasers sign confidentiality agreements so that discounts will not be revealed and others cannot ask for similar treatment; D. Drake and M. Uhlman, *Making Medicine, Making Money* (Kansas City: Andrews and McMeel, 1993), 51.

24. A. Regalado, "Who Gets Health Care? Rationing in an Age of Rising Costs—Message in a Bottle: To Sell Pricey Drug, Lilly Fuels a Debate over Rationing," *Wall Street Journal*, September 18, 2003:A1.

25. H. S. Warren, A. F. Suffredini, P. Q. Eichacker, and R. S. Munford, "Risks and Benefits of Activated Protein C Treatment for Severe Sepsis," *N Engl J Med* 2002; 347:1027–30.

26. Regalado, "Who Gets Health Care?"; L. Kowalczyk, "Rationing of Medical Care under Study," *Boston Globe*, September 14, 2003:A1. On the ethics of bioethicists accepting this sort of funding, and in effect becoming part of Lilly's public relations campaign, see C. Elliott, "Not-so-Public Relations," *Slate*, December 15, 2003; slate.msn.com/id/2092442/ (accessed January 26, 2005).

27. The principal source for this account is Greider, *The Big Fix*, 10–12. For another account, mentioning somewhat different figures, see A. Dembner, "A Cure for Fraud: Weston Doctor Saves Taxpayers Millions by Blowing Whistle," *Boston Globe*, October 7, 2001.

28. D. L. Bartlett and J. B. Steele. *Critical Condition: How Health Care in America Became Big Business—and Bad Medicine* (New York: Doubleday, 2004), 65.

29. C. Haddad and A. Barrett, "A Whistle-Blower Rocks an Industry: Doug Durand's Risky Documentation of Fraud at Drugmaker TAP is Promoting Wider Probes," *Business Week*, June 24, 2002:126.

30. To cite one example mentioned previously, General Motors discovered that it was paying Medco's mail order site $181.22 for ninety capsules of generic ranitidine, when consumers could log onto the Costco discount website and get one hundred of the capsules for $22; Martinez, "Generic Drugs by Mail."

31. M. Petersen, "Bayer Agrees to Pay U.S. $257 Million in Drug Fraud," *New York Times*, April 17, 2003:C1.

32. M. Freudenheim, "Records Show Merck Unit Favored Its Parents' Drugs," *New York Times*, January 8, 2003; M. Freudenheim, "Documents Detail Big Payments by Drug Makers to Sway Sales," *New York Times*, March 13, 2003:C1.

33. B. Martinez, "Drug-Benefit Managers Win Round—Enforcement of Maine Law Forcing Disclosure of Deals with Makers Is Delayed," *Wall Street Journal*, March 11, 2004: D6; B. Martinez, "Medco May Face Turbulence from U.S. Suit," *Wall Street Journal*, November 26, 2004:C1; J. Appleby, "Drug Manager Accused of Cheating New York," *USA Today*, August 5, 2004:1B; M. J. Feldstein, "20 States Are Investigating Drug-Sale Firm," *St. Louis Post-Dispatch*, July 28, 2004:A1.

34. As this book was in its final copyediting, two major PBMs announced a development that can be viewed as a victory for the free market. Medco and Caremark announced their acceptance of a new purchasing model, in which they would reveal to corporate buyers how much the drugs cost and how much of the savings was passed on. This new transparency model was forced on the PBMs by an alliance of fifty-six of their largest corporate clients; Fuhrmans V. "Managers of Drug benefits Aregee to More Transparency in Pricing," *Wall Street Journal*, July 24, 2006: B6.

35. The scenario of a rapacious international drug company exploiting the poor in developing nations underlies John Le Carré's novel, *The Constant Gardener* (New York: Pocket Books, 2001) and the motion picture later adapted from it. The novel depicts several murders contracted for by company operatives to cover up the deaths of numerous research subjects in studies of a new tuberculosis drug in Africa. Le Carré informs the reader that the drug and these activities are all fictional, and certainly in my own research I have found no suggestion that the industry engages in murder. (As later chapters will make clear, less crude means usually suffice to bring the industry most of what it desires.) Nevertheless Le Carré insists, "As my journey through the pharmaceutical jungle progressed, I came to realize that, in comparison with the reality, my story was as tame as a holiday postcard" (558).

36. W. Bogdanich and E. Koli, "2 Paths of Bayer Drug in 80's: Riskier Type Went Overseas," *New York Times*, May 22, 2003:A1. The reporters' revelations were characterized by Dr. Sidney M. Wolfe of Public Citizen Health Research Group as "the most incriminating internal pharmaceutical industry documents I have ever seen." Since Dr. Wolfe tends to be an outspoken critic of the pharmaceutical industry, such an assertion coming from him is worth noting.

37. L. McGinley and S. Hensley, "Leading the News: Drug Makers Aim to Protect Patents," *Wall Street Journal*, May 3, 2002:A3.

38. E. Silverman, "Drug Maker Promotes Generics for Workers: Novartis Draws Fire on Cost-cutting Bid," *Newark Star-Ledger*, October 15, 2004.

4

PATENTS, GENERIC DRUGS, AND ACADEMIC SCIENCE

Within a few years, every one of these supposedly sacrosanct tenets of "basic academic values" had been violated. They were trampled in the stampede to stake a claim in what science reporter Nicholas Wade called "the genetic El Dorado."

—Linda Marsa, on the outcome of the Pajaro Dunes conference, March 1982, to set ethical guidelines to govern agreements between universities and business around new genetic technology[1]

Even if you are a hard-digging reporter looking for the one [academic medical] clinic that's objective and has not taken company money and has credibility, it's like looking for a needle in a haystack. You're likely to find a clinic that is either directly or indirectly on the company's payroll.

—Peter Rost, vice president of marketing at Pfizer, on the difficulties faced by journalists trying to obtain unbiased information about research on new drugs[2]

THE HYTRIN STORY

While Abbott Laboratories prided itself on a long history of research and innovation, its creative well seemed to have run dry in the mid-1970s. Abbott had not brought out any really new drugs for some years. The best thing to come along now was Hytrin (terazosin), a drug for high blood pressure. And Hytrin was basically a me-too version of prazosin, manufactured by Pfizer. Abbott chemists changed a part of the molecule, prazosin became terazosin, and Abbott was granted a series of patents on its new drug in 1977. But the tinkering with the molecule did have one beneficial effect. The new drug had to be taken only once a day while prazosin had to be taken twice.

It took another ten years for Abbott to complete the studies required to earn FDA approval for Hytrin as a drug for high blood pressure. In 1993, however, the drug took off in a new direction. There are many drugs good for treating high blood pressure. There are relatively fewer drugs that relieve the symptoms of an enlarged prostate in older men, without requiring surgery. It turned out that drugs in the prazosin-terazosin family do both. Many older men who have enlarged prostates have high blood pressure too, and for them such a drug is a "two-fer." Other men have only prostate trouble, but the drugs do not lower their blood pressure enough to cause any troublesome symptoms at the dose needed to relieve the prostate distress. By the mid-1990s, Hytrin was earning Abbott $500 million a year—about a fifth of its total revenue. But its patent was set to expire in 1995.

As any smart company would, Abbott set about the task of "evergreening" Hytrin. Anticipating the problem, the company had already filed requests for six more patents on its drug, covering such things as particular crystalline forms of the drug, their manufacturing process, and a time-release capsule form. If these patents were granted, Abbott could use them to keep generic drug makers at bay. If the patent requests were turned down, Abbott could still sue generic makers and perhaps delay the entry of competitors into the field, even if Abbott eventually lost the suits. Since Hytrin was earning the company more than a million dollars a day, it was profitable to pay the legal fees to file all these patent requests and (later) numerous lawsuits.

Perhaps Abbott expected that these patent applications would be viewed as legitimate protection of their intellectual property rights; perhaps not. In most instances these applications are eventually refused and serve only to delay, not to prevent, a generic version of the drug coming onto the market. But once in a while a big firm gets lucky. AstraZeneca, in its effort to "evergreen" its blockbuster drug Prilosec, filed a patent on a subcoating in the pill that protects the active ingredient. Critics scoffed, noting that many other drugs had similar subcoatings. But after ten months of hearings, a federal judge in New York ruled in 2002 that the subcoating patent was valid and that three of four generic firms had infringed upon the patent. AstraZeneca's stock value promptly took off.

Meanwhile, Abbott's competition was lining up. Two relatively small manufacturers of generic drugs, Zenith Goldline Pharmaceuticals and Geneva Pharmaceuticals, had filed with the FDA for permission to market their versions of terazosin when the Hytrin main patent ran out. Geneva got there first with its 1993 filing date, and Zenith followed eighteen months later. For these companies the dollar figures were much lower but just as compelling. When Geneva finally began to sell generic terazosin, for instance, it made up to eleven million dollars a month—considerably less than what Abbott had made from brand-name Hytrin, yet still amounting to about a 50 percent increase in the company's total sales. Four other generic companies eventually filed with the FDA for terazosin as well.

Of the six firms vying for generic rights, Geneva held an advantage. It had gotten to the FDA first with its filing. Under the Hatch-Waxman Act, the first company to market a generic version of a drug could be granted a six-month exclusive right to the generic market—a deal that Congress apparently thought would sweeten the pot, encourage generic competition, and so work to bring down the costs of drugs for the consumer.

Abbott proceeded to sue all the generic firms for patent infringement. At this point the company unwittingly handed Geneva another advantage. Abbott's high-priced lawyers slipped up. They filed papers to block a tablet form of terazosin but somehow failed to file the right documents to prevent a capsule form, which is what Geneva planned to make.

On February 2, 1998, lawyers for Abbott and Zenith squared off in federal patent court in Washington, D.C., to argue the claims of patent infringement. After the morning session the two sides repaired to the plush Hay-Adams Hotel and lunch in a private dining room. Over the meal Zenith's lawyers proposed that Abbott and Zenith bury the hatchet and become partners in introducing a generic terazosin. No, replied Kenneth Griesman, the lawyer for Abbott. His company, he said, preferred a "straight numbers deal" (according to court records later unearthed by the *New York Times*).

What the "straight numbers deal" was to consist of became clear (but not public) nearly two months later. On March 31, Abbott agreed to pay Zenith $2 million dollars a month not to produce its generic terazosin, up to a maximum of $42 million dollars. Griesman now had to go after the more serious contender, Geneva. According to the deal he had just concluded with Zenith, they could go to market with their terazosin if another generic company entered the market. And because Geneva had priority in the FDA filings, Geneva owned the Hatch-Waxman six-month exclusive rights. Keeping Geneva off the market automatically ensured that no other company could sell a generic terazosin for that six-month period.

On March 30, Geneva got the green light from the FDA to go ahead with their generic version. Their general counsel, Jeremiah McIntyre, called Griesman. The call, documents later revealed, was a bluff. Geneva had run into technical difficulties and was not at the moment prepared to mass-produce terazosin. But McIntyre wanted to see if Abbott would do business. And he found he had something of an upper hand, as Griesman now finally became aware of the slip-up over Abbott's failure to block the capsule form. So the horse trading began.

Geneva had predicted that it could make $84 million in profits in the first year of sales. So McIntyre started by demanding $7 million a month to stay off the market. No way, countered Griesman; Abbott had done its own calculations and had figured that with other generic competitors, Geneva's profits would be a good deal less. But Abbott was prepared not to get finicky over the details; Greisman made a counteroffer of $2 to $3 million a month. After some haggling, the two agreed the next day on $4.5 million a month. According to the deal (which did not have to be disclosed in court, as Geneva, unlike Zenith, was not settling its lawsuit with Abbott), Abbott would pay Geneva until a higher federal court overruled its patent claims, or until another patent expired in 2000, whichever came sooner.

In the end, Geneva pocketed $101 million from the deal—which it voluntarily walked away from in 1999. Geneva pursued its suit against Abbott in court and won; its generic terazosin went on sale in August, 1999. Abbott's CEO, Miles White, sent a note to his team: "I'd like to take this opportunity to recognize the truly outstanding work of our legal team, which successfully defended Hytrin's patent protection against challenges for nearly four years. This has been one of the most important contributions to Abbott's success in this decade." Abbott had messed up in not filing to block the capsule form, had lost all its court battles, and had had one of its patents stripped off the registry at the FDA. But its four years of maneuvering protected about $2 billion in Hytrin sales.

White might have been less pleased with some of the fallout from these deals. First, the Federal Trade Commission (FTC) started looking into the Abbott-Geneva deal. In March 2000, the FTC accused those two firms of violating antitrust laws. They got off by signing an agreement not to do it again. But in the meantime, consumers' groups had filed class-action suits against all three firms, seeking repayment for the extra money paid for Hytrin during the years it kept generics off the market.[3]

The Hytrin story introduces another aspect of the "free market" controversy—the competition between brand-name and generic drugs. We saw previously that the pharmaceutical industry regards patent protection as part and parcel of the free market, while many economists would see patents as violations of the free market.

Economists Dean Baker and Noriko Chatani, in a report prepared for the Center for Economic and Policy Research, suggested that we need to view patents in the pharmaceutical industry as a way government can stimulate research on new drugs: "It is important to recognize that the choice between patent-supported research and direct funding through the public/non-profit sectors is not a choice between the market and the government, but rather a choice between two different forms of government intervention." They claim that if it turns out, on careful study, that the patent road is a very inefficient way to pay for innovations in pharmaceuticals, then we should all feel very comfortable with doing away with drug patents and seeking a different way to pay for the necessary research.[4]

The rhetoric of the industry, as we have seen, is very different. The language of "intellectual property" has been adopted as a way of making the implicit argument that a company has a right to patent protection and that reducing the period of patent protection, or otherwise making it easier for other firms to compete, amounts to a form of thievery. It is important that we understand that this is rhetoric and not necessarily a close analysis of the legal or the moral basis of patents. If, on the other hand, the industry can afford extremely generous lobbying in Congress, it amounts to the same thing—Congress will pass the patent laws that the industry wishes, regardless of whether the public interest is served.

THE HATCH-WAXMAN ACT

In 1984 Congress passed a law that was intended to stimulate the generic drug industry. The broad bipartisan support the legislation enjoyed is indicated by the name by which it is commonly known, Hatch-Waxman,[5] after Senator Orrin Hatch (R-Utah) and Representative Henry Waxman (D-Calif.).

The main feature of Hatch-Waxman has performed completely as intended. Generic drug makers had previously been required to test their drugs in clinical trials, as if they were brand-new drugs just now seeking FDA approval. Under Hatch-Waxman, the only requirement was to show that the drug was bioequivalent to the comparable brand-name drug—that is, that the generic acted the same way in the human body, and that the same dosage led to the same levels in the bloodstream.

But other features of Hatch-Waxman have turned out to be an unintended windfall for the brand-name drug companies. Perhaps the most noxious provision has been the automatic thirty-month delay in FDA approval of the generic form in any case where the brand-name company sues the generic company for patent infringement. The framers of the bill apparently envisioned that such lawsuits would be rare, and would involve substantive and serious claims about patent violations. But the mere existence of the thirty-month extension has proven an incentive for the brand-name company to patent every conceivable aspect of its drug and to file frivolous lawsuits. After all, as we saw with Claritin and Hytrin, when you are selling a million dollars' or more worth of a drug each day, you can afford to spend a lot on attorneys and court costs.

Another problematic provision of Hatch-Waxman was the law's way of sweetening the pot for the first generic drug maker to step up to the plate. That competitor was given its own six-month period of exclusivity, during which no other generic could enter the market. This means in practice that the real drop in price when a drug goes off patent occurs not with the appearance of the first generic version of the drug, but rather six months later. At first, when there is no danger of the initial generic being undercut by other companies, the generic version may be priced just slightly below the cost of the brand-name drug. The intent of the law was that during this six-month period, the first generic maker (that presumably took some risks and underwent some expenses in order to successfully copy the brand-name drug) would get a nice extra profit as a reward for its efforts; and the brand-name company could continue to price its own drug fairly high, thereby sweetening the pot for them as well. But as we also saw in the Hytrin case, the six-month exclusivity period tempts the brand-name company to play underhanded games. If the first generic version can somehow be kept off the market, the company knows that no other generic company can leap in during that time.

Today, most critics of the industry agree that Hatch-Waxman should be amended to fix these problems. In the previous chapter we saw how large corporations, state governors, and labor leaders formed a coalition in 2001 to push for just such an amendment. But the bipartisan support the initial legislation enjoyed in 1984 has fallen by the wayside. Even Representative Waxman was noted in 2002 to be less than enthusiastic about an amendment to the law—out of fear that the version that emerged from the present Congress would favor the big pharmaceutical companies even more strongly.[6]

PATENTING THE SUN?

Today, one commonly sees in the media that university scientists have discovered the gene for some important bodily function or disease and have immediately rushed to patent it. This gives most people some unease. First, it seems weird that one should be able to patent an aspect of human biology. Second, it might seem strange to some people that scientists employed by a university (especially if it is a public university) should seek to patent a product rather than make it available for the general good of humankind. In the early 1950s when Dr. Jonas Salk invented the polio vaccine, he was asked why he had not tried to patent this lifesaving discovery, which surely could have made an immense fortune. Salk appeared startled at the question and replied, "How could you patent the sun?"[7] His answer precisely captured one mindset about these matters—first, that a responsible medical scientist would not seek to make personal profit off a discovery; and second, that there were some areas of medicine and of nature that were simply off limits for patents and private ownership.

Dr. Salk's attitude, it turns out, reflects poorly on the true history of the relationships between the pharmaceutical industry and academic physicians during the early years of the twentieth century. Some medical schools issued strict guidelines that implied that research money received from the industry was tainted. But other academic physicians freely accepted pharmaceutical support and became active consultants for the firms, without suffering any discernible moral rejection or concern from their peers.[8] Dr. Soma Weiss, for instance, was regarded as a rising star at Harvard, one of the outstanding academic internists of the late 1930s and early 1940s.[9] Weiss authored a review article on drug development in the *New England Journal* in 1939, in which he especially praised two drugs, Benzedrine (an amphetamine) and Paredrinol (an amphetamine-related vasoconstrictor that raised blood pressure), while giving scant attention to any risks or side effects. Both drugs were products of Smith, Kline, with which company Weiss had consulted widely and from whom he had received a number of research grants. Such an article did not appear to detract in any way from Weiss's reputation, nor did Weiss—who was as highly regarded for his exemplary morals as for his technical skill as an investigator and clinician—apparently have any concerns that it might affect him negatively.[10]

Leading academic physicians of the period between the World Wars were somewhat worried about the harm that might be done to their reputations by collaborating closely with industry. But they were swayed more strongly by their commitment to the cause of well-designed research trials as an alternative to anecdotal testimonials. Dr. Joseph Earle Moore, professor at Johns Hopkins and prominent syphilis expert, wrote in the early 1930s that the manufacturer of a promising new drug had two choices: "He can either ship small quantities of the drug to several hundred Dr. Whose-and-whats in small towns throughout the country, subsequently foisting the drug upon the medical public on the grounds of such reports as, 'I have treated three patients with your drug and think it is better than [a competitor product]'; or he may make a serious effort to interest one of the six or eight larger . . . clinics in the country in carrying out a detailed and respectable trial."[11] The academic physicians knew that the drug companies were far from disinterested, but the sums of money changing hands were small and any excess income was plowed back immediately into research.

The issue of patenting medical discoveries was somewhat more complex. Some universities, along with the AMA, argued that it was unethical for physicians and scientists to patent their discoveries and to seek to profit from them. Universities countered, first, that only by patenting important discoveries could they retain legal control and fight off poor-quality imitations; and second, that modern research was expensive and that patent and licensing arrangements could bring in necessary funds for further discoveries. On such a basis, for instance, the University of Toronto patented the process for extracting insulin in the 1920s and entered into an exclusive licensing agreement with the Eli Lilly company. A committee of the American Association for the Advancement of Science indicated its approval of such patents in 1934.[12]

BAYH-DOLE AND CHAKRABARTY

Whatever the attitude of academic leaders toward patents and commercial support, their world changed dramatically in 1980, due both to a law passed by Congress and a decision of the U.S. Supreme Court.

The new law was called Bayh-Dole, after the bipartisan pair of senators who sponsored it. At the time it was passed, many viewed it as an uncontroversial win-win situation.[13] Initially the bill was pushed by the Carter administration, facing a serious economic slump and hoping that stimulating technology transfer would turn the economy around. One study in the late 1970s had shown that of twenty-eight thousand patents held by the federal government and its scientists, only 5 percent had been licensed to manufacturers—suggesting a huge, untapped market for new scientific discoveries if only the transfer from laboratory to industry could be streamlined.[14]

Under Bayh-Dole and later laws, universities and the NIH can patent scientific discoveries and grant exclusive licenses to firms to manufacture the resulting products. The law also had what appeared to be a safety valve for consumer concerns, a reasonable-pricing requirement. Specifically, if an NIH discovery were patented and licensed to a drug company, the company had to place the drug on the market at a reasonable price; if not, the government could exercise "march-in rights" and the company would forfeit its exclusive license.

Even with the safety valve, a few critics took a dim view of the Bayh-Dole bill and urged that it be rejected or modified. Some criticized the bill as a giveaway of the taxpayers' money.[15] Admiral Hyman Rickover testified against Bayh-Dole, to the chagrin of his former navy protégé Jimmy Carter. "'Based on 40 years' experience in technology and in dealing with various segments of American industry,' he gravely intoned, 'I believe the bill would achieve exactly the opposite of what it purports.' It would throttle technological development, hurt small business, stifle competition, and cost the taxpayers plenty while promoting 'greater concentration of economic power in the hands of large corporations.'"[16] Another early critic was then Representative (later Vice President) Al Gore, who feared that the bill would lead to a loss of public control over publicly financed discoveries.[17] Nevertheless, these voices remained in the minority and the bill became law.

Also in 1980, the U.S. Supreme Court decided the case of *Diamond v. Chakrabarty*. Ananda Chakrabarty, a microbiologist working for General Electric, had bred a new strain of the bacterium *Pseudomonas* that fed on materials in crude oil—hoping to create a bacterial solution to oil spills. At first the Patent Office refused to issue a patent because this bacterium was a life form, a product of nature by their existing guidelines rather than a human invention. The Court ruled that a new form of life could still be a human discovery and was patentable. This opened the doors for gene sequences, gene products, and numerous other genetic discoveries all to be patented.[18]

Despite the provisions of Bayh-Dole and subsequent laws, the large drug firms showed a marked aversion to doing business with NIH until 1995. In that year the NIH dropped the reasonable-pricing requirement altogether. Between 1993 and 1999, the NIH negotiated 619 formal research-and-development agreements with drug firms, and 515 of those occurred after dropping the reasonable-pricing clause. Efforts in Congress to reinstitute and strengthen reasonable-pricing requirements have been effectively fought off by industry lobbyists.[19] The way thus remains open for the pharmaceutical industry to make huge profits off drugs that have already had their research costs mostly paid by U.S. taxpayers, even if some of the taxpayers cannot afford the drugs as a result. The experience with taxol suggests, however, that even before the NIH dropped the reasonable-pricing requirement, it provided no very effective safeguard for the consumer.

THE TAXOL STORY

Taxol, a compound derived from yew trees, is considered a major success story for treating breast and ovarian cancer, some of the most feared diseases of women.[20] The NIH's National Cancer Institute (NCI) spent two decades and more than thirty-two million dollars doing research on taxol and determining how it could be effectively and safely used as an anticancer drug.

Merrill Goozner, in his book *The $800 Million Pill*, generally describes pharmaceutical research and development as depending heavily on prior work done with government funds. He is careful to note that the program at the NCI that discovered taxol was prompted at first by the success of a private drug firm. Botanists at Eli Lilly heard accounts from folk doctors in Madagascar about the healing properties of a local plant, the rosy periwinkle. Eventually the company extracted from that plant the drugs vincristine and vinblastine, which for decades were a mainstay of cancer chemotherapy. NCI was thus prodded to develop a comprehensive attempt to search through all known natural plant derivatives for anticancer properties. Unfortunately, of the one hundred fourteen thousand plant-derived chemicals eventually screened by NCI, only a handful were sufficiently promising to go to clinical trials.[21]

In 1962, botanists from the U.S. Department of Agriculture, working with NCI, identified an extract in the bark of the Pacific yew tree, a low- and slow-growing evergreen that the timber companies were used to burning as trash when they clear-cut a forest. Chemist Monroe Wall at the Research Triangle Institute in North Carolina identified the active ingredient in 1967 and named it taxol. The compound then went largely unnoticed until 1979, when Susan Horwitz, a molecular pharmacologist at Albert Einstein College of Medicine in New York, published a paper on taxol's ability to prevent cell division. NCI scientists then showed that taxol was effective against colon and mammary tumors in mice. Severe reactions limited taxol's first trials in human patients, but by 1986, research at Johns Hopkins School of Medicine was starting to show some promising early results against ovarian cancer.

The NCI now faced squarely the supply problem—it took the bark from several yew trees to supply enough taxol to treat one patient. Deciding at this point that it was time for private industry to show its role, the NCI put the taxol project out for bids, and the drug firm Bristol-Myers (now Bristol-Myers Squibb) won. As it turned out, though, the key discovery of a process to manufacture taxol synthetically in large quantities was made by another university investigator, Robert Holton at Florida State, with NCI funds. Bristol-Myers then licensed Holton's discovery. The NCI continued to fund much of the cost of clinical trials of taxol, with the company supplying the drug.

The NCI contract gave Bristol-Myers exclusive rights to market the drug for five years, and included a fair-pricing clause. There has been some subsequent controversy about how the market price for taxol was chosen. One version is that the NCI gave Bristol-Myers a list of fifteen cancer drugs and demanded that taxol be comparably priced. The list, according to consumer advocates, was an invitation to overcharge. The cheapest drug on the list was levamisole, at six dollars a pill; but the same drug, when used to control worms in sheep, costs six cents a pill. Critics charged that the drug firm was given the green light to charge the same prices as if it had developed taxol without any help from the federal research budget.

Another account of the pricing (from an investigation by the *Washington Post*) suggested that Bristol-Myers basically fooled the NCI team.[22] They indicated a price and the NCI negotiators accepted. But the NCI thought that price was to represent the retail price for an average dose, while the company meant the price to represent the direct-from-manufacturer price of a dose for an especially small woman.

Regardless of how everyone got there, when taxol was finally on the market, it was the most expensive cancer drug. A single dose came in at a cost of $1,800; a full course of treatment commonly cost $10,000 for women with ovarian cancer and $20,000 in cases of breast cancer.

The company told a different story. Bristol-Myers Squibb CEO Peter Dolan wrote a letter to company employees, posted on the firm's website, claiming that the company invested nearly one billion dollars in taxol. This sum represents the cost of both figuring out how to manufacture a compound that occurs in nature in very small quantities and also to test it on a wide array of other cancers. Of course, once NCI had shown that the drug worked for a few cancers, and Bristol-Myers Squibb had exclusive marketing rights, they stood to make a hefty profit if they could show that the same drug was useful for other cancers too.

The NCI, in giving Bristol-Myers Squibb its exclusive license, assumed that taxol (as a naturally occurring compound) was not patentable and that after the five-year period generic versions could be marketed. In 1993, an executive of the company assured a House of Representatives committee that no patents were either possible or being sought. But as the five-year period ended, Bristol-Myers Squibb did in fact seek patents—on the delivery system, not on the drug itself—and proceeded to sue all firms that applied for permission to manufacture generic equivalents. When that tactic failed, Bristol-Myers Squibb was sued by a small California drug company, American BioScience, who demanded that the larger firm file information about its patents with federal regulators. Eventually, the attorneys general of twenty-nine states filed suit against Bristol-Myers Squibb for violation of antitrust laws in preventing generic competition. The attorneys general claimed that the suit filed by American Bioscience was a sham and that the small firm was collaborating secretly with Bristol-Myers Squibb, knowing that by filing that suit they effectively delayed any other generic competition for thirty months under the provisions of the Hatch-Waxman Act.

Bristol-Myers Squibb eventually settled the lawsuit brought by the states without admitting wrongdoing. The attorneys general estimated that during the time that Bristol-Myers Squibb fought off generic versions of taxol, effectively keeping the drug out of the hands of many indigent patients, the company gained revenues of at least $5.4 billion. In January 2003, the figure at which Bristol-Myers Squibb had agreed to settle the states' lawsuit was announced as $135 million.[23]

How typical is the taxol story? According to the pharmaceutical industry, it is an aberration, since in most cases the industry itself does the lion's share of the research on which new drugs are based.[24] According to industry critics, a vast proportion of basic drug research is done by the academic sector and the NIH. Linda Marsa writes, "In 1991 alone, the NIH, or researchers supported through extramural grants, had 121 drugs under development—more than any single drug company. In that same year, the FDA approved 327 new drugs and products, yet only 5 of them were considered a significant advance, 9 were targeted to 'severely debilitating or life-threatening illness,' and 2 were for the treatment of AIDS. All 5 of the therapies deemed an important therapeutic gain, 6 of the 9 drugs for treatment of serious ills, and both AIDS drugs were devised with federal funds."[25]

MARCH-IN RIGHTS?

Since the "march-in rights" retained by the federal government according to Bayh-Dole had never been exercised, most people by the turn of the century had forgotten they even existed. Peter Arno and Michael Davis wrote in the *Washington Post* in 2002 to argue that given the large number of drugs that had been discovered in part as a result of federal funding, Bayh-Dole constituted a potent tool to force drug makers to reduce prices to "reasonable" levels.[26] This interpretation of Bayh-Dole was challenged. No less an authority than former Senator Birch Bayh weighed in to state that reducing high drug prices had never been an intent of Bayh-Dole. Rather, the concern had been over a drug company that received an exclusive license to market a useful drug and then failed to bring the drug into production. Only in that case should the Feds exercise the march-in rights, to ensure that the public had access to the new drug—at whatever price the company decided to charge.[27]

The strongest test to date of the government's intent to use "march-in" occurred with the AIDS drug Norvir, manufactured by Abbott, in 2004. The company saw sales figures decline as AIDS doctors stopped using Norvir as a first-line anti-AIDS medicine and began instead using it in lower doses as a supplement to other drugs. Abbott responded by quintupling the price it charged for Norvir, despite the fact that the drug had already achieved total sales of one billion dollars, what many considered an adequate return on Abbott's research investment.

A nonprofit group, the Consumers Project on Technology, petitioned the NIH to hold hearings on whether this price increase was reasonable and whether Abbott's license should be overruled. AIDS advocacy groups had previously been loath to attack the pharmaceutical industry directly, generally adhering to the argument that without high profits for AIDS drugs, development of new breakthroughs would be slowed. But the extreme nature of this latest price increase also galvanized some of the AIDS groups into action against Abbott.[28] On August 4, 2004, the NIH agreed with Senator Bayh's interpretation and ruled that it had no powers under Bayh-Dole to interfere with drug pricing.[29]

ACADEMIC SCIENCE FOR SALE?

The taxol story shows that one unfortunate consequence of the Bayh-Dole and subsequent acts has been the high prices charged for drugs, even those that were discovered in large part through taxpayer funding. These laws, combined with the Chakrabarty decision, have also had deleterious effects on many aspects of academic science, turning the late Admiral Rickover into a prophet in the minds of some critics of today's university scene.

One negative effect has been the substitution of business values for scientific values and the resultant alteration in the way scientific research is conducted. The ideals of science demand that scientists report their findings and try to replicate the findings of other scientists. Scientists are expected to facilitate the process of replication of key experiments by sharing their data and in some cases their materials with their fellows. All this changes when patenting is the name of the game. Scientists withhold research results from public announcement while the university seeks a patent for the discovery. Scientists refuse to share data and materials with those who have now, in effect, become their business competitors.[30]

A more basic concern is the fundamental direction of scientific research itself. Since Bayh-Dole was passed, the United States has gone through a long period in which privatization and "shrinking big government" have become popular political watchwords. While the NIH budget itself, in recent years, has been growing, the proportion of clinical research funded by private industry has exceeded the publicly funded portion, as can be seen in figure 4.1.[31]

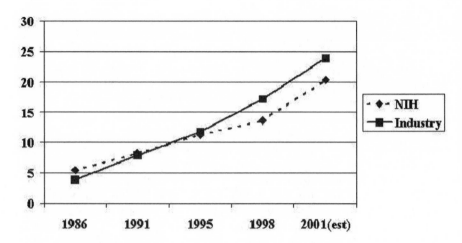

Figure 4.1. Research and development spending by NIH and U.S. pharmaceutical industry, 1986–2001 ($ billions).

The message seems clear—we the public are telling the academic community that we are less and less willing to pay for science out of the public purse; and since the academy can now make big money off the marketing of its scientific research, we want the universities to turn to that alternative source of funds. How, then, would university administrators and scientists act? It would be quite logical for there to be a systematic turning away from the sorts of research questions that represent pressing public concerns, unless those questions also involve a chance for hefty profits in the marketplace. At the same time, one might well expect to see university scientists eager to do research on questions that promise immediate spin-off products that can be sold in the marketplace, even if the problems solved by these breakthroughs are of quite minor importance.

Two major books published in 2003 take basically different approaches to this set of problems. Derek Bok, former president of Harvard, believes generally that Bayh-Dole has had a positive impact in increasing the universities' search for marketable and useful applications of research and sees no evidence that it has fundamentally shifted the attention of the basic sciences away from the fundamental problems in their fields. Bok sees the necessary task as cleaning up around the edges rather than as completely reversing Bayh-Dole.[32]

Sheldon Krimsky, a professor at MIT, sees a much less favorable picture. He argues that academic science has been far too eager to sell its integrity and far too ready to deny that any integrity has been lost. He sees the major loss of scientific values in precisely the place that Bok believes the values have been protected—that the sorts of questions that scientists choose to study are now driven much more by the search for profits in the marketplace as opposed to the public need. Krimsky argues that no sufficient reform will occur until certain roles are kept strictly separate:

- those who produce knowledge in academia and those who have a financial stake in the knowledge;

- those who have fiduciary interest in protecting human research subjects and those with a financial stake in products being tested; and
- those who assess therapies versus those with a financial stake in the success or failure of the products.[33]

The Office of Technology Assessment, a former nonpartisan agency of the U.S. Congress, predicted both of these problems succinctly in a 1988 report: "It is possible that the university-industry relationships could adversely affect the academic environment of universities by inhibiting free exchange of scientific information, undermining interdepartmental cooperation, creating conflict among peers, or delaying or impeding publication of research results. Furthermore, directed funding could indirectly affect the type of basic research done in universities, decreasing university scientists' interests in basic studies with no potential commercial payoff."[34]

It is important to keep historical perspective and to realize that these forces did not necessarily originate with Bayh-Dole in 1980. As long ago as the late 1960s, for instance, a leaking offshore oil well left a huge oil slick in California's Santa Barbara Channel. "Yet California state officials couldn't find a knowledgeable campus scientist to advise them on the cleanup or to testify against the oil companies. The reason? Every single expert they contacted was already the recipient of research money from the companies responsible for the spill."[35]

Nevertheless, the environment created by Bayh-Dole and Chakrabarty have clearly hastened and expanded these commercialization forces. Perhaps the poster child for the new university is the University of California-Berkeley and the contract between its Department of Plant and Microbial Biology and the drug firm, Novartis. In 1998, Novartis agreed to pay the department twenty-five million dollars over five years, thereby paying for roughly a third of the department's total research budget, in exchange for the first rights to license any new research discoveries. Novartis also gained the right to name two of the five members of the committee to decide how the research funds would be distributed.[36]

Bok, who believes that on balance Bayh-Dole has been a good thing, still worries that the Berkeley-Novartis deal has set a bad precedent. On one hand, Bok argues, the deal seems not to have created undue bias within the department. But the Berkeley department was selected by Novartis for this sort of contract precisely because it was a national leader. Because of its national stature, there is less chance the Berkeley department will be unduly influenced, because it can easily get grant funding elsewhere. But once a precedent is set, Bok fears, weaker departments will try to follow suit and will be more vulnerable to undue influence.[37] Krimsky does not believe that we will have to wait that long for deleterious consequences. After the contract was announced, he notes, the California Senate held hearings. The dean of the relevant college was asked: What if a faculty member who had signed the confidentiality agreement discovered a serious danger to public safety in some product that the department and Novartis were jointly developing? Would UC-Berkeley defend him if he spoke out and the company tried to suppress or punish him by legal means? The dean's answer was clear—the university had no obligation to defend a scientist who violated the contract even in the face of a clear public interest.[38] For Krimsky, this single answer was enough to show that the contract is contrary to the basic interests of academic science.[39]

CONCLUSION: PATENTS AND THE PUBLIC INTEREST

The following is a scenario that could occur any day, if it has not happened already. A small team of university scientists has an idea for a novel way of combining the use of several popular drugs with genetic testing. They have realized a basic fact about the way that a set of human genes interact with each other and with these medicines. They can envision a clinical application of their theory that would allow the much more effective use of these drugs and the avoidance of most life-threatening side effects.

They approach a small biotechnology company, realizing that capital will have to be invested to take their idea from its current theoretical stage to human application. The company, in turn, consults its patent attorney. The word is grim. In the mad rush to patent everything, and with the U.S. Patent Office apparently abandoning its traditional criteria for what is patentable and what is not, virtually every conceivable gene product or fragment has been patented by someone. These patent owners have no idea how to make any practical use of these "inventions," yet the patents are on the books all the same. Now that the firm has a new idea that would make good use of these gene sequences for a practical clinical outcome, the company discovers that it would have to negotiate licensing fees with thirty patent holders in order to have access to all the genetic tests and materials that would eventually be needed—since the discovery hinges on the interactions among many genes, not the detection of a single gene. The lawyer says that this is basically an impossible task. Even if the company were to raise several million dollars of initial capital, all that money would be spent doing the legal negotiations and securing the licensing agreements—before a single dollar could be spent on research and development. No one is going to invest capital in the project when its chances of long-term success are so restricted. In effect, the lawyers say that this project is a loser right out the door. Better not even to go down that pathway.

This scenario shows that patents, in our present state of scientific development, may be doing the opposite of what they are supposed to do. Instead of promoting scientific and technological advance for the public good, they may be thwarting that advance. Jon Merz and colleagues gave a specific example of this phenomenon when they studied genetic testing for the iron-overload disease, hemochromatosis. They argued that the current pattern of genetic patents was thwarting the spread of useful genetic tests and causing centers to offer less satisfactory and more limited tests instead of developing better ones.[40]

Some of the problem arises from shifts in the practices of the Patent Office. By law, a patent should be issued when an invention is useful, novel, and nonobvious. The discovery that led to the Chakrabarty decision in the Supreme Court illustrates these criteria rather well. Using a bacterium to clean up an oil slick was certainly a novel and highly practical idea. And a good deal of work was done to create the bacterium, since no oil-eating *Pseudomonas* existed already formed in nature. Allowing a patent on such a product seems a far cry from letting universities or companies patent thousands of gene sequences as part of a roulette game to see which one will someday be useful. And it seems a far cry from allowing a drug company to patent every feature of a pill or capsule, including its color, as a way of fending off generic competition. As we saw in the last chapter, to justify all this activity on the grounds that somehow it contributes to a "free market" rings hollow.

Yet we have not yet gotten to the major claim of the industry—that its high profits are justified because it plows that money back into research, thus leading to major breakthroughs like Gleevec. So far we have seen reasons to doubt that as large a proportion of the creative scientific work is done by industry scientists as is often claimed. The next chapter will look at the research-and-profits connection in more detail.

NOTES

1. L. Marsa, *Prescriptions for Profit: How the Pharmaceutical Industry Bankrolled the Unholy Marriage between Science and Business* (New York: Scribner, 1997), 133. The reference is to science writer Nicholas Wade, formerly of the journal *Science*, now with the *New York Times*. (Marsa made no reference to a specific column by Wade, nor was Wade himself able to direct me to the original source; e-mail communication, Nicholas Wade to H. B., April 4, 2004.)

2. T. Lieberman, "Bitter Pill," *Columbia Journalism Review* 2005; 44:45–51, quote p. 49.

3. All facts of the Hytrin story are taken from S. G. Stolberg and J. Gerth, "Keeping Down the Competition: How Companies Stall Generics and Keep Themselves Healthy," *New York Times*, July 23, 2000.

4. D. Baker and N. Chatani, *Promoting Good Ideas on Drugs: Are Patents the Best Way? The Relative Efficiency of Patent and Public Support for Biomedical Research* (Washington, D.C.: Center for Economic and Policy Research, 2002); www.cepr.net/promoting_good_ideas_on_drugs.htm (Accessed 8/27/04).

5. A good basic summary of this law can be found in M. Angell, *The Truth about the Drug Companies: How They Deceive Us and What to Do about It* (New York: Random House, 2004), 178–82.

6. C. Adams and G. Harris, "Drug Makers Face Battle to Preserve Patent Extensions," *Wall Street Journal*, March 19, 2002:A24.

7. Marsa, *Prescriptions for Profit*, 50.

8. Historian of science Nicholas Rasmussen succinctly summarized the practices he had identified among relatively distinguished academic physicians in the years between the World Wars, that would today be viewed as ethically questionable: "These clinical collaborators were often willing to refrain from disclosing their company sponsorship in their publications, to allow the sponsoring firm to design their research protocols in detail, to allow the sponsoring firm to discontinue or to decide not to publish a study in the event of unfavourable results, and even, in some cases, to edit or write their journal papers for them"; N. Rasmussen, "The Moral Economy of the Drug Company: Medical Scientist Collaboration in Interwar America," *Soc Stud Sci* 2004; 34:161–85, quote p. 165; for more details see N. Rasmussen, "The Drug Industry and Clinical Research in Interwar America: Three Types of Physician Collaborator," *Bull Hist Med* 2005; 79:50–80.

9. On Weiss's career and stature generally see K. M. Ludmerer, *Time to Heal: American Medical Education from the Turn of the Century to the Era of Managed Care* (New York: Oxford University Press, 1999), 28–29.

10. Rasmussen, "The Drug Industry and Clinical Research in Interwar America."

11. Quoted in H. M. Marks, "Notes from the Underground: The Social Organization of Therapeutic Research," in: *Grand Rounds: One Hundred Years of Internal Medicine*, ed. R. C. Maulitz and D. E. Long (Philadelphia: University of Pennsylvania Press, 1988), 297–336; quote p. 306–7. On the elitist and classist biases suggested by this comment, see T. J. Kaptchuk, "Powerful Placebo: The Dark Side of the Randomized Controlled Trial," *Lancet* 1998; 351:1722–25.

12. Rasmussen, "Moral Economy of the Drug Company."

13. Marsa, *Prescriptions for Profit*, 97.

14. M. Goozner, *The $800 Million Pill: The Truth behind the Cost of New Drugs* (Berkeley: University of California Press, 2004), 126.

15. Marsa, *Prescriptions for Profit*, 97–98.

16. Marsa, *Prescriptions for Profit*, 98.

17. Marsa, *Prescriptions for Profit*, 141.

18. Marsa, *Prescriptions for Profit*, 99. On the ethical issues involved in this extension of patents to genetics and human life, see D. Magnus, A. Caplan, and G. McGee (eds.), *Who Owns Life?* (Amherst, NY: Prometheus Books, 2002).

19. K. Greider, *The Big Fix: How the Pharmaceutical Industry Rips Off American Consumers* (New York: PublicAffairs, 2003), 54.

20. The facts in the taxol story are taken from Greider, *The Big Fix*, 52–54; M. Petersen and M. W. Walsh, "States Accuse Bristol-Myers of Fraud on Taxol," *New York Times*, June 5, 2002; M. Petersen, "Bristol-Myers Squibb to Pay $670 Million to Settle Lawsuits," *New York Times*, January 8, 2003.

21. Goozner, *The $800 Million Pill*, 185–91.

22. The *Washington Post* investigation was summarized by Greider, *The Big Fix*, 53, without giving a specific reference to the original source.

23. At the same time the company agreed to pay $535 million to resolve similar lawsuits involving its anti-anxiety drug, BuSpar; the settlement did not put an end to ongoing investigations of possible antitrust violations by the Federal Trade Commission; Petersen M. Bristol-Myers Squibb to pay $670 million to settle lawsuits. *New York Times*, January 8, 2003.

24. S. Taurel, "Hands Off My Industry," *Wall Street Journal*, November 3, 2003:A14.

25. Marsa, *Prescriptions for Profit*, 264.

26. P. Arno and M. Davis, "Paying Twice for the Same Drugs," *Washington Post*, March 27, 2002:A21.

27. M. Groppe, "Birch Bayh Opposes Price Limits on Drugs Developed with Federal Aid," Gannett News Service, Washington, May 25, 2004; D. Brown, "Group Says U.S. Should Claim AIDS Drug Patents," *Washington Post*, May 26, 2004:A4.

28. Brown, "Group Says U.S. Should Claim"; G. Harris, "Price of AIDS Drug Intensifies Debate on Legal Imports," *New York Times*, April 14, 2004:A1.

29. Associated Press, "U.S. Won't Override AIDS Drug Patents," *New York Times*, August 5, 2004.

30. D. Blumenthal, "Academic-Industrial Relationships in the Life Sciences," *N Engl J Med* 2003; 349:2452–59; E. G. Campbell, K. S. Louis, and D. Blumenthal, "Looking a Gift Horse in the Mouth: Corporate Gifts Supporting Life Sciences Research," *JAMA* 1998; 279:995–99; J. E. Bekelman, Y. Li, and C. P. Gross, "Scope and Impact of Financial Conflicts of Interest in Biomedical Research: A Systematic Review," *JAMA* 2003; 289:454–65.

31. The data for figure 4.1 were taken from R. A. Rettig, "The Industrialization of Clinical Research," *Health Aff (Millwood)* 2000; 19:129–46 (through 1998), and updated to 2001 with data obtained from the website www.phrma.com.

32. D. Bok, *Universities in the Marketplace: The Commercialization of Higher Education* (Princeton, NJ: Princeton University Press, 2003), 139–56.

33. S. Krimsky, *Science in the Private Interest: Has the Lure of Profits Corrupted Biomedical Research?* (Lanham, MD: Rowman & Littlefield, 2003), 227.

34. U.S. Congress, Office of Technology Assessment, *New Developments in Biotechnology: U.S. Investment in Biotechnology.* (Washington, D.C.: U.S. Government Printing Office, July 1988), 113; quoted in Krimsky, *Science in the Private Interest*, 31. It is unfortunate that the Office of Technology Assessment itself became a victim of the push toward privatization and shrinking government, as various administrations found its critical voice increasingly inconvenient and embarrassing.

35. Marsa, *Prescriptions for Profit*, 142.

36. Bok, *Universities in the Marketplace*, 151.

37. Bok, *Universities in the Marketplace*, 151–53.

38. Krimsky, *Science in the Private Interest*, 37.

39. In 1992, the Scripps Research Institute, a nonprofit research center in La Jolla, California, signed a ten-year, $300 million contract with the Swiss pharmaceutical company Sandoz, granting the company exclusive rights to commercialize any discoveries. Since Scripps received $100 million annually in research funding from the U.S. government, the NIH director, Dr. Bernadine Healy, testified in Congress that this would effectively transform Scripps into a "subsidiary of a foreign drug company." Scripps had already established similar deals with other firms, including Johnson & Johnson, but refused to furnish government investigators with copies of their contracts. A later federal investigation showed that 94 of the 130 patents that Scripps had filed over a decade, many of which it licensed to private companies, had actually resulted from federally sponsored research. Scripps claimed this miscalculation was merely a bookkeeping oversight. Richard Lerner, the president of Scripps, had negotiated a $60,000 annual consulting fee with Johnson & Johnson. In 1992 he also made more than $160,000 selling stock in Cytel Corporation, a subsidiary of Sandoz; Marsa, *Prescriptions for Profit*, 257–62.

40. J. F. Merz, A. G. Kriss, D. G. B. Leonard, M. K. Cho, "Diagnostic Testing Fails the Test: The Pitfalls of Patents are Illustrated by the Case of Haemochromatosis," *Nature* 2002; 415:577–79.

5

RESEARCH AND PROFITS

If one were to awaken any one of a thousand drug executives in the dead of night and ask him where all those profits went, the answer would undoubtedly be "Research." For most of the witnesses at the [Kefauver Senate] hearings who used it tirelessly—and, as far as that goes, for many who heard it—the word seemed to have the force of an incantation.

—Richard Harris, 1966[1]

One of the most commonly repeated claims by the pharmaceutical industry—today as in the 1960s—is that if the industry were not as profitable as it is, it could not fund the research that will be very likely to produce new breakthrough drugs in the future. We now need to assess the claim that there is a direct relationship between the industry's profits and its ability to conduct research.

Public Citizen's assessment of the ten drug firms among the *Fortune* 500 companies in the United States showed that they were substantially more profitable than any other industry in 2002. That recession year was a bad year for U.S. industry overall; the *Fortune* 500 companies suffered a decrease of 66.3 percent in profits. The drug companies had a bad year also, but for them, a bad year was a 3.5 percent drop-off in profits. Nor was 2002 unique; the pattern of drug company profits exceeding industry averages goes back at least thirty years.[2]

It is true that drug companies must bring in *revenue* to fund research and development; but that is not the same as saying that they need to make high *profits*. Using the figures in the Public Citizen 2002 report illustrates the difference. There are three ways to calculate profits: as a percentage of revenue, of assets, and of equity. Using these three methods, drug company profits are (respectively) 5.5, 6.1, and 2.7 times the average for all *Fortune* 500 firms. Let's adopt the 2.7-times figure as the most conservative way of assessing profits. Let's imagine further that the largest ten drug firms were content to make *only twice as much profit* as the average *Fortune* 500 company. This would mean that the portion of revenue that was allocated to profits would be reduced to 74 percent of its present level. The 2002 figures for the ten companies are:

- Total revenues: $217,467,000,000
- Profits: $35,896,000,000
- Research and development (R&D, calculated as 14.1 percent of revenue): $30,663,000,000
- Marketing and administration (calculated as 30.8 percent of revenue): $66,980,000,000[3]

If the companies were satisfied with 74 percent of their present level of profit, they could make do with profits of only $26,260,000,000. The remaining money could then be reallocated to research and development and would increase expenditures in that category by 32 percent over present levels.

In this example, we see that if the companies decided to do so, they could increase spending on research and development by nearly one-third. In the process they would not reduce by one penny the sums now spent on marketing (which many industry analysts view as excessive), and they would still remain at least twice as profitable as the average *Fortune* 500 company. This example would seem to make clear that there is no essential connection between the current high industry profitability and the amount available to invest in research. If drug prices were to be cut severely and revenue fell accordingly, there would come a time when research funding was threatened along with profits. That time appears far away at present, and no such trend has been seen in the industry at any time over the past three decades.

There is another way to look at the relationship among revenues, profits, and R&D investment. The industry rhetoric suggests that it engages in research solely because of public-spirited motives. A more realistic assessment is that the industry is profit driven—just what we would expect in a capitalist society—and spends money on research precisely because that is where its future profits come from. The industry organization is called the Pharmaceutical *Research* and Manufacturers of America because that is the nature of their business. Companies take every opportunity to point out that they are different from the generic drug makers, because those firms simply manufacture already discovered drugs and do not invest in any research to find new drugs. It is not especially charitable or public spirited to find firms investing in R&D if R&D is their business. A corollary of this is that the firms will decide upon the amount of R&D investment based on the implications for overall profitability. If the firms thought they could be more profitable by investing even more in R&D, presumably they would.[4] If they thought they'd make just as much profit by investing less in R&D, they would presumably do that instead. There is no reason to expect that the goal of improving the public health, *apart from* the impact that goal has on company profits, primarily motivates the industry.

THE DEBATE

The dispute over the true costs of research and development, and the relationship of those costs to profits, is hard to settle because of the dramatic mismatch between research costs claimed by industry advocates and costs calculated by industry critics. A handy summary of the issues appears in a sequence of publications: a 2001 report on research costs by the advocacy group and industry critic, Public Citizen; a response to that report by PhRMA, and finally a Public Citizen rebuttal.[5] Public Citizen took issue with the industry claim that the average cost of bringing a new drug to market was then approximately $500 million (an estimate since raised to $800 million).[6] In its defense, PhRMA produced estimates from two private consulting firms, Lehman Brothers Healthcare and the Boston Consulting Group, and the Public Citizen rebuttal addressed the methodology of these reports as well as that of an earlier published article by DiMasi's group at Tufts University.[7] The main points of contention are:

- Industry estimates often use before-tax figures while critics claim that the considerable tax breaks enjoyed by the industry as a result of its research should be factored in. Public Citizen estimated, for instance, that if one divides aggregate R&D spending by all new drugs approved for market between 1994 and 2000, one obtains the figure of $179 million per drug before tax deductions; this drops to $118 million after taxes. Public Citizen cited a Congressional Research Service 1999 report that calculated that the pharmaceutical industry is taxed at an effective rate of 16 percent, compared to 27 percent for all other industries.
- Business estimates of the costs of research often include an opportunity cost for the use of capital. This can amount to half the calculated cost of research. Public Citizen's rejoinder was that while this may be standard business accounting practice, in fact the company does not "pay" the opportunity cost in any real sense. According to industry figures, nearly half of the reputed costs consist of this theoretical entity rather than actual cash expenses. To those of us not in the accounting business, it seems odd to say that a latte for which I paid three dollars actually costs me six dollars, because to the three dollars in cash that I paid out for the latte I have to add the lost opportunity to buy something else that cost three dollars with the same money.
- Public Citizen argued that the industry estimates attached unrealistically high costs to clinical trials. The Congressional Research Service report estimated that taking a drug through Phases I, II, and III of clinical trials on humans cost an average of $10 million, $20 million, and $45 million, respectively. Lehman Brothers estimated that *each* of the three phases of research incurred costs of $169 million.
- Presumably, research costs drug companies so much because most of the compounds initially tested never pan out as useful drugs. Considerable money may be spent testing a chemical before one finds that it has no useful effect, or causes unacceptable toxicity, or both. The cost of bringing a successful drug to market therefore includes the cost of testing however many

failures the company had to run through to find the one success. But even DiMasi, an industry defender, noted that nearly one-third of the "failures" abandoned by the companies were not scientific but rather economic failures.[8] That is, they could have been quite acceptable drugs based on what was known about their effects. The companies elected to terminate research on them not because of unfavorable results, but rather because economic forecasting suggested that higher profits could be made by investing elsewhere.

• Public Citizen made no effort to sift out marketing costs that might be hidden among the research costs claimed by the industry. Their rebuttal noted, however, that the industry routinely allocates the cost of Phase IV, or postmarketing, trials to its research budget, despite the fact that many Phase IV trials are considered by critics to be nothing other than marketing ploys ("seeding trials") in which practitioners are paid "research fees" merely for prescribing the drug.[9] For instance, Merck documents, made public as a result of Vioxx litigation, showed that the Advantage trial, published in 2003 to compare the safety of Vioxx and naproxen with regard to stomach bleeding, was viewed by the company's own staff as scientifically unnecessary. The trial was a seeding trial, designed by the marketing department to introduce six hundred physicians to the use of Vioxx. Merck scientists were then forced to reclassify several deaths, first thought to be heart attacks, as noncardiac, lest the trial show that Vioxx caused excess heart deaths.[10]

What happens when others, outside the industry, try to estimate the costs of research on new pharmaceuticals? Merrill Goozner, in his critical book, *The $800 Million Pill*, cites the Global Alliance study, which calculated the total cost of developing a new antituberculosis drug at $115 to $240 million. Goozner argues that this estimate is in sync with the Tufts University calculations of DiMasi and colleagues, because the estimated costs leave out the R&D costs that we will be discussing shortly, aimed more at market position and advantage than at genuine discovery. "In short, if the industry-funded academic economists at Tufts had factored out the half of industry research that is more properly characterized as corporate waste, their numbers would have been similar to that of the Global Alliance."[11] A group from the European Society of Cardiology estimated that research trials of cardiovascular drugs could be conducted at university centers for approximately one-tenth to one-twentieth the cost of the standard industry-sponsored trial, since the industry routinely channels its clinical trial funding through numerous for-profit middlemen, each one tacking on a hefty surcharge.[12]

Millions of patients benefit daily from the fruits of research conducted by pharmaceutical companies, and few of even the industry's harshest critics would wish personally to forego the benefits of that research. The industry claims that any diminution, however slight, in its profits would immediately be translated into less of this research; and the predictable consequences of less research would be an increase in human suffering. By calling the latter assertion into question, we do not necessarily deny the reality of the former observation. We can recognize both that pharmaceutical research has many good social consequences and also that among the companies' goals, profit maximization rather than disinterested public service takes the front seat.[13]

THE TRUE RISKS OF RESEARCH

Research is a risky enterprise. How risky it can be is shown by the plight of the pharmaceutical industry early in 2003, when several companies found their stock prices taking a hit for the first time in memory. The companies were then facing a substantial decrease in future profits, as many "blockbuster" drugs were all due to go off patent and face generic competition. According to the ideal business plan, a company facing the loss of a profitable blockbuster drug would now have a new blockbuster drug ready to roll out, with many years of patent protection left. But the pipeline of new drugs suddenly seemed to have run dry. The industry had focused most of its research efforts over the previous decade in two areas—me-too drugs, that is, variants on already successful drugs, and the promises of the new genetics. Many had predicted that genetic research would, by the first decade of the twenty-first century, usher in a new era of "designer drugs." These drugs would be highly effective and safe because they would be tailored to the genetics of each individual patient. Genetic testing would reveal how each patient's body metabolized a drug, and the companies would make not one drug, but a set of drugs to suit each different genotype and its specific biochemical needs. The problem was that when 2003 rolled around, there were very few "designer drugs" in sight (with a few exceptions like Gleevec, which was based on a knowledge of the specific genetic traits of cancer cells). It now seemed that their advent would be delayed at least ten more years. In retrospect, the American pharmaceutical industry seemed to have put its research eggs in the wrong basket in the decade of the 1990s, and now faced a serious crunch in profits as a result.[14]

But it is also true that the plight of the industry in 2003 was largely unprecedented in recent history. Since research is risky, and producing new drugs depends on research, one might have expected that the financial record of the industry between, say, 1970 and 2000 would be one of periodic ups and downs. One might have expected also that the occasional drug company would go bankrupt if it invested heavily in a line of research that proved to be a dead end. Instead, the companies uniformly showed a high rate of profits throughout this period. And while there were many mergers, they generally involved a very successful company buying out another successful company, not a successful company buying out a failing company. The industry appears to have taken a great deal of the financial risk out of research, for the better part of a forty-year period. How could it do this?

One obvious way to reduce research risks is to focus on me-too drugs. A me-too drug is a chemical that is virtually identical to an existing drug but with very slight differences. Because of the differences, the company can claim that the me-too drug is chemically unique; because of the similarities, there is a very high probability that the new drug will act in the human body in ways very similar to the old, already proven drug, thereby greatly reducing the riskiness of R&D. One common criticism of the pharmaceutical industry is that it makes too many drugs that are potentially marketable and profitable but that promise no significant therapeutic advantage over drugs already on the market. Garattini, for example, set out to evaluate the state of affairs in his native Italy (which, because of the international nature of the pharmaceutical trade, is probably reasonably typical of the rest of the world). Between 1984 and 1992, the Italian Ministry of Health approved more than one thousand prescription drugs. Of these, 244 were new chemical entities, while 581 were copies of existing products. Of the 244 new chemical entities, only 22 (9 percent) could be considered truly innovative drugs. Another 24 percent were me-too drugs that at least claimed to have some advantages over existing drugs; fully 47 percent were simple me-too drugs offering no claimed advantages.[15]

Criticism of me-too drugs must be tempered, however. FDA Commissioner David Kessler and colleagues wrote an article in the *New England Journal of Medicine* in 1994 to blow the whistle on some shady promotional practices of the industry. But the FDA team also defended the industry from charges that they deliberately set out to create me-too drugs. Often, they noted, the FDA received simultaneous new drug applications from multiple companies for drugs in the same class due to the fact that scientists in all these companies had been working along parallel lines. Even when a company directly tries to copy a chemical entity that is already someone else's successful drug, the goal is seldom to create a me-too drug, but rather the hope that by modifying the molecule in some way, the new drug will be more effective, or better tolerated, or both.[16] To give just one example, an early drug for diabetes, phenformin, caused so many toxic reactions that it had to be taken off the market. Years later, its cousin, metformin, turned out to be very well tolerated by the vast majority of patients and also to have numerous advantages. Today metformin is a mainstay of diabetes management. But, had metformin been introduced immediately after phenformin, the company would probably have been accused of marketing "merely" a me-too drug.

It is probably not rational policy to eliminate all research of the me-too variety, for at least two reasons. First, it is relatively easy for "one other effective drug already on the market" to turn into "no effective drugs on the market," since the presumed drug of choice might be shown to have serious toxic effects and need to be withdrawn. Seldane was the first nonsedating antihistamine, and Claritin appeared at first to be its me-too competitor. When dangerous interactions between Seldane and commonly used antibiotics were discovered, suddenly Seldane was out of the picture and Claritin was the new number one drug in its class. Admittedly this is not the best example, as Claritin has turned out to be much less effective than first claimed. But the principle applies equally well to more effective drugs.

A second reason to allow a certain amount of me-too research is that "effective drug" does not mean "equally effective for all patients." Almost always physicians find, by trial and error, that some of their patients do poorly on one drug in any given class and do well on a competitor drug, even though the two drugs are chemically quite similar. There is no clear answer to the question of how many drugs in any therapeutic class *should* be marketed so as to allow for the optimal chances of switching drugs to meet individual patient idiosyncrasies. Almost always it seems advantageous to have at least three or four drugs available in any given class. But one might have to do research on twenty or thirty different compounds to find those three or four drugs that are both safe and effective.[17]

We should, therefore, avoid attacking all me-too drugs. In some cases, such drugs have considerable utility and were not the deliberate aim of the company's research policy. Yet it remains true, overall, that the industry produces a great many me-too drugs for each instance of a true therapeutic advance. It is incredibly one-sided to look only at the Gleevecs in assessing the risks and the benefits of pharmaceutical industry research. It appears by any analysis that the industry puts a fair proportion of its R&D resources into the search for drugs that differ relatively little from molecules already on the market. A focus on such drug "discoveries" considerably reduces the financial risks associated with pharmaceutical research.

The most extreme instances of nearly risk-free research occur as part of the "evergreening" process by which a company seeks to extend the life of a blockbuster drug that is about to go off patent and to face generic competition. Many drugs consist of a mixture of two molecules that are mirror images of each other, called isomers. Frequently, in biological systems, only one of the two isomers is active. The other usually causes no harm and is, in effect, so much filler. There is little reason in such a case for the company to expend a lot of effort to isolate the effective isomer and to eliminate the ineffective half of the mixture.

The circumstances change, however, when the drug is about to go off patent. The company can obtain a patent on a drug that consists of the active isomer only, just as if it had discovered a brand-new molecule. Therefore, by an odd coincidence, a company seems to "discover" a purified, single-isomer form of its old drug just as that compound is within a year of two of losing its patent protection. When AstraZeneca's top-selling heartburn drug, Prilosec, the famed "purple pill," was about to go off patent, the company filed numerous patent infringement lawsuits to keep generics at bay, and then launched the "new purple pill," Nexium, along with a huge marketing campaign designed to convince both physicians and patients that Nexium was far superior to Prilosec. In actuality, Nexium is the active isomer of Prilosec, and in head-to-head studies the two drugs behave almost identically, as one would expect. In a similar move, when Forest Laboratories' antidepressant Celexa was about to face generic competition, it spawned Lexapro, its active isomer.[18] There is, obviously, very little financial risk in "discovering" the active isomer of an existing drug.

Another way to avoid the financial risks of research is to let others assume the risks. The pharmaceutical industry banked on the success of designer drugs and the genetic testing procedures that would make them possible, but invested relatively little in the basic research to develop this technology. Instead, many biotechnology start-up companies were created during the 1990s, each one around a small group of scientists with a promising idea. Most of the ideas came to nothing and many of these companies failed—fueling the 2001 biotechnology stock slump. A biotechnology company whose idea promised the creation of a marketable drug was, from a financial point of view, a David compared to the Goliath of a large pharmaceutical company. It was much easier, and cheaper, for the pharmaceutical company to buy out the occasional biotech firm that had a marketable product, than to pay for all the basic research from the get-go.

It was even easier for industry to deal with research done in universities and at the NIH. Virtually all such research is published and is openly available. It is becoming more common today for universities to patent promising laboratory discoveries; but universities patent these discoveries to make money, and the drug companies are happy to oblige, paying large sums for licenses that give them the exclusive right to produce the drugs. This works to both parties' benefit. The sums that seem large to the university administrator are peanuts compared to what it would have cost for the industry to undertake all the basic research strictly on its own. One study conducted in 1991 and cited in a report by the Office of Technology Assessment of the U.S. Congress showed that a quarter of drugs produced by industry could not have been developed at all, or only after substantial delay, had it not been for publicly funded preliminary work.[19] Later studies around the turn of the century documented that as many as one-third of today's cancer drugs were developed almost totally by federally funded research, even though the profits from their sales go exclusively to private industry. Industry is then free to charge for these drugs whatever the market will bear—even if the end result is that many U.S. taxpayers whose dollars supported the basic research to develop the drugs cannot afford them, as proved to be the case with taxol.

Research risks are also reduced if the industry can lobby for favorable tax or regulatory breaks in exchange for doing the research. This appears to have happened, for instance, with regard to pediatric drug research. Child health advocates became concerned through the 1990s that many drugs potentially useful in children had never been tested in that age group, and so optimal doses and safety had not been determined. The industry had calculated that the pediatric market was not big enough to justify the added expense of this research. Congress responded to this concern by allowing drug firms an extra six months of patent protection in exchange for testing the drugs in children. Given that a blockbuster drug can be worth millions of dollars in profits per each extra day that it remains on patent, this regulatory break suddenly shifted the risk, making it economical for companies to do pediatric research and claim the patent extension, even for drugs that have little practical use in pediatrics. The pediatric "loophole" is now seen as one of the factors delaying generic competition and keeping drug prices high.[20]

THE NEW ECONOMICS OF RISK AVERSION

Finally, companies can reduce the financial risk of drug research by dropping research on drugs that are therapeutically but not economically promising. This practice is quite contrary to the public-service rhetoric of the industry and points out that the marketing arm of the industry exercises considerable control over the research arm. Numerous case examples have shown over the years that when a company has a potential blockbuster drug, it will continue to do research on and aggressively market the drug even in the face of new research evidence that the drug may be ineffective or unsafe—the COX-2 group of NSAIDs (such as Celebrex and Vioxx) being only the latest example. The contrary is also true. A drug may show great therapeutic promise and be quite safe, but the company drops the research project because it has calculated that sales will never be strong enough to recoup the development costs. The most striking example of research risk aversion is the development of medications to treat diseases prevalent in developing nations, whose health systems cannot afford to pay U.S.-type prices for new drugs. The fact that there has been no new drug introduced for treatment of malaria in about thirty years, despite the huge toll this disease continues to take in the developing world, is frequently cited as an example of marketing concerns dominating research. But this same phenomenon can also occur with drugs intended for the domestic market. While Gleevec now seems one of the most striking success stories in recent pharmaceutical develop-ment, and one of the stories that most closely adheres to the rhetoric of the industry, critics charged that the company at one point dragged its feet on research into this drug, calculating that the potential market among sufferers of only certain rare types of cancer was too weak to justify continued investment.[21]

In the twenty-first century, pharmaceutical companies have become ever more captive to the demands of Wall Street. Even a small dip in profitability, no matter how healthy the company's long-term portfolio, is enough to send shivers through investors. The end result is less and less willingness to run any risks at all in order to perform research on promising new drugs.

One example is the development of new antibiotics. An increasing number of bacteria are becoming more resistant to the antibiotics now in use. At least part of the reason for increasing antibiotic resistance is the behavior of physicians, who have in turn relied for most of their prescribing information upon pharmaceutical marketing. Physicians routinely prescribe antibiotics for viral illnesses, which cannot respond to antibiotics, and use more expensive broad-spectrum antibiot-ics, the type most likely to produce resistance problems, instead of the older, cheaper antibiotics.[22]

The industry, however, is not interested in discovering new antibiotics. It costs the company as much to discover and test out a new antibiotic as it does a new cholesterol-lowering drug. But patients who have to take the cholesterol drug ev-ery day for life might take the antibiotic only for one or two weeks. Moreover, the company may only have to run one set of trials to show that a drug lowers choles-terol but multiple sets of trials to get an antibiotic approved—if they want to show that the antibiotic is effective for several different infectious diseases, which is critical for sales. So the companies have for the most part decided that antibiotic R&D just doesn't pay.[23]

Another example: In January, 2004, the *Wall Street Journal* reported that St. Jude Children's Hospital had just spent forty million dollars of its charitable dona-tions to build and open a state-of-the-art drug-testing facility.[24] For some years the hospital's scientists had been making valuable discoveries, pointing toward new, effective drugs and vaccines. A promising new AIDS vaccine was among those discoveries. When they then went out looking for drug firms that wanted to do the follow-up research needed to take the drug from the test tube to the mass-produc-tion stage, they encountered a cool reaction. Unless there was nearly certain proof that the new drug would work, and then would sell a billion dollars' worth a year, the companies simply were not interested. St. Jude's decided they had no choice but to develop their own in-house pharmaceutical lab so that their scientists could test the new drugs more extensively. According to the *Journal*, many other research hospitals and medical centers were going in the same direction.

The data we have reviewed in the last two chapters show problems with the industry's self-portrayal of the relationship between its profits and its research efforts. The data do not support the argument that the current high level of profits is required to fuel the research machine. Rather than profits in the service of research, we too often find research in the service of profits. The companies have powerful incentives to investigate the drugs that will sell best, not the drugs that are most vitally needed for human health. The companies spend much less on drug research than they claim, and could perhaps do high-quality research for even less money. Far from being leaders in research, the industry often waits for academic or government scientists to make the key discoveries, and even then the companies are notably averse to risk.

We have, however, only begun to scratch the surface of the problems posed by relying so much on the pharmaceutical industry to fund the U.S. drug research enterprise. We must next look at the quality of the research that is conducted and at how much of the research data is transmitted to the scientific community.

NOTES

1. R. Harris, *The Real Voice* (New York: MacMillan, 1966), 76.

2. Public Citizen, "2002 Drug Industry Profits: Hefty Pharmaceutical Company Margins Dwarf Other Industries," Public Citizen Congress Watch, June 2003, www.citizen.org/congress/reform/drug_industry/corporate/articles.cfm?ID=9923 (accessed March 8, 2005).

3. The trend shown here, to spend considerably more on marketing than on research, is not new. A 1958 exposé reported that the pharmaceutical industry at the time spent four times as much on promotion as it did on research; R. Carter, *The Doctor Business* (Garden City, NY: Doubleday, 1958), 137.

4. In fact, this has happened more recently. Despite falling profits across the industry in the years between 2003 and 2005, investments in R&D have gone up. Apparently the companies believe that the threat posed by a drying-up pipeline of new drugs requires additional R&D investment despite harder economic times. See the epilogue for more discussion of these trends.

5. The Public Citizen rebuttal, which summarizes the key issues from the earlier documents, can be found at www.citizen.org/print_article.cfm?ID=6514 (accessed December 31, 2003).

6. J. A. DiMasi, R. W. Hansen, and H. G. Grabowski, "The Price of Innovation: New Estimates of Drug Development Costs," *J Health Econ* 2003; 22:151–85.

7. J. A. DiMasi, R. W. Hansen, and H. G. Grabowski, and L. Lasagna, "Cost of Innovation in the Pharmaceutical Industry," *J Health Econ* 1991; 10:107–42.

8. DiMasi, et al., "Cost of Innovation."

9. D. A. Kessler, J. L. Rose, R. J. Temple, R. Schapiro, and J. P. Griffin, "Therapeutic-Class Wars—Drug Promotion in a Competitive Marketplace," *N Engl J Med* 1994; 331:1350–53; J. La Puma, C. B. Stocking, W. D. Rhoades, et al., "Financial Ties as Part of Informed Consent to Postmarketing Research: Attitudes of American Doctors and Patients," *BMJ* 1995; 310:1660–63; G. Harris, "As Doctors Write Prescriptions, Drug Company Writes a Check," *New York Times*, June 27, 2004:1.

10. A. Berenson, "Evidence in Vioxx Suits Shows Intervention by Merck Officials," *New York Times*, April 24, 2005:1; J. R. Lisse, M. Perlman, G. Johansson, et al., "Gastrointestinal Tolerability and Effectiveness of Rofecoxib versus Naproxen in the Treatment of Osteoarthritis: A Randomized, Controlled Trial," *Ann Intern Med* 2003; 139:539–46.

11. M. Goozner, *The $800 Million Pill: The Truth behind the Cost of New Drugs* (Berkeley: University of California Press, 2004), quote p. 264. Goozner in turn cites *The Economics of TB Drug Development* (The Global Alliance for TB Drug Development, October, 2001), 66.

12. J.P. Bassand, J. Martin, L. Ryden, and M. Simoons, "The Need for Resources for Clinical Research: The European Society of Cardiology Calls for European, International Collaboration," *Lancet* 2002; 360:1866–69. The current trend in the United States is to shift industry-sponsored trials out of academic medical centers and into the for-profit sector; T. Bodenheimer, "Uneasy Alliance—Clinical Investigators and the Pharmaceutical Industry," *N Engl J Med* 2000; 342:1539–44.

13. Economist Joseph Newhouse tries to defend the industry argument that higher profits enable research investment. However, in doing so, he seems to grant the basic point that these decisions are based on profit maximization, not on a commitment to science; J. P. Newhouse, "How Much Should Medicare Pay for Drugs?" *Health Aff (Millwood)* 2004; 23:89–102.

14. T. Ginsberg, "Party May Be Over for Big Pharma," *Philadelphia Inquirer*, February 16, 2005.

15. S. Garattini, "Are Me-Too Drugs Justified?" *J Nephrol* 1997; 10:283–94.

16. Kessler et al., "Therapeutic-Class Wars."

17. Abraham's review of a number of nonsteroidal anti-inflammatory drugs (NSAIDs) tested by companies in the 1970s and 1980s is eloquent testimony that very similar chemicals might turn out to have vastly different toxic effects and levels of effectiveness when subjected to clinical trials or to animal testing to identify cancer risk; J. Abraham, *Science, Politics and the Pharmaceutical Industry: Controversy and Bias in Drug Regulation* (London: UCL Press, 1995).

18. N. Swidey, "The Costly Case of the Purple Pill," *Boston Globe Magazine*, November 17, 2002. Recall from chapter 1 that Clarinex was a slight variation on this theme; instead of being the active isomer of Claritin, it was the active metabolite (a compound that the body produced in the process of breaking down Claritin).

19. D. Drake and M. Uhlman, *Making Medicine, Making Money* (Kansas City: Andrews and McMeel, 1993), 71.

20. M. Angell, *The Truth about the Drug Companies: How They Deceive Us and What to Do about It* (New York: Random House, 2004), 248.

21. A. S. Relman and M. Angell, "America's Other Drug Problem," *New Republic* 227 (December 16, 2002): 27–41.

22. The use of inappropriate and unnecessary antibiotics in such infections has even been described as a "drug addiction" problem among physicians; J. S. Abramson and L. B. Givner, "Bacterial Resistance Due to Antimicrobial Drug Addiction among Physicians: Time for a Cure!" *Arch Fam Med* 1999; 8:79–80.

23. R. Nelson, "Antibiotic Development Pipeline Runs Dry: New Drugs to Fight Resistant Organisms Are Not Being Developed, Experts Say," *Lancet* 2003; 362:1726–27.

24. S. Begley, "Lab Work: Researchers Try to Cut New Path to the Pharmacy," *Wall Street Journal*, January 12, 2004:A1.

6

SUPPRESSION OF RESEARCH DATA

Q (From Senate panel, early 1960s): Isn't it true that the costs of research for the pharmaceutical industry are high because so many initially promising drugs turn out to be failures?

A (Dr. Dale Console, formerly medical director of Squibb): "This is true, since it is the very essence of research. The problem arises out of the fact that they market so many of their failures."[1]

The late theologian and pioneer medical ethicist Joseph Fletcher once explained to me why he thought science was superior to theology. As a visiting professor at the University of Virginia Medical Center in the 1970s, Fletcher encountered a professor of neurology walking down the hall, grinning from ear to ear. What had made him so happy? Fletcher asked. The neurologist replied, "I just found out that something I had thought was true for the last thirteen years is really false."

Fletcher claimed that he had never seen a fellow theologian act that pleased when one of his pet theories was knocked down. This, to him, meant that science was the more intellectually honest pursuit.

Fletcher was perhaps naive in imagining that his neurologist colleague's reaction was typical among scientists. But he was surely right about the central point. The ethical conduct of science requires that the pursuit of truth be the highest priority. The personal interests of the scientist or the institution funding the research must always take second place. Negative findings must be published with the same enthusiasm as positive findings—lest other scientists be led down useless blind alleys.

The pharmaceutical industry's pursuit of profits can most seriously and directly undermine scientific values when companies try to suppress valid research that has unfortunate commercial implications for the company's products. Suppression of undesirable research results therefore constitutes one of the most serious ethical breaches that occurs at the medicine-industry interface. Unfortunately, I could extend this chapter for the length of the book if I gave all the possible examples, at least a few of which were briefly mentioned in the introduction. We will consider three illustrative incidents: the Nancy Olivieri case; the case of Betty Dong, named "Thyroid Storm" from a *JAMA* editorial; and the major trials of the COX-2 drugs.

THE OLIVIERI CASE

Dr. Nancy F. Olivieri of Toronto, an internationally respected hematologist (blood specialist), has become a poster child of sorts for two abuses of scientific research—attempts by the pharmaceutical industry to intimidate scientists to prevent them from publicizing information that could hurt the sale of drugs, and the failure of universities and teaching hospitals to defend the scientific integrity of their own faculty members and instead ally themselves with the industry that promises lucrative grants and contracts.[2]

The Facts of the Case

In early 1993, Dr. Nancy Olivieri was considered the major expert in Toronto on the care of patients with thalassemia major, a severe form of inherited anemia. She held clinical appointments at both the Hospital for Sick Children and the Toronto Hospital, caring for both children and adults with thalassemia, and held a faculty appointment at the University of Toronto. She wished to study a promising new drug called deferiprone, or L1.

Thalassemia patients need regular blood transfusions, but the anemia prevents their body from using the iron in the transfused blood to make new, normal blood. The result is a steady buildup of iron, causing damage to the liver. The standard treatment for iron overload is deferoxamine, which has to be given intravenously and causes numerous side effects. An oral medicine that would effectively prevent the damage caused by iron overload would be a great breakthrough for these unfortunate patients, and L1 had seemed to have potential based on preliminary studies.

Dr. Olivieri proposed a research trial to the Medical Research Council, Canada's major national scientific funding body, and was rejected. The council told her, however, that she might be more successful if she reapplied under a special program that required matching funds from industry. One of Dr. Olivieri's colleagues at the Hospital for Sick Children, Dr. Gideon Koren, was a clinical pharmacologist with contacts with a drug company, Apotex. Apotex did a large business manufacturing generic drugs but wanted to branch out and start developing its own new drugs. The company had a strong relationship with both the hospital and the university and had been having discussions with University leaders about a donation of more than twenty million dollars to build a new research center. Apotex agreed to sponsor Dr. Olivieri's research and acquired the commercial rights to sell L1. With the Apotex support in hand, Dr. Olivieri went back to the Medical Research Council and this time successfully got funding. She started two research studies to test the safety and effectiveness of L1 in thalassemia patients. Because of Dr. Koren's expertise in drug research, as well, perhaps, as a modest payback for his help in securing the agreement with Apotex, she involved him as a coinvestigator.

The contract Dr. Olivieri signed with Apotex for one of the two studies contained a confidentiality clause giving Apotex the right to control all communication of the results for one year after completion of the study.

In early 1996, Dr. Olivieri identified a serious problem among patients enrolled in one of the trials. Patients who initially had had a good response to L1 later began to get iron buildup again. Dr. Olivieri immediately notified Apotex and also consulted with the research ethics review board at the Hospital for Sick Children. She was worried that the informed consent she had obtained from the parents of these patients, to allow their participation in the research, was no longer valid unless she told them about this new risk associated with L1. She saw no reason to stop the research trial, however. Maybe more study would show why the drug seemed to stop working or how to predict the patients in whom it would not work. Furthermore, many of the patients in the study were simply unable to take deferoxamine, so L1 was really their only chance of avoiding the dangers of iron buildup. Since L1 was still working for many of the patients, Dr. Olivieri felt that she was obligated to continue to offer it, while making sure all patients were fully informed of any risks. Dr. Koren and the other members of the research team agreed with Dr. Olivieri.

Apotex didn't see it that way. The company, through its senior vice president for scientific affairs, Dr. Bernard Spino, informed Dr. Olivieri that they disagreed with her interpretation of the data and therefore saw no reason to inform the patients of any problem. When Dr. Olivieri told Apotex that she had been instructed by the ethics review board to inform the patients of the risk, Apotex abruptly cancelled both contracts and shut down the research studies (as they had a right to do under the contract). The timing of the action suggested that Apotex did this primarily to prevent the disclosure of the information to the patients and the general public, since if there was no research study going on any more, the research ethics board no longer had jurisdiction. At the same time Dr. Spino reminded Dr. Olivieri of the confidentiality clause in the contract, and threatened her with immediate legal action if she disclosed her conclusions about loss of effectiveness of L1.[3]

L1 was being used in several other countries and was the subject of other research trials. Dr. Olivieri felt that it was important that physicians be warned of the risk she had found. When Apotex refused to notify physicians who were using L1, she decided she had no choice but to publish her data through professional conferences and journals. She informed Apotex of every step she took to spread this information, at the advice of the legal counsel she had obtained through the Canadian organization that provides malpractice defense for physicians. Dr. Spino continued to write letters threatening legal reprisals and calling her conclusions erroneous. Dr. Koren continued to express his support for Dr. Olivieri's interpretation of the data until she invited him to cosign a report to a professional journal, at which time he begged off, pleading that it would be too difficult for him to get into a fight with Apotex when he still hoped to secure Apotex funding for other research projects he was responsible for. Dr. Olivieri's other major coinvestigator, Dr. Gary Brittenham of Cleveland, continued to back her fully.

One legal authority who later reviewed the Apotex contracts that Dr. Olivieri had signed claimed that those contracts were legally unenforceable. They forbade *any* disclosure of information, preventing the physician from telling patients about newly discovered risks. But the legal duty of informed consent overrides any such contract provision.

Dr. Olivieri was at fault for having signed such a contract in the first place. She later admitted that she did not realize the full import of what she was signing, and at the time, neither the Hospital nor the University had in place a policy advising or demanding faculty not to sign such contracts. (The University of Toronto first claimed that they did have such a policy, and charged that Dr. Olivieri had violated university policy by signing the contracts. Two years later, the university announced a new policy that included language prohibiting faculty from signing a contract with a nondisclosure clause. In that way the university tacitly admitted that it had previous not had any such policy.) As soon as Dr. Olivieri realized what the confidentiality clause meant, she concluded that her ethical duty to her patients and research subjects outweighed any supposed duty she might have under her contract. Nor did she jump to this conclusion; she consulted with the ethics review board at the hospital and received their assurances that she had interpreted her ethical duty correctly.

Even though the studies had been officially stopped, Dr. Olivieri had been able to get L1 to continue to give to the patients who seemed to be responding to it, under a program called Emergency Drug Release. She continued to monitor those patients for possible organ damage just as they had been in the research trial. This required liver biopsy—inserting a thin needle into the liver, taking out a small sample of tissue, and examining it under the microscope. In February 1997, the biopsy specimens showed that a number of the L1 patients were developing fibrosis, scarring that could lead to serious liver disease. Dr. Olivieri and her colleagues concluded that it was most likely that L1 itself was causing this fibrosis. This led to a new round of denials and threats from Apotex. Apotex demanded that Dr. Olivieri send them the original biopsy slides, which they then sent to a pathologist they had hired, who decided that there was no sign of fibrosis. Apotex then again called Dr. Olivieri's claims unsupported and threatened her once again with legal action. (Despite all these threats, Apotex never filed a lawsuit.)

Apotex defended the safety and effectiveness of L1 by quoting from a report that was presented at an international hematology conference in Malta. This report cited data on thalassemia patients receiving L1 and showed that it was effective for all of them and did not mention any risk of fibrosis. One of the coauthors of this report was Dr. Koren. For the first time, Dr. Olivieri realized that while he had been telling her and her colleagues that he agreed with her interpretations of the data, he had simultaneously been telling Dr. Spino and Apotex that he thought Dr. Olivieri was off base. The Malta report used early data from Dr. Olivieri's research study. But the report did not mention Dr. Olivieri's name, was published without her knowledge, and did not reveal that any of the authors had received funding from Apotex. Later Dr. Koren and several of his research fellows published these same data in a journal, again concealing both Dr. Olivieri's role in the study and the company funding of their work. Apotex used that journal article as further evidence that L1 was safe and effective.

Meanwhile Apotex and Dr. Spino were spreading allegations that Dr. Olivieri had been wrong about the risks of L1 because she didn't know how to conduct proper research. Ideally, the Hospital for Sick Children and the University of Toronto would have come to her defense. Institutions concerned to protect the integrity of the scientific process would have seen that the ability of a scientist to conduct ethical research and publish her results was being endangered by industry pressure. Several faculty at the university defended Dr. Olivieri. But the university leadership quickly concluded that this was a hospital matter and so the university should stay out of it (despite the fact that the hospital is officially affiliated with the university, and that all involved parties, even Dr. Spino, were university faculty).

The hospital, for its part, apparently decided that its best course of action was to join with Apotex in accusing Dr. Olivieri of misdeeds. Two disciplinary inquiries were held at the hospital. In each case, Dr. Olivieri was not informed of the specific charges that she was supposed to answer and was denied effective due process. At both hearings erroneous information about her was given to the boards of inquiry, and she had no chance to refute it. The boards concluded that she had been guilty of wrongdoing, and these conclusions were then spread about in a highly public manner. Other scientists at the hospital became disgusted with the way Dr. Olivieri was being treated and started to circulate petitions in her defense. Beside being rebuffed by hospital administrators, these supporters of Dr. Olivieri soon found that they were also the targets of anonymous character assassination and administrative harassment.[4]

Despite this maltreatment, Dr. Olivieri enjoyed a few advantages not shared by other scientists who found themselves at the wrong end of attention from the pharmaceutical industry. Her international reputation assured that the case would garner publicity and that she would have distinguished outside defenders.[5] While Apotex hoped she would quickly cave in to their threats because the cost of hiring legal counsel could quickly impoverish her, Dr. Olivieri was fortunate in gaining the wholehearted legal support of the Canadian Medical Protective Association— even though technically her case might not properly have come under their jurisdiction since she was not being sued for medical malpractice. Finally, while the Hospital for Sick Children seemed intent on wrecking her career, her colleagues in adult medicine at the Toronto Hospital continued to stand by her.

In January 1999, the Hospital for Sick Children summarily removed Dr. Olivieri from her post as head of the hemoglobinopathy program at the hospital and imposed a gag order on her and one of her chief defenders, prohibiting them from publicly discussing the case. These actions finally woke up the University of Toronto. The dean of the medical school had been getting messages from authorities in the United States and Britain defending Dr. Olivieri's reputation and asking why she was being persecuted. Further, universities pride themselves in believing in "academic freedom," and telling faculty members they cannot publicly discuss important issues is the opposite of academic freedom. The president of the university interceded and mediated a resolution whereby Dr. Olivieri was reinstated as director of her program. The Hospital for Sick Children was required to assure her legal defense from any further actions Apotex might take. The university paid a price for this intervention. Apotex broke off discussions with the university about donations for the new research center. In 1999 Apotex did finally make a donation to the university for a smaller amount than originally suggested, though it was still in the range of five to ten million dollars.

A Double Standard?

One aspect of the case that especially struck the Canadian Association of University Teachers board of inquiry was the apparent double standard when the hospital and the university dealt with faculty and staff who were on different sides of the pharmaceutical industry's favor. We have seen just how Dr. Olivieri was treated. In two separate actions taken at the hospital, she was denied basic due process and the hospital did nothing to protect her reputation from unjustified smears. The university said that this was a matter for the hospital to deal with, despite Dr. Olivieri's status as a university faculty member.

What about Dr. Koren, who continued to receive Apotex money and who seemed a likely conduit for more pharmaceutical grants in the future? We have already seen that he served in effect as a double agent, telling Dr. Olivieri that he shared her concerns about the risks of L1 while at the same time working with Apotex and Dr. Spino to discredit her work.

The character assassination of Dr. Olivieri at the Hospital for Sick Children included anonymous letters sent to various hospital staff. These first attacked Dr. Olivieri herself, and then later also attacked her few defenders. Some language in the letters led the Olivieri camp to suspect that Dr. Koren was the author. He was confronted by the hospital administration and vehemently denied the charge. The hospital then hired a private investigator, who spent several fruitless months partly because she was deliberately misled by Dr. Koren. Meanwhile the Olivieri contingent hired their own private investigator and eventually proved by DNA evidence that Dr. Koren had sent the anonymous letters. Faced with this evidence he finally admitted his role.

The hospital then held a disciplinary hearing against Dr. Koren. Unlike the case with Dr. Olivieri, the hearing was handled with great concern for due process; Dr. Koren was fully informed of the charges against him and had opportunities to present his defense. When Dr. Olivieri's group approached the authorities with some of the evidence they had gathered implicating Dr. Koren, the hospital trustees directed them "not to take any unilateral steps which might damage the reputation of one of your colleagues"—a concern that seemed strikingly absent in Dr. Olivieri's case.[6]

The final outcome of the hearing against Dr. Koren was that he was found guilty of "gross misconduct" that provided "sufficient grounds for dismissal."[7] He was, however, not dismissed. He was given some months of leave without pay, and allowed to resign from two administrative posts. The journal article written by Dr. Koren, using Dr. Olivieri's data without her knowledge or permission, constituted a serious violation of scientific integrity in authorship; yet the university and the hospital never brought any charges against Dr. Koren on those grounds.

Dr. Spino, even though his salary was paid by Apotex, remained a faculty member at the University of Toronto. Therefore, one of the university's faculty members had been systematically violating the academic freedom of another. Despite that, the university never took any disciplinary action against Dr. Spino and indeed renewed his faculty appointment. It is hard to escape the conclusion that faculty members who potentially can bring large sums of drug company money into the university in the future are treated in one way, while a faculty member who has incurred the wrath of the drug industry, and therefore is unlikely henceforth to be a good source of lucrative industry grants, is treated by a different standard.

THE "THYROID STORM" STORY[8]

Regular readers of *JAMA* must have been surprised at the issue of April 16, 1997. The average *JAMA* editorial is about a page to a page-and-a-half, two pages perhaps on the outside. That day's editorial, titled "Thyroid Storm," by deputy editor Drummond Rennie, ran for six pages.[9] Something had happened, and Dr. Rennie and his fellow editors thought that a brief summary would be insufficient. Only by following all the details of the story could the medical community appreciate its true importance. And the story was indeed a convoluted one, like the mouse's "tale" out of *Alice in Wonderland*.

When a patient suffers from an elevated level of thyroid hormone, symptoms may arise very gradually or quite dramatically, depending on how fast hormone levels increase. A slower onset is by far the more common. The unusual case in which levels rise rapidly and symptoms assume a particularly malignant character is called "thyroid storm."

The story for which Rennie chose this suggestive title concerns Betty J. Dong of the University of California at San Francisco (UCSF), where Dr. Rennie also holds an appointment in the Institute of Health Policy Research. Dong has a doctoral degree in pharmacy. In 1986, Dong and others published a letter in another journal showing that a number of different thyroid replacement medicines—which patients take when their body's natural thyroid hormone level is too low—acted quite differently. In medical jargon, they were not bioequivalent. Dong and her colleagues recommended two brand-name thyroid preparations as being the most reliable and predictable in their effects. One of these was Synthroid, manufactured by Flint Laboratories, the most popularly prescribed brand of the drug that is known generically as levothyroxine.

The following year Flint approached Dong about doing a further study of the bioavailability of Synthroid compared to three other thyroid preparations. A positive study result for Flint could mean even greater dominance of the $600 million annual market in thyroid replacement drugs. Dong, on her part, had every reason to believe that the study would confirm her earlier findings and show Synthroid to be superior. She and Flint signed a contract specifying the precise study protocol and how the data would be analyzed. As the study began, Flint was taken over by Boots Pharmaceuticals. Boots pursued the study and performed regular site visits, which showed that the study was well conducted and that any problems were minor.

Nonetheless, the relationship between Boots and Dr. Dong's team began to go sour. As the study was going on, the state of Massachusetts was considering adding Levoxyl, a rival thyroid drug, to its approved formulary. Hoping to show that Synthroid and Levoxyl were not bioequivalent, Boots asked Dong for the preliminary data from her study. Dong and her colleagues refused this request because they would then have to prematurely reveal which research subject was taking which drug—and keeping everyone "blinded" to drug assignment was a critical part of the research design. Boots kept asking for the preliminary data and Dong kept refusing.

By late 1990, Dong's team had finished their study and, as agreed, sent all the results to Boots. It was now clear that all four drugs were bioequivalent. Synthroid did not have the advantage that so many physicians had assumed for years.

Boots now performed an abrupt about-face. A study that had, according to all the site visits, been well conducted and in line with a previously developed protocol, now appeared to be riddled with errors. Boots's medical services director, Dr. Gilbert Mayor, criticized virtually every aspect of the study, hinted that there were ethical problems and financial conflicts of interest, and complained about Dong's purported misdeeds to the chancellor, vice chancellor, and several department heads at UCSF. The university looked into the complaints and decided that only the most minor errors had occurred during the research; the company's response, they said, was pure and simple harassment, designed to suppress research findings they did not like. (Unlike the University of Toronto and the Toronto Hospital for Sick Children, UCSF at this stage was not willing to hang one of its faculty out to dry just to protect future largesse from the pharmaceutical industry.) UCSF also found that all ethical guidelines had been complied with. In August, 1994, UCSF told Boots that to prevent publication of the study results, as the company demanded, would constitute an unprecedented intrusion into academic freedom.

Dong and six colleagues made numerous revisions in their paper between 1991 and 1994, trying to mollify Boots, but finally decided to go ahead and publish when it became clear that no honest presentation of their data and conclusions would satisfy the company. In April 1994, *JAMA*'s editorial offices received the manuscript along with a letter from Dong describing the dispute with Boots. She requested that several people she knew to be thyroid experts and also to be paid consultants of Boots not be asked to review the manuscript. *JAMA* sent the paper out to five expert reviewers and discovered that several of them were also paid Boots consultants. In fact, Rennie reported, the journal had considerable trouble identifying suitable experts in thyroid disease who were competent to review the paper and were *not* paid consultants of Boots. Nonetheless the paper was somewhat revised and then accepted for publication, scheduled to appear in the issue of January 25, 1995.

Meanwhile, Boots adopted a more sinister interpretation of Dr. Dong's motives. From their vantage point, the study results seemed tailor-made to serve the interests of their rival, the manufacturer of Levoxyl, Daniels Pharmaceuticals. So they concluded that Dong's study produced the unfavorable results because she had been bought off by Daniels. They hired private investigators, who discovered no financial link between Daniels and Dr. Dong.

On January 13, twelve days before the scheduled publication, Dong abruptly wrote to *JAMA* and asked that the paper not be printed. Boots had invoked a clause in the contract she had signed back in 1987, giving them the right to prevent publication of any data from the study without the company's written permission. In the past, the UCSF attorneys had assured Dong that such contracts had never prevented publication and that the language was routine boilerplate that she could simply ignore. (In 1997, Dong told journalist Daniel Zalewski that she had originally objected to signing the contract with the offending language in it, but that she had been advised by a UCSF patent officer not to worry about it—"that no pharmaceutical company would have the gall to violate so flagrantly the norms of academic research."[10]) In 1993, UCSF began to review all research contracts for its faculty and to forbid the signing of any contract with that language; but back in 1987 there had been no such process in place. Now Boots was threatening to sue Dong and UCSF for damages if sales of Synthroid suffered in any way as a result of the article. A recently appointed UCSF attorney, Shelly Drake, reversed the position that had been taken by his predecessors. He noted that Dong had in fact signed the contract with that language in it and feared that under those circumstances he could not defend Dong in court.

By this time Boots had successfully prevented publication of this study for a little more than four years. According to Dong and colleagues' calculations, $356 million were wasted each year that physicians continued to prescribe brand-name drugs because they did not know that the generic drugs were just as good.

One reason Boots dug in its heels in 1994–1995 was that the firm was being considered for purchase by yet another company, BASF AG, and the status of Synthroid as a leading drug could easily affect the selling price of the firm. In March, 1995, BASF AG bought Boots for $1.4 billion and combined that firm with their Knoll Pharmaceutical subsidiary. The new company, Boots/Knoll, notified *JAMA* that they intended to take the same hard line on preventing publication.

As it turned out, the new firm took more than a hard line; they tried to do a complete end run. In June, 1995, an article appeared in a new journal called the *American Journal of Therapeutics*, by Boots' Dr. Gilbert Mayor—who also happened to be an associate editor of the journal.[11] The paper consisted of the data that had been gathered by Dong and colleagues, without giving Dong's team any credit, and reanalyzed the data so as to reach exactly the opposite conclusions. Mayor's paper managed to cast doubt on Dong's findings and conclusions without mentioning Dong by name or even admitting that her paper existed. The goal of publishing in this manner was presumably to make it impossible for any other journal to publish Dong's paper. Medical journals have strict rules against duplicate publications; and Boots/Knoll could argue that any later publication of Dong's study was merely a duplication of the data that had now been published by Mayor and his colleagues.

Boots/Knoll, however, encountered unforeseen difficulties. First, the company was embarrassed to read a detailed exposé of the whole affair splashed over the pages of the *Wall Street Journal*.[12] The *WSJ* article led the FDA to inquire into some of the company's Synthroid labeling, arguing that the company did not have adequate data to support some of its claims—and wondering why, if the Dong data existed, the company had not submitted them to the FDA. Under this new pressure, Boots/Knoll shifted ground and began to negotiate with UCSF over allowing publication.

The end result was an odd assembly of articles in the April 16, 1997 issue of *JAMA*. The journal published the Dong study exactly as it had been set in proof two years previously.[13] Boots/Knoll had two letters to the editor—one giving the company's version of the events, the other continuing its arguments that the study was flawed and the authors' conclusions erroneous.[14] Dong and coworkers were allowed to reply to both letters and defend their work. Boots/Knoll was later subjected to a class-action lawsuit on behalf of thyroid patients who claimed to have been harmed by the delayed publication, which the company eventually settled for more than a hundred million dollars.[15]

COX-2 DRUGS

John Abramson, in proposing that government hearings be held to address "the commercial distortion of our medical knowledge," suggested that the first case to be investigated ought to be the overprescribing of COX-2 drugs such as Celebrex and Vioxx.[16] These expensive drugs, costing roughly ten times as much as a reasonable therapeutic substitute such as ibuprofen, never performed well on the measure that was supposed to be their strong suit, the avoidance of gastrointestinal bleeding. Eventually they were shown to have serious heart risks. Yet they immediately zoomed to the top of the industry's bestseller charts.

Carolanne Dai and her colleagues reviewed national prescribing data to see what sorts of patients received COX-2 drugs between 1999 and 2002. They argued that the one group of patients for whom these drugs might have made some sense were those needing an anti-inflammatory drug and who were at especially high risk of serious gastrointestinal bleeding. Only about 3 percent of prescriptions for COX-2 drugs were written for patients in this high-risk category. Yet at their height, COX-2 drugs managed to capture about 61 percent of the total market for anti-inflammatory drugs.[17] Similarly, the Kaiser health plans in California, using a risk tool developed by scientists at Stanford, found that only about 5 percent of patients were appropriate candidates for COX-2 drugs.[18] In other words, the vast majority of prescriptions written by U.S. physicians for COX-2 drugs were arguably irrational, even before the serious risks of heart disease were widely known.[19]

In theory, the COX-2 drugs were intended to be improved versions of a much larger class of drugs called the nonsteroidal anti-inflammatory drugs (NSAIDs), including ibuprofen and naproxen. The good news about NSAIDs is that they reduce pain and inflammation in conditions like arthritis, by inhibiting chemicals called prostaglandins. The bad news is that prostaglandins in the stomach help to protect against ulcers. The same drugs that interfere with prostaglandins in other tissues also interfere with prostaglandins in the stomach, so increased ulcer risk is one of the most important side effects of NSAIDs.

In the 1990s, scientists discovered that a drug might relieve pain but not cause ulcers if it inhibited an enzyme called cyclooxygenase-2 but not cyclooxygenase-1. This led to the creation of the new class of drugs that blocked only cyclooxygenase-2 (COX-2 for short), unlike the nonselective NSAIDs that blocked both.

COX-2 drugs like celecoxib (Celebrex) and rofecoxib (Vioxx) were released with great fanfare and quickly became popular, in part because of direct-to-consumer advertising. They were great money makers for Pharmacia and later Pfizer, which manufactured Celebrex, and Merck, the maker of Vioxx. Unfortunately, the scientific data accumulated after the drugs were on the market did not match the high expectations. Some studies showed that while COX-2 drugs caused fewer ulcers than the older NSAIDs, the differences were small.[20] Some studies even suggested that there was a slight excess of heart attacks among patients taking the COX-2 drugs. By the turn of the twenty-first century, even though the COX-2 drugs continued to be top sellers, clouds were gathering on their horizon.[21]

Toward the end of 2000, two large-scale studies of COX-2 drugs were published in widely respected medical journals. The CLASS study, involving Celebrex, appeared in *JAMA*, and a short while after, the VIGOR study, using Vioxx, was published in the *New England Journal of Medicine*. At first blush these studies largely put all the controversies to rest. They appeared to show without doubt that COX-2 drugs were superior to NSAIDs in preventing ulcers and other serious bleeding complications, while at the same time laying to rest any fears about cardiovascular risks from these drugs.

It turns out that neither CLASS nor VIGOR actually proved what they set out to prove and what they were widely thought to have proved. The CLASS story is the more interesting, complicated, and worrisome of the two.

CLASS

On September 13, 2000, the Celecoxib Long-term Arthritis Safety Study (CLASS) was published in *JAMA*. Sixteen authors were listed, of which (according to the article's financial disclosure) six were employees of Pharmacia and all the rest were paid Pharmacia consultants. The lead author, Dr. Fred E. Silverstein, was a professor in the Department of Medicine, University of Washington.[22] Other authors were affiliated with such centers as University of Illinois–Chicago, Harvard Medical School, Vanderbilt University, and Johns Hopkins. The study had been carried out at 386 clinical sites in the United States and Canada and involved a total of 8,059 research subjects. In sum, CLASS appeared in a prestigious medical journal with a prestigious battery of authors and gave every promise of being highly important scientific research.[23]

The subjects had one of two forms of arthritis, rheumatoid arthritis or osteoarthritis. They were randomly assigned to receive one of three drugs—celecoxib, or one of the two older NSAIDs, ibuprofen and diclofenac. The study followed all subjects and identified those who developed significant ulcers, stomach bleeding, or related complications, as well as heart attacks and other cardiovascular complications. The subjects, according to the article's abstract, were treated for six months.

The results appeared highly favorable for Celebrex. Despite the fact that a relatively high dose of Celebrex had been used, there were significantly fewer ulcer complications in the Celebrex subjects compared to those taking either of the other NSAIDs. There were no differences seen in the number of heart attacks or cardiovascular events.

As is typically done with major research papers, the editors of *JAMA* asked some independent experts to comment on CLASS. This editorial was written by Drs. David H. Lichtenstein and M. Michael Wolfe of the Section of Gastroenterology, Boston University School of Medicine. Lichtenstein and Wolfe were generally less enthusiastic about the COX-2 drugs and pointed out details in the study that cast some doubt on the major conclusions. They mentioned, for instance, that the six-month follow-up period was relatively short, since the average patient may need to take these drugs over many years. In the end, however, they agreed that, "The results of this important study by Silverstein et al. provide promising data to suggest that celecoxib and possibly other COX-2 selective NSAIDs are effective in reducing, but not eliminating, the risk of symptomatic ulcers." They also acknowledged the absence of excess heart disease risk.[24]

Dr. Michael Wolfe, one of the writers of the *JAMA* editorial, next encountered the data from CLASS in February 2001. Dr. Wolfe was a member of the FDA's arthritis advisory committee, and by law, Pharmacia had to turn all its data on Celebrex over to the FDA. Dr. Wolfe had gone over CLASS with a fine-tooth comb when he wrote his editorial—or so he thought. What he saw at the FDA, however, left him "flabbergasted," as he later told Susan Okie of the *Washington Post*.[25]

Instead of six months of follow-up data, Wolfe found one year of information. In the second six months of the study, a disproportionate number of ulcer and bleeding complications had occurred in subjects using Celebrex. According to the data in the FDA files, CLASS showed ultimately that Celebrex had no advantage over the other two NSAIDs. The material published in *JAMA* the previous September looked suspiciously like a highly selective culling of the research data—publishing the information that made the company's drug look good while concealing unfavorable data. Dr. Wolfe later told Okie, "I am furious. . . . I wrote the editorial. I looked like a fool."[26]

Another physician to express concern over the CLASS publication was Dr. James M. Wright, professor of clinical pharmacology at the University of British Columbia. Dr. Wright is managing director of Therapeutic Initiatives at his university, created by Canada's Ministry of Health to issue bimonthly bulletins to physicians and pharmacists in British Columbia about new drugs. The bulletin had already issued a skeptical report about the COX-2 drugs, and so Dr. Wright and his staff were on the lookout for further data.

Dr. Wright told Candis McLean of *Report Magazine* that he first became suspicious of CLASS when he contacted the authors of the *JAMA* article seeking further information, and was told that the data were unavailable. Dr. Wright's team then read, in February 2001, that the drug company's request for new labeling, stating that Celebrex had been proven to be safer than other COX-2 drugs, had been denied by an FDA advisory committee (the one upon which Dr. Wolfe sat). Dr. Wright knew that the labeling request required the company to submit all its raw data to the FDA. His group managed to track down the complete CLASS data on an obscure portion of the FDA website. Dr. Wright, it turned out, had been the beneficiary of the work of the consumer lobby, Public Citizen's Health Research Group. The group had lobbied heavily to stop the FDA from relabeling Celebrex with the more favorable assessment, and it was largely as a result of their pressure that the FDA put the complete CLASS data on its public website. "We would still be in the dark," Dr. Wright commented, had it not been for the consumer group.[27]

Dr. Wright's team still had the task of combing through all one thousand pages of the CLASS data. Anyone coming to the website without the benefit of the extra staff help would probably have given up long before he downloaded it all. It was only after sifting through all the raw data that the Canadian team discovered, as Dr. Wolfe had previously, that only six months' instead of twelve months' worth of data had been published.

The editor of *JAMA*, Dr. Catherine D. DeAngelis, told the *Washington Post* that she had had no inkling the previous September about the missing data when she made the decision to publish Dr. Silverstein's paper. "I am disheartened to hear that they had those data at the time. . . . We are functioning on a level of trust that was, perhaps, broken."[28]

On November 21, 2001, *JAMA* published two letters to the editor complaining about the publication of partial data from CLASS—one by Dr. Wright and three of his colleagues from British Columbia, the other from Drs. Jennifer B. Hrachovec and Marc Mora, members of the Pharmacy and Therapeutics Committee of Group Health Cooperative in Seattle.[29] Drs. Hrachovec and Mora noted that the truth about CLASS was very little known among physicians, nearly nine months after Dr. Wolfe's moment of enlightenment at the FDA advisory committee.

Dr. Silverstein and his colleagues were now given an opportunity to reply to these criticisms. The authors admitted, "In retrospect, we acknowledge that we could have avoided confusion by explaining to the *JAMA* editors why we chose to inform them only of the 6-month analyses, and not the longer-term data that were available to us when we submitted the manuscript." But they then proceeded to defend the integrity of their publication: "We submitted only this information because the authors believed the 6-month data were the most scientifically and clinically valid. The data after 6 months were so confounded as to be difficult to interpret for assessing a drug-related causal [stomach] toxicity."

Silverstein and his colleagues then went on to explain that there was a very high dropout rate during the last half of the study. That and other data suggested that after six months, they had in effect lost all the subjects from the study who were susceptible to developing ulcers, leaving only a core of subjects who were relatively resistant to ulcers. The authors argued that the population being studied after six months differed in a fundamental way from the population they had enrolled at the beginning. For all these reasons they viewed the final six months' worth of data as contaminated.[30]

How compelling are the issues raised by Dr. Silverstein and the other CLASS authors? Several reasons cause one to be highly skeptical of their explanation. First, and most important, the routine way to handle the problem they identified is to discuss it openly in the section of the paper dealing with research methods. One would say something like, "We had originally intended to carry the study on for twelve months. However, we discovered after six months that such-and-such problems had arisen. We accordingly tried to correct for those problems by doing such-and-such corrections in the way we analyzed the data." Ideally, the paper would have presented the six-month and twelve-month data side by side, and the authors could then have argued why they felt that the six-month data were more valid. That way the reader would have no reason to worry that anything had been withheld. By coming up with their methodological concerns only after being caught, Dr. Silverstein and his colleagues cast grave doubts on the validity of their position.

There are yet other reasons to be skeptical of the offered explanation. The authors claimed that the last-six-month data were "so confounded as to be difficult to interpret." But the two groups writing letters to the editor, from Seattle and British Columbia, had no problem at all interpreting the complete CLASS data as shown on the FDA website, and concluding that Celebrex had no superiority to the other drugs. Dr. Silverstein's group also suggested that the problem was that there had been too many subjects dropping out later in the study, so that too few people were left who were susceptible to ulcers. But the problem that actually arose was that *too many* of the patients in the celecoxib group developed ulcers during the second six-month period, eliminating the apparent advantage that the drug had shown during the first six months.[31]

The controversy over CLASS continued to bubble up in the pages of medical journals—but in Britain and Canada, not in the United States. In November 2002, Dr. Wright published his own analysis.[32] He combined the entire twelve months of CLASS data with the results of the other COX-2 study (VIGOR). By combining data from both studies in what is called a meta-analysis, Dr. Wright was able to pool the experiences gained from about sixteen thousand patients who had either taken one of the two different COX-2 drugs or one of several different NSAIDs.

Dr. Wright found that patients taking the COX-2 drugs had slightly fewer serious ulcers, and slightly more deaths, than those taking the NSAIDs, but that in neither case was the difference statistically significant (that is, the difference could have arisen by chance). One statistically significant difference was noted, however. More "serious adverse events"—death, hospital admission, and life-threatening or disability-threatening occurrences—occurred in subjects taking the COX-2 drugs than those taking regular NSAIDs.

Dr. Wright concluded that with the studies published so far, one could not determine with certainty whether COX-2 drugs were dangerous. He went on to describe the large-scale study that would be needed to put these issues finally to rest. He predicted that any such study would *not* be a drug-company-funded trial, because the potential outcome would be too embarrassing for any manufacturer of COX-2 drugs to take the chance. In this he was wrong. The makers of both Vioxx and Celebrex thought it economically worth the risk to conduct a large-scale, long-term study of each drug, in hopes of being able to gain FDA approval for a new use—prescribing a COX-2 drug as a preventive for colon cancer. When the Vioxx study had to be stopped prematurely, due to excess deaths from cardiovascular disease, Merck decided to withdraw their drug from the market in September 2004.[33]

How much did Pharmacia's reputation suffer as a result of its apparent role in suppressing key data? An editorial in the *BMJ* in June 2002 estimated that thirty thousand reprints of the original CLASS publication had been purchased, presumably to be distributed by detail people selling Celebrex. Sales of Celebrex had risen from $2.6 billion in 2000 to $3.1 billion in 2001. One of the editorialists attended an osteoarthritis workshop in Basel, Switzerland, in December 2001, and found that very few of the fifty-eight physicians attending had heard about the problems with the original CLASS paper and thought that the *JAMA* report was trustworthy.[34] Pharmacia's promotion apparatus, it appears, had done a masterful job in assuring that the partial news about Celebrex was widely disseminated to the medical community both in the United States and internationally, while the full news about Celebrex remained the property of a small group of scientific experts. And one is led to wonder, in hindsight, if that had not been the master plan in publishing the six-month data from CLASS all along.

The CLASS story presents extremely depressing news for practitioners who aspire to scientific prescribing. Most physicians, I believe, are aware at some level and to some degree that the information they receive from drug detail people is commercially biased. If you were to ask these physicians how they would get the ideal scientific evidence on which to base their practice if they cannot depend on the detail people, they would answer that they would have to somehow find the time and the skill to read the complete research studies in major medical journals independently and critically assess those studies for their quality. The amount of time and energy it takes to do this is an excuse that many physicians use, quite understandably, for relying on detail people instead.

CLASS shows how the "ideal" might still not work, because of the extent to which commercial bias has been allowed to creep into even the (apparently) best papers in the best journals. Dr. M. Michael Wolfe thought that he had carried out the ideal process of critical evaluation—his editorial contained an entire page of analysis of the strengths and weaknesses of the CLASS paper as originally published—and yet he, too, was in the end misled about the safety of the COX-2 drugs. It is wildly unrealistic to expect the average physician to expend the time and energy that Dr. Wolfe did in analyzing CLASS. It is even more wildly unrealistic to expect that average physician to wait six months and then get on the FDA website to see if the originally published study indeed contained all the data—assuming that a consumer's lobby in the meantime has filed a lawsuit to force the FDA to publish the material on its website. Exactly to what lengths must a physician go today to assure that she is basing her prescription decisions on sound science? If we add up how many improbable events all had to line up for the true story of CLASS to emerge, we are forced to ask how many similarly flawed research papers appear in medical journals and are simply never found out.

VIGOR

The Vioxx Gastrointestinal Outcomes Research (VIGOR) study lacks the sensational, dog-ate-the-homework quality of CLASS.[35] Nonetheless it is an equally instructive example of how drug-company-funded research can hide more than it reveals.

From the company's point of view, the VIGOR study came out better than CLASS. There turned out to be fewer serious ulcer complications in the group taking Vioxx, and this difference was statistically significant. So no data had to be "lost" from VIGOR in order to get the major result that the company wished to promote.

The major questions about VIGOR have to do instead with the issue of cardio-vascular risk. Dr. John Abramson, in his book, *Overdosed America*, gave perhaps the most detailed analysis of VIGOR for the purposes of the average reader (physi-cian or layperson). Abramson's book was published in September 2004, so he must have ceased writing no later than the early months of 2004. This means that he drew all of his conclusions well before he could have known anything about Vioxx being taken off the market.

Dr. Abramson became suspicious when he noted that the VIGOR authors said that they had counted cardiovascular complications in subjects assigned to both the Vioxx and standard NSAID groups, but for some reason elected not to report them as part of the study. He eventually found some of the raw VIGOR data, along with the FDA's assessment of it, on the same website that reported on the FDA advisory committee from February 2001. When he returned to the text of VIGOR, Dr. Abramson immediately noted something interesting. Steroid drugs are known to cause an increased risk of ulcers. The vast majority of people for whom physi-cians will prescribe a drug like Vioxx are *not* at that time also taking steroids. But more than half the subjects in the VIGOR study *were* taking steroids, because many of them had rheumatoid arthritis, for which steroids are often required. If one looked at the subset of subjects in VIGOR who were not taking any steroids—the group most comparable to the normal patient population—it turned out that Vioxx did *not* cause statistically significantly fewer ulcers than other NSAIDs. So the "right answer" that the drug company obtained through VIGOR was appar-ently obtained only by including in the study a highly atypical population of pa-tients. Abramson commented, "This may have been the most important finding in the study, but it remained hidden in plain sight and is still virtually unknown."[36]

Dr. Abramson then turned to the data on the FDA website to fill in what the authors of VIGOR had not seen fit to include in their paper. He soon found out that the serious cardiovascular complications totally eliminated any supposed ad-vantage of Vioxx due to ulcer prevention. Vioxx takers in VIGOR had twenty-one fewer serious ulcers, but had twenty-seven more serious cardiovascular complica-tions (like heart attack and stroke). After looking at all the numbers, and compar-ing notes with the FDA statisticians who had reviewed the same data, Abramson came to the dramatic conclusion, "The results of the VIGOR study show that for every 100 people with a history of cardiovascular disease treated with Vioxx instead of naproxen there were between *seven and 11 additional serious cardiovascular complications each year.*"[37]

Those with a history of cardiovascular disease, of course, are the patients at highest risk already—even though arthritis, the reason most physicians prescribed Vioxx most often, occurs disproportionately in the elderly, many of whom are at higher risk for cardiovascular disease. Among all the VIGOR subjects, not just the ones at highest risk, the likelihood of a serious cardiovascular complication is still nearly twice as high when taking Vioxx as when taking naproxen, the comparison NSAID—and this difference is highly statistically significant.[38]

It is important to step back and to realize what Drs. Abramson and Wright, be-tween them, have said. Looking independently at the CLASS and VIGOR data, as they were published in 2000, each discovered a statistically significant increase in serious cardiovascular complications (or serious adverse events generally) among those who took the COX-2 drug. What if this fact had been emphasized and disseminated back in 2000, when the data first became known, instead of in 2004, when Vioxx was taken off the market? Extrapolating from a large data set from Kaiser Permanente in California, critics later estimated that during the time that Vioxx was on the market, somewhere between "88,000–140,000 excess cases of serious coronary heart disease probably occurred in the USA."[39]

Neither CLASS nor VIGOR, on careful analysis, turns out to be very useful, as long as one's aim is to understand the scientific truth about the relative advantages and risks of COX-2 drugs in real-life patients. Both studies turned out to be tremendously useful as marketing tools for their respective companies. They appear to illustrate one of the most worrisome trends in today's pharmaceutical industry—the tendency of research to become subverted to the much-better-funded marketing function.[40]

Research that is driven by marketing rather than by scientific aims would seem, in the end, to be low quality research. Even among the industry's most severe critics, few have suggested that the quality of the research conducted by the pharmaceutical companies is generally deficient. In the next chapter, however, we will find reason to question the quality of at least some industry research.

NOTES

1. R. Harris, *The Real Voice* (New York: Macmillan, 1964), 78–79.
2. The Olivieri case was widely discussed both in the popular press and in medical journals. Here I rely especially on a detailed report of the case written by Professors Jon Thompson, Patricia Baird, and Jocelyn Downie under a commission from the Canadian Association of University Teachers (CAUT); J. Thompson, P. Baird, and J. Downie, *The Olivieri Report: The Complete Text of the Report of the Independent Inquiry Commissioned by the Canadian Association of University Teachers* (Toronto: James Lorimer, 2001). Several of the key figures in the case refused to participate in the inquiry, charging that the CAUT was well known to be heavily biased in Olivieri's favor, making it likely that the report was simply a put-up job. Nonetheless I find the report persuasive for several reasons. It is long (540 pages) and thoroughly documented, and contains details not available elsewhere. While the professors were given their charge by CAUT, they proceeded independently of CAUT and in a few instances even criticized CAUT for its previous actions in the case. Similarly, they included criticism of some of Dr. Olivieri's own behavior at the early stages of the case and indicated errors in judgment that compounded her problems.

A later account, considerably more critical of Dr. Olivieri's actions and based partly on interviews unavailable to the CAUT investigators, is M. Shuchman, *The Drug Trial: Nancy Olivieri and the Science Scandal that Rocked the Hospital for Sick Children* (Toronto: Random House Canada, 2005). Unfortunately I only received this volume after this book had reached the final copyediting stage. Shuchman paints Olivieri in a much less flattering light, but her major allegation is that Olivieri was scientifically wrong, and Apotex and Koren were right, about the drug L1. She claims that the Olivieri-Brittenham study relied on non-blinded assessment of technically poor liver biopsy specimens; later studies (including at least one not sponsored by Apotex) using larger samples and better methods found no evidence for fibrosis. Shuchman adds that subsequent clinical experience with L1 in Europe has shown that the drug has definite side effects but that liver toxicity is not a major problem. Dr. Olivieri replied by sending *CMAJ* a detailed list of "inaccuracies and omissions in Shuchman's story" (which they declined to publish), and noting that Dr. Shuchman's husband was coauthor of a 2003 paper with Gideon Koren, one of Olivieri's major foes at the hospital; N. Olivieri, "A Response from Dr. Nancy Olivieri," *CMAJ* 2006, 174:661–62.

3. A minor note in the case is the fact that Dr. Olivieri was conducting two different research trials for Apotex under two separate contracts. Contract #1 contained the confidentiality clause; but the risk of loss of effectiveness of the drug emerged in Research Trial #2. That contract had no confidentiality clause. Therefore Apotex had no contractual right to demand that Dr. Olivieri remain silent (even if such a confidentiality clause is enforceable at all, since it could be argued that the physician's duty to inform research subjects of risks overrides any commercial contract). But neither Dr. Olivieri nor Apotex seems to have noticed this quirk at the time; the fact only received attention when the CAUT inquiry unearthed it several years later.

4. The *Journal of Medical Ethics* devoted its January 2004 issue to a series of papers addressing various aspects of the Olivieri case. For the University of Toronto's defense of the later actions it took to correct problems, see L. E. Ferris, P. A. Singer, and C. D. Naylor, "Better Governance in Academic Health Sciences Centres: Moving beyond the Olivieri/Apotex Affair in Toronto," *J Med Ethics* 2004; 30:25–29.

5. Indeed, her case received some unlooked-for publicity when John le Carré included events adapted from the Olivieri case in his novel, *The Constant Gardener* (New York, Pocket Books, 2001). The later motion picture of the same name omitted most mention of pharmaceutical industry practices.

6. Thompson, et al., *The Olivieri Report*, 396.

7. Thompson et al., *The Olivieri Report*, 401.

8. The two sources for the Betty Dong story are D. Rennie, "Thyroid Storm" [editorial], *JAMA* 1997; 277:1238–43; and R. T. King, "Bitter Pill: How a Drug Firm Paid for University Study, Then Undermined It," *Wall Street Journal*, April 25, 1996:1. See also M. Shuchman, "Consequences of Blowing the Whistle in Medical Research," *Ann Intern Med* 2000; 132:1013–5; D. Zalewski, "Ties That Bind: Do Corporate Dollars Strangle Scientific Research?" *Lingua Franca* 1997; 7 (June–July): 51–59.

9. Rennie, "Thyroid Storm."

10. Zalewski, "Ties That Bind," 56.

11. G. H. Mayor, T. Orlando, and N. M. Kurtz, "Limitations of Levothyroxine Bioequivalence Evaluation: Analysis of an Attempted Study," *Am J Ther* 1995; 2:417–32.

12. King, "Bitter Pill."

13. B. J. Dong, W. W. Hauck, J. G. Gambertoglio, et al., "Bioequivalence of Generic and Brand-Name Levothyroxine Products in the Treatment of Hypothyroidism," *JAMA* 1997; 277:1205–13.

14. C. H. Eckert, "Bioequivalence of Levothyroxine Preparations: Industry Sponsorship and Academic Freedom," *JAMA* 1997; 277:1200–1201; M. K. Spigelman, "Bioequivalence of Levothyroxine Preparations for Treatment of Hypothyroidism," *JAMA* 1997; 277:1199–1200.

15. M. Shuchman, "Consequences of Blowing the Whistle in Medical Research," *Ann Intern Med* 2000; 132:1013–15.

16. J. Abramson, *Overdosed America: The Broken Promise of American Medicine* (New York: HarperCollins, 2004), 258. This was a notably prescient statement as it was written some time before Vioxx was pulled from the market.

17. C. Dai, R. S. Stafford, and G. C. Alexander, "National Trends in Cyclooxygenase-2 Inhibitor Use Since Market Release: Nonselective Diffusion of a Selectively Cost-Effective Innovation," *Arch Intern Med* 2005; 165:171–77.

18. B. Meier, "Medicine Fueled by Marketing Intensified Trouble for Pain Pills," *New York Times*, December 19, 2004: 1.

19. Dr. Robert Goodman's "No Free Lunch" website, an activist site dedicated to opposing pharmaceutical industry influence over medicine, offers a tongue-in-cheek "CAGE" questionnaire (modeled after the questionnaire of the same name used as a quick screen to detect alcohol abuse) to determine whether the physician is "drug company dependent." The "C" item on the questionnaire is: "Have you ever prescribed Celebrex?" www.nofreelunch.org (accessed February 5, 2005).

20. B. M. Spiegel, L. Targownik, G. S. Dulai, and I. M. Gralnek, "The Cost-Effectiveness of Cyclooxygenase-2 Selective Inhibitors in the Management of Chronic Arthritis," *Ann Intern Med* 2003; 138:795–806.

21. Because of all the publicity Vioxx received in the fall of 2004 when it was removed from the market, it is important to note that scientific studies showing a possible risk to heart disease and stroke had been appearing in the literature for several years prior to that date. Examples include: D. Mukherjee, S. E. Nissen, and E. J. Topol, "Risk of Cardiovascular Events Associated with Selective COX-2 Inhibitors," *JAMA* 2001; 286:954–59; E. Wooltorton, "What's All the Fuss? Safety Concerns about COX-2 Inhibitors Rofecoxib (Vioxx) and Celecoxib (Celebrex)," *CMAJ* 2002; 166:1692–93; H. K. Choi, J. D. Seeger, and K. M. Kuntz, "Effects of Rofecoxib and Naproxen on Life Expectancy among Patients with Rheumatoid Arthritis: A Decision Analysis," *Am J Med* 2004; 116:621–29.

22. Later, when I tried to contact Dr. Silverstein for more information, I found that his dominant web location was as a senior partner in Frazier Healthcare Ventures, a venture capital firm; www.frazierhealthcare.com/showpage.asp?page=0 (accessed February 5, 2005).

23. F. E. Silverstein, G. Faich, J. L. Goldstein, et al., "Gastrointestinal Toxicity with Celecoxib vs Nonsteroidal Anti-inflammatory Drugs for Osteoarthritis and Rheumatoid Arthritis: The CLASS Study: A Randomized Controlled Trial. Celecoxib Long-term Arthritis Safety Study," *JAMA* 2000; 284:1247–55.

24. D. R. Lichtenstein and M. M. Wolfe, "COX-2-Selective NSAIDs: New and Improved?" [editorial], *JAMA* 2000; 284:1297–99.

25. S. Okie, "Missing Data on Celebrex: Full Study Altered Picture of Drug," *Washington Post*, August 5, 2001:A11.

26. Okie, "Missing Data on Celebrex."

27. C. McLean, "The Real Drug Pushers," *Report Newsmagazine* (Edmonton, Alberta), March 19, 2001. www.report.ca (originally accessed 2003; unable to access in 2005).

28. Okie, "Missing Data on Celebrex." I would have imagined that submitting a manuscript to a journal claiming to have done a six-month study, when one had actually done a twelve-month study, would amount to research fraud, equivalent to falsifying data, and cause the journal to later rescind the publication. I attempted to get from the *JAMA* editors an explanation of why such a decision had not been made in the case of CLASS. I was informed that all such discussions are confidential within the editorial board.

29. J. M. Wright, T. L. Perry, K. L. Bassett, and G. K. Chambers, "Reporting of 6-month vs. 12-month Data in a Clinical Trial of Celecoxib" [letter], *JAMA* 2001; 286:2398–2400; J. B. Hrachovec, and M. Mora, "Reporting of 6-month vs. 12-month Data in a Clinical Trial of Celecoxib" [letter], *JAMA* 2001; 286:2398.

30. F. Silverstein, L. Simon, and G. Faich, "Reporting of 6-month vs 12-month Data in a Clinical Trial of Celecoxib" [authors' reply], *JAMA* 2001; 286:2399–2400.

31. For a somewhat different account of why the last six months of CLASS data were suspect, by a different coauthor, see S. Gottlieb, "Researchers Deny Any Attempt to Mislead the Public over *JAMA* Article on Arthritis Drug," *BMJ* 2001; 323:301.

32. J. M. Wright, "The Double-Edged Sword of COX-2 Selective NSAIDs," *CMAJ* 2002; 167:1131–37.

33. M. Kaufman, "Merck Withdraws Arthritis Medication: Vioxx Maker Cites Users' Health Risks," *Washington Post*, October 1, 2004:A1; A. W. Mathews, "Vioxx Recall Raises Questions about FDA's Safety Monitoring," *Wall Street Journal*, October 4, 2004: B1; E. J. Topol, "Failing the Public Health—Rofecoxib, Merck, and the FDA" [perspective], *N Engl J Med* 2004; 351:1707–79.

34. P. Juni, A. W. Rutjes, and P. A. Dieppe, "Are Selective COX 2 Inhibitors Superior to Traditional Non-steroidal Anti-inflammatory Drugs?" [editorial], *BMJ* 2002; 324:1287–88.

35. C. Bombardier, L. Laine, A. Reicin, et al., "Comparison of Upper Gastrointestinal Toxicity of Rofecoxib and Naproxen in Patients with Rheumatoid Arthritis. VIGOR Study Group," *N Engl J Med* 2000; 343:1520–28.

36. Abramson, *Overdosed America*, 33.

37. Abramson, *Overdosed America*, 35 (italics in original).

38. Abramson, *Overdosed America*: 35. After the manuscript for this book was mostly completed, the *New England Journal of Medicine* made headlines by releasing an editorial "expression of concern"; G. D. Curfman, S. Morrisey, and J. M. Drazen, "Expression of Concern: Bombardier et al., 'Comparison of Upper Gastrointestinal Toxicity of Rofecoxib and Naproxen in Patients with Rheumatoid Arthritis,'" *New England Journal of Medicine* 2005; 353:2813–14. This appeared in print in the December 29 *Journal* but was posted on the web on December 8. The editorial stated that, tipped off by some documents released in the then-pending Vioxx lawsuits, the *Journal* had discovered that the VIGOR authors erased data from the computer disk on three heart attacks that had occurred among patients receiving Vioxx and called on the authors to issue a clarification. This lost data represented a face-saving way for the editors of the *Journal* to disown VIGOR; as Abramson has shown, they had already been exposed as complicit with the VIGOR authors in downplaying the known cardiovascular risks and playing up the largely nonexistent ulcer benefits. By contrast, as of that date, the editors of *JAMA* had never officially expressed any concern about the six months' worth of data "lost" from CLASS.

39. D. J. Graham, D. Campen, R. Hui, et al., "Risk of Acute Myocardial Infarction and Sudden Cardiac Death in Patients Treated with Cyclo-oxygenase 2 Selective and Non-selective Non-steroidal Anti-inflammatory Drugs: Nested Case-control Study," *Lancet* 2005; 365:475–81; quote p. 480.

40. M. Petersen, "Madison Ave. Plays Growing Role in Drug Research," *New York Times*, November 22, 2002:A1.

7

THE QUALITY OF PHARMACEUTICAL RESEARCH

MES HAS DRAFT COMPLETED, WE JUST NEED AN AUTHOR.

> —Memo from Medical Education Systems (MES) of
> Philadelphia, a communications firm, to the drug firm
> Parke, Davis and Co., seeking a purported physician author
> for a ghostwritten paper on off-label uses of Neurontin[1]

SHODDY RESEARCH?

Pharmaceutical industry research, we have seen, raises concerns about its true costs and about the tendency of industry to suppress unfavorable data. A less-commonly-heard criticism of the industry is that it all too often conducts shoddy research, so that the dollars invested by the industry produce much less public benefit than industry rhetoric would suggest. Given the ability of industry to fund research at a level that exceeds that of the NIH, and by implication, to hire the best brains in the business, the charge of shoddiness might sound astounding at first blush. So let us look at some of the historical record as well as at more recent events.

Following the Kefauver Senate hearings and the thalidomide scandal in the early 1960s, new laws (the Kefauver-Harris Amendments) were enacted requiring that companies demonstrate that new drugs were effective as well as safe. There was a retroactive provision—companies now had to prove to FDA panels that drugs that had been introduced between 1938 and 1962 were effective, or else remove the drugs from the market. Silverman and Lee commented on this process in 1974:

> Perhaps most disconcerting were the disclosures that much of the drug company's vaunted research had been shoddy; that much of its well publicized scientific evidence

consisted only of testimonials; that well over half its therapeutic claims were unsupportable; that many industry spokesmen and physicians were content to determine drug efficacy by a popularity vote [that is, companies presented sales data as if those proved that a drug worked]; that many medical journals seemed less anxious to inform physicians than to protect advertisers, and had been publishing supposedly scientific reports that could not withstand the scrutiny of experts; and that thousands of physicians had often been prescribing drugs without adequate proof of their value.[2]

These problems with industry research led FDA Commissioner James Goddard to deliver an unusually harsh speech to the Pharmaceutical Manufacturer's Association in 1966:

I can say I have been shocked at the quality of many submissions to our IND [investigational new drug] staff. The hand of the amateur is evident too often for my comfort. So-called research and so-called studies are submitted by the cartonful and our medical officers are supposed to take all this very seriously. I cannot, however. As their chief I have told them that unprofessional INDs should be cancelled immediately. If the sponsoring company is imprudent enough to waste stockholders' money on low quality work, then that company must bear the consequence of such waste. The Food and Drug Administration will not waste public money reviewing it.[3]

John Abraham, studying commercial bias in scientific research, looked in detail at the approval process for several nonsteroidal anti-inflammatory drugs (NSAIDs) in the 1970s and 1980s. He came upon several examples that call into question not only the presence of bias but also the quality of the basic research. Perhaps the most striking example involved the now commonly used drug Naprosyn. In 1976, Syntex, the drug's manufacturer, was required to test the drug for cancer risks using an animal model. Syntex contracted with another company, IBT Laboratories, to carry out a twenty-two-month study in rats. The FDA scientific auditor who reviewed the IBT data discovered numerous fundamental problems with the study. Some animals appeared to have died multiple times, and other animals were reported to have been weighed alive after their recorded dates of death. The auditor concluded that the study was irreparably flawed.

According to the standard industry rhetoric, that no company would ever engage in shoddy research because it fears to lose its good reputation among scientifically minded physicians, Syntex should immediately have disowned the flawed IBT study and have conducted its own, high-quality carcinogenesis research. Instead, at the FDA hearing held to consider whether Naprosyn should be withdrawn from sale because its safety had not been adequately demonstrated, a Syntex scientific vice president presented a reanalysis of the IBT rat study. He claimed that the errors were simple recording errors, mostly due to misidentifying the rats in adjoining cages, and that it was possible to go back and reconstruct with confidence what the IBT scientists meant to record. The FDA auditors went back to work on this new data analysis and concluded that even if one made all the generous assumptions needed to "reconstruct" the data, things still did not make enough sense to draw any valid conclusions.

If the FDA had followed its own rules at this point, Naprosyn should have been withdrawn from the market. Perhaps leery of withdrawing a drug that had so far show no serious, unanticipated toxic effects in humans, based solely on a flawed study in rats, the FDA instead accepted Syntex's new suggestion that the drug remain on the market while they completed a second carcinogenesis study. (Syntex only admitted to the need for a brand-new study after its "reconstruction" gambit failed.) The new study was of reasonable quality and was negative for any risk of cancer. Hardly anyone remembers this Naprosyn episode, because the drug has been used for years (now being available without a prescription) and no suggestion of any cancer risk has ever arisen in practice. Of course, at the time Naprosyn was undergoing testing as a new drug, no one could be sure that it was low risk.[4]

Another example from the same era suggests that the problems with NSAIDs were not isolated examples. In 1980, Ciba-Geigy was trying to gain approval of the drug sulfinpyrazone (Anturane) for preventing deaths after a heart attack. The Anturane Reinfarction Trial Research Group published its findings in the *New England Journal of Medicine*. The data sounded impressive—sulfinpyrazone cut the death rate by 32 to 74 percent in 1,558 patients followed for sixteen months after their first heart attack.[5] An FDA advisory committee urged quick approval, and physicians were itching to start prescribing the drug. So there was considerable outrage when the FDA refused to approve it.

The FDA's Dr. Robert Temple had noted that some subject deaths were not counted in the final report. The investigators had divided cardiac deaths into three subcategories and had attributed only some subcategories of deaths to the drug. But these subcategories had not been called for in the initial study design. When the FDA staff reanalyzed the data and considered all cardiac deaths, there was no advantage shown in the patients taking sulfinpyrazone compared to those taking a placebo. It now appeared that on first analyzing the data, the investigators found no advantage to their drug, and then proceeded to invent the subcategories as a way of reclassifying deaths to show that the drug worked.[6] FDA historian Philip Hilts commented, "It was never determined whether the errors in the study resulted from mistakes or fraud."[7]

THE INCREASING COMMERCIALIZATION OF RESEARCH

In 1991, the drug industry devoted 80 percent of the money spent on clinical trials to work done in academic medical centers. The companies needed the academic centers for several reasons. They lacked the expertise in-house to design and carry out large clinical trials. The university teaching hospitals promised the patient volume from which to recruit subjects. And the companies wanted the added prestige of having the names of distinguished medical centers and academic investigators on the resulting publications.

By 1998, things had changed markedly. The share of industry dollars going to academic medical centers had fallen to 40 percent.[8] (By 2004, the share had dropped even lower, to 26 percent.[9]) A review in 2002 calculated that as a result of this outsourcing of research, the overall number of physicians involved in clinical research had grown by 600 percent in the previous ten years.[10] It seems fair to assume that the number of physicians who have received intensive training in research methods, or the ethics of research, did not increase by those proportions.

The companies had decided they could get the research done faster outside of academia. The industry estimated in 2000 that for every *day* of delay in getting FDA approval for a new drug, the company loses about $1.3 million.[11]

Academic medical centers have several reasons to be slow in conducting trials. Numerous committees have to review trials, including institutional review boards charged with protecting the rights and safety of research subjects. Investigators are seldom full-time in research; they often have to teach and see patients as well.

Thus, money that used to flow into academic centers now went to contract-research organizations (CROs) and site-management organizations (SMOs). Dr. Thomas Bodenheimer, surveying the scene in 2000, noted that ultimately a large clinical drug trial might involve four layers.[12] At the lowest notch might be a private physician who is paid to recruit patients into the trial and perhaps to gather some rudimentary data. Next up the ladder is an SMO that organizes a network of similar physicians' offices, facilitates recruitment, and delivers patient data to the CRO. The next rung up is the CRO, organizing the entire trial, obtaining human subjects approvals, coordinating the trial protocol and facilitating data collection. Finally at the top is the manufacturer's scientific team, who will eventually analyze the assembled data.

As everything else has moved from the academic medical center into the for-profit world, so too has the institutional review board function. There are now for-profit institutional review boards serving the needs of the CROs and companies. Of course, whether these review boards make a profit and stay in business depends on whether they please their corporate sponsors, who above all else want to move with haste. One might be somewhat skeptical about the thoroughness and diligence of these review boards in discerning possible risks to research subjects, or in demanding a more stringent level of informed consent.

Taking the research function out of the hands of the academic medical center and putting it into this collection of for-profit entities has indeed hastened the research process overall, and tightened the control of the company over the research enterprise—allowing, as we shall see, a much closer relationship between the marketing and the research divisions of the firm. Since each of the new layers of the research enterprise is looking out for its own slice of the profit, this system has arguably increased the cost of research considerably. Dr. Jean-Pierre Bassand and some colleagues with the European Society of Cardiology estimated that while the industry commonly spent five to ten thousand euros per research subject to conduct its clinical trials, these studies could be carried out at academic institutions for five hundred euros.[13]

One could view the shift of research from the academic medical center to the for-profit sector in two ways. From the industry view, the problem is that the universities and their teaching hospitals have simply not kept up with the times. But it might also be argued that the academic way of doing research is slower precisely because there is a greater assurance of quality. To put haste above all other criteria for success in research is virtually a guarantee that one will settle for a lower standard.

Anthropologist Jill A. Fisher studied the process of outsourcing clinical trials in the southwestern United States. She noted the roles of the physician-investigator and the research coordinator, and how the CRO approaches each of them. The physician-investigator is the private practitioner who is supposed to make his or her office a research site; the research coordinator is a staff person, sometimes a nurse but often a person with even less training, who is assigned the day-to-day tasks of recording data and generally ensuring that the research proceeds on track and according to protocol. Fisher found that the message used to "sell" the physicians on research participation was a dual one—they were already fully trained to do research because they had a medical degree, and "any idiot can do it" (therefore any staff person who had time available could take on the research-coordinator position). The message stressed the profits to be made from research participation by understating the work involved.

Typically, the investigators and research coordinators would be invited to a weekend orientation meeting to introduce the research protocol. The physicians would be dismissed on Saturday and the research coordinators would stay through all of Sunday. The end result was that often the physicians had a very shaky idea of what the research was all about and what was required, and they could offer little practical assistance to their coordinators should problems arise. For their part, the coordinators often became extremely committed to the research—no less so because they realized that all the responsibility rested on their shoulders—and devoted extra time and energy to seeing the project through as an act of altruism and in support of the ideal of scientific advancement. In effect, the success or failure of the research protocol rested on what was almost sweatshop labor, as the coordinator might be among the lowest-paid persons in the entire research enterprise, and might receive a very small portion (if any) of the funds that flowed into the practice.[14]

CROs, therefore, may represent a relatively lower standard of research quality. What about the lowest standard of all? If one doesn't like the data produced by a research study, one can simply make up new data. When Braithwaite was researching corporate crime in the pharmaceutical industry in the early 1980s, he found that this practice was so prevalent that it had its own insider phrase: "the practice is called 'making' in the Japanese industry, 'graphiting' or 'dry labelling' in the United States."[15] While one would hope that out-and-out fraud remains rare in industry research, the following two case studies are not exactly reassuring. They highlight the fact that there may be a direct correlation between the increasing commercialization of research, and the temptation to cut corners.

THE STORY OF TWO CROOKED PHYSICIANS

At first blush, Drs. Robert Fiddes and Richard L. Borison would seem to be at the opposite ends of the medical food chain. Fiddes was a local medical practitioner in Whittier, California, with no academic credentials. Borison had a Ph.D. in pharmacology in addition to his M.D. degree, and was chair of the Department of Psychiatry and Health Behavior at the Medical College of Georgia.

But they had at least two things in common. The first was a thirst for a lifestyle somewhat more lavish than the average income in their field would support. Dr.

Fiddes and his wife drove matching BMWs and were planning to build their dream house on the beach in the Cayman Islands. Dr. Borison included authentic suits of armor among his collection of antiques and was planning to build his own castle to house them.

The other thing they had in common was that both ended up serving jail time for the way they accumulated their wealth.

Let's start with Dr. Fiddes. In the 1990s, as drug firms started pulling away from academic medical centers and looking to the private sector to conduct drug studies, Fiddes organized the Southern California Research Institute. Eventually he landed contracts to conduct more than one hundred seventy research studies, earning millions of dollars. For a number of years, neither the drug firms paying for the research nor the government agencies to which the firms submitted the research findings found any reason to question Dr. Fiddes's operation. Then, in June 1996, the office manager of another local clinic told government investigators what she had heard from Research Institute employees and put the investigators in touch with Susan Lester, a former worker for Fiddes. From Lester and the documents she provided, the investigators eventually pieced together a picture of massive fraud. Fictitious patients were enrolled in research trials. Bottles of blood and urine with already-known lab values were kept in the refrigerator, to be substituted for the real samples from patients who did not qualify for the studies. Employees who raised questions were told that this was simply how it was done in the world of pharmaceutical research and that their jobs would be at risk if they complained further.

When Fiddes was finally caught, he blamed everyone but himself, saying that the companies demanded such impossible levels of performance in their research contracts that no one could possibly keep getting their business and do so honestly. But he also claimed that the fraudulent activities had been carried out by his employees without his knowledge. He ended up pleading guilty in 1999 and served a fifteen-month sentence in a Los Angeles detention center.[16]

Now back to Dr. Borison. While studying for his Ph.D. in pharmacology at the University of Health Sciences in Chicago, he became friendly with a fellow student, Bruce I. Diamond. Dr. Borison meanwhile had begun his M.D. studies at the University of Illinois–Chicago, finishing his M.D. in 1977. In 1981 both Borison and Diamond joined the faculty of the Medical College of Georgia in Augusta. They were recruited at least in part because of their outstanding research productivity. By the time Dr. Borison had finished his residency, he had already published eighty-five articles in medical journals, and he and Diamond had collaborated on more than fifty research projects. They continued to do joint research and in 1994 opened a drug-testing site across the street from the medical school in an office park. Diamond and Borison owned a firm called PharmEd Inc. to receive research contracts from drug companies. But the new offices had neither the name "PharmEd" nor "Medical College of Georgia" on the door, which remained unmarked except for "Suite 7." The office used Medical College employees, supplies, and stationery, and the workers there simply assumed it was a branch of the College, though it eventually turned out that the College administration knew nothing about its existence. In addition, although all research conducted by faculty at the College was supposed to be submitted to the school's research ethics review board for approval, Borison and Diamond submitted none of their research protocols to that board. Instead, they sought approval from other ethics boards, including one as far away as Olympia, Washington. Apparently no drug company giving contracts to Borison and Diamond wondered why they were bypassing their local ethics board, even though the companies (as representatives later testified) had been led to believe they were signing contracts with the Medical College of Georgia, not Borison and Diamond's private firm. Nor did the companies become suspicious when they were asked to send checks to the private firm rather than to the College.

Borison and Diamond had one attribute that might have prompted drug companies not to look too hard at any questionable practices. They were superb recruiters of research subjects. Somehow Borison and Diamond managed to get more people enrolled in their studies more quickly than almost any other investigators. With Borison being such a good recruiter, drug firms were loathe to ask rude questions about, for instance, why he had been chastised by the FDA in 1986 for research in which he claimed that brand-name Thorazine acted differently from the generic version of the drug in psychiatric patients. He had claimed that the study had been conducted at the local VA hospital during a time when both the brand-name and the generic drug were available for use. The FDA checked and found that there had been no such time period when both drugs were available.

In 1996, Borison and Diamond, always searching for more recruits for their studies, opened a branch office in Charlotte, North Carolina. The drug company Sandoz at the time had hired a firm, Quintiles Transnational Corporation, to help audit Sandoz's studies of an experimental drug for Alzheimer's disease. John Stokes, a Quintiles inspector, showed up at the Charlotte office and started asking Diamond some questions. He wanted to know in particular how Dr. Borison had managed to sign a number of patient records in Charlotte on a day that he was actually two hundred miles away in Augusta. Diamond called up Stokes's superiors at Quintile to complain, and the next day Stokes was informed that he was off the case.

Finally, Borison and Diamond ran afoul of the same problem that brought down Dr. Fiddes—talkative former employees. One of their staff, Angela Touey, gave up her position as a drug studies coordinator to attend graduate school. A while later, in the fall of 1995, she took a job with a VA hospital neurologist, Dr. David Hess. Hess found that Touey had virtually no idea how to run a proper research study, and moreover, she gave accounts of what had happened at her previous job that were wildly out of line with acceptable practices. Hess eventually pieced together some information about the Borison-Diamond operation and notified VA and school officials.

The investigation then set in motion found that back in 1988, Borison and Diamond had begun their career in fraud by entering into a contract to do a study and asking the firm to pay the money into their own company, PharmEd, instead of to the Medical College. Later, when the two opened their office across the street, Diamond (who had no medical degree) routinely signed prescriptions for and forged the name of Dr. Borison on patient records and other documents, and employees without proper training were routinely interpreting lab tests and electrocardiograms. It was charged that one reason why the two did such a great job of recruiting was that they routinely falsified test results to make subjects appear eligible for studies when they were not. In the Sandoz study of the Alzheimer's drug, for instance, the protocol stated that the drug would be tested only in patients with moderate or mild disease; but patients with severe disease had their test results fudged to allow them to enroll.

Diamond and Borison resigned their positions at the College in early June 1996, a week after the administration started asking them questions about Dr. Hess's charges. That same month, they moved $3.41 million in assets out of a Georgia bank to a bank in South Carolina. In December 1997, Diamond started to negotiate a plea bargain in which he agreed to testify against Borison and to receive a five-year sentence, a $125,000 fine, and a ban from any future work in medical research. Dr. Borison was to stand trial in September, 1998 but abruptly decided to plead guilty and also received a five-year sentence.[17]

UPDATING THE RECORD

Are these historical examples of poor-quality industry research simply yesterday's news? Evidence that this is not the case comes from a 2003 report from the Office of the Inspector General (OIG) of the Department of Health and Human Services, on the FDA's performance in approving new drug applications from industry. The OIG report basically concluded that the FDA needed additional staff to be able to keep up with the desired pace of review. In passing, however, the OIG report noted that many company submissions have to be sent back because of problems with the data analyses and presentations.

Critics of the FDA commonly call attention to the "revolving door" by which former FDA staff end up employed by the pharmaceutical industry. The industry gains its own in-house window into the workings of the FDA and how best to massage the drug approval process to the company's advantage. If the industry employs the best scientists, and also has insider knowledge of FDA procedures, one would think they could get things right the first time when they prepare scientific data as part of a new drug application. The problem, according to the OIG, was not that the FDA arbitrarily changed the rules all the time; the rules were standard and easily discoverable in advance. So the OIG of DHHS is on record as recently as 2003 claiming that a good deal of the research that emanates from the pharmaceutical industry is subpar for purposes of FDA review.

Still, allegations of poor-quality research by private companies must not be blown out of proportion. Recent reviews of both clinical and basic-science studies published in respected journals have shown a significant problem in quality. If you develop a grading system that lists all the ingredients that ought to be found in a top-quality scientific research study, hardly any of these papers gets a score of 100 percent and the average study ends up scoring no better than 50 or 60 percent.[18] The bottom line, it appears, is that careful science is very hard to do and a good result depends on luck as well as on skill. So if company research falls below ideal quality standards, that might not distinguish industry research from research done in universities and government labs. However, given the inflated industry rhetoric, concerns over quality of research are still worth pointing out. And the problem is not merely that research falls below a defined standard of quality. The deeper problem is the strong financial incentive to ignore the poor quality so long as the result favors the industry's drug. (By contrast, as we saw in the previous chapter, the industry will viciously attack a well-designed and well-run study if the outcomes show its drug in a bad light.)

RESEARCH AS MARKETING

Another way to reduce quality is to forget that one is doing scientific research and to imagine that one is doing something else instead. When the average pharmaceutical company spends about 25 percent of its revenues on marketing and only about half of that on research, it is easy for the marketing division to imagine that the research division is merely one of its branch offices. When the goals of marketing take over from the goals of proper scientific research, the result is shoddy from a scientific point of view and shoddy from the point of view of a medical profession that relies on accurate, dispassionate data to know how best to treat patients. The 1980 Anturane trial is a good example. The result is far from shoddy from the point of view of the marketers (though the 1980 Anturane trial backfired from a marketing point of view as well, since the FDA failed to approve the drug for sale).

Subsuming research under marketing could represent a gradual, unintended drift, or it could be deliberate company policy. Some recent evidence suggests that incorporating the marketing agenda into research from the beginning is a growing trend in the industry.[19]

Good science requires what is commonly called the "honest null hypothesis." A high-quality research study is designed to be as likely to confirm the hypothesis that the investigators do *not* believe to be true, as it is to confirm the hypothesis that the investigators happen to favor. A good research study starts with the balance pan weighted equally between the two outcomes. A shoddy research trial starts with the scientist's thumb on one pan of the scale. If you view research as simply a different form of marketing, it seems no more than prudent to design the trial so as to be as certain as possible that the results will help "sell" the drug.

Drs. Lisa Bero and Drummond Rennie, in one paper, and Daniel Safer in another, have provided extensive analyses of the various ways that research can be bent to meet marketing goals.[20] Safer focuses on his own field of psychopharmacology, but comparable examples could be found from other areas of medicine. Combining these two papers yields the following list of ways to conduct a clinical trial to meet the needs of industry marketing. Some of these have to do with research publication rather than the actual conduct of the research, but these authors argue that the research process should be seen as including the publication of results as well as the gathering and analyzing of data.

1. *Asking too narrow a question*: Research is supposed to be *clinical* research and answer questions that would help guide therapy. A study that asks what effect an antidepressant has on the electrocardiogram, but not whether the

patients actually suffer any ill effects, is an example of a research question that is more or less irrelevant, but which can be used by marketers to create the impression that one drug is safer than its competitor. This problem is called "surrogate endpoints." The endpoint of real interest in our example is whether a drug has a positive or negative effect on the patient's heart in a way that affects either length or quality of life, such as causing more heart attacks. What the drug does to the electrocardiogram tracing may or may not be related to this real endpoint; often only a further research study would answer that question. Since it is almost always cheaper and quicker to do a study of surrogate endpoints instead of real ones, this strategy is very tempting for the industry.

2. *Playing tricks with randomization*: A randomized controlled study is considered the gold standard for most studies involving drugs. Bero and Rennie report numerous instances of studies that claimed to be randomized trials that either were not when one read the fine print or that included no information on what method of randomization the authors used. One study was titled, "Preliminary Results of a Controlled, Randomized, Regimen-Comparative Trial," and presented data from only one patient.

3. *Inappropriate dosing*: This is one of the oldest ploys, and it may be becoming less common simply because more people know to look out for it; yet Safer was still able to cite numerous recent examples. If you want to show that your drug works better than your competitor's, you simply give the research subjects a low dose of the competitor's drug and the full dose of your own. On the other hand, if you want to prove that the competitor's drug has more side effects than your product, conduct a study in which a very low dose of your own drug is compared to the full dose of the competition. (This is how Schering-Plough went about proving that Claritin was nonsedating.)

4. *Inappropriate comparisons*: Bero and Rennie mention studies that compare the manufacturer's drug with a placebo and then go on to claim that the study proves that the drug is superior to a drug made by a competitor. Only a study that directly compared the two drugs could properly draw that conclusion.

5. *Lack of blinding*: A randomized study, to be properly unbiased, should be "double-blind"—neither the subjects nor the investigators should know who is getting which treatment at the time that measurements are being made. Many studies claim to be double-blind but fail to specify just what method was used to insure blinding, and even more studies fail to test to see whether they were actually successful in maintaining the blind. (For example, if a drug with frequent and obvious side effects is tested against placebo, it may be very easy for the majority of subjects to detect whether they are getting the drug or the placebo.)

6. *Invent your own scale*: Studies often report data in the form of scores on symptom scales. Creative scientists can invent special scales for their studies that artificially highlight the good points of the study drug and obscure its less favorable features. Safer reported that using such special scales, several groups were able to demonstrate that one antipsychotic drug was essentially free of Parkinson's-like side effects, whereas using any of the more standard, widely used research scales revealed that this drug regularly produced such side effects.

7. *First shoot the arrow, then draw the target*: The practice of first gathering the data, then looking back to see what turned out to be favorable for one's drug, is called "data dredging." In a proper research study one specifies in advance what results one is going to look for. In a poor study, one might, for instance, have set out to show that depressed patients treated with your new drug are significantly less depressed after twelve weeks. You do the study and find that at twelve weeks, your patients are no different from those getting the other drug. But you go back and sift through the data and find that at eight weeks, patients on your drug had slightly better quality of sleep. So you report your data as proving that your drug produces better quality sleep in depressed patients after eight weeks of treatment, as if that is what you intended to study from the beginning. Data dredging is frowned upon by serious scientists because it is highly likely to uncover associations that occur purely at random. The Anturane reinfarction trial was a classic example of data dredging.

8. *Don't ask, don't tell*: Sometimes you have to ask very detailed questions to elicit all the side effects produced by a drug—especially if the side effect is embarrassing, such as diminished sexual function. Safer recounts how many studies make antidepressants (for instance) sound as if they produce very few side effects simply because the questions avoid any detailed probing.

9. *Protocol violations and poor record keeping*: Summers and colleagues published a paper purporting to be a randomized, controlled trial of the drug tacrine, showing that the drug was effective in treating Alzheimer's dementia. Despite the fact that the paper appeared in the prestigious *New England Journal of Medicine*, an FDA audit later showed that the authors had violated their own protocol in so many ways that the study was not a randomized trial at all but in fact a series of uncontrolled anecdotes.[21] Moreover, the record keeping was so poor that the auditors could not tell which patient had been on which drug during different parts of the study.

10. *If you get good results, publish and publish again*: The literature is full of data that seem to represent several different trials, which on further investigation turn out to be the same study published in four or five different places. Journal editors try hard to weed out any duplicate publication, but persistent folks who know the ropes can evade detection. The company naturally figures that if you see that five "different" studies all say their drug is great, you are more likely to believe it.

11. *Sales pitch in the article's abstract*: The abstract of a scientific paper is supposed to be a summary of the key points of the research study, not an advertisement for a product. Writers of industry-sponsored papers commonly violate this guideline, knowing that the vast majority of physicians (if they bother to read anything at all) will read the abstract and skip most or all of the full article. The abstract therefore may highlight all the good news about the drug and conveniently leave out any undesirable findings; or the abstract may include gratuitous advice to use the drug as one's first choice in treating certain patients. Bero and Rennie noted some examples of conclusions stated in the text of the article that were not supported by the actual data. Gøtzsche reported that among 196 published trials on NSAIDs, fully 42 percent contained doubtful or invalid conclusions.[22] Studies

reported in drug-company-sponsored journal symposia—which we will discuss in a later chapter on medical journals—are especially likely to contain unsupported conclusions.

12. *Lying with statistics*: Safer found many instances of playing fast and loose with statistical analyses. It is quite common for industry-sponsored research to report its results using whatever numbers make the difference between your drug and the competitor's drug seem most dramatic, even if that way of reporting the numbers is misleading. One example is reporting insignificant differences in the form of relative risks without giving the confidence intervals. Suppose that you state that your drug has a relative risk of 0.81, compared to another drug, of producing a certain side effect. You fail to report, however, that the confidence interval is 0.66–1.12. This might easily occur with a small number of research subjects, and shows that the difference between the two drugs could easily have occurred by chance alone, as the confidence interval includes the number one. You have reported a statistically insignificant result in such a way as to imply that your drug is clearly superior to the competition.

13. *Refuse to publish unfavorable results*: In the absence of a mandatory trials registry, drug companies are required to notify no one that they have begun a trial, so if they don't like the results, that trial can simply disappear off the face of the earth. This provides an additional incentive for companies to try to force investigators to suppress scientifically valid data that showed the company's product in an unfavorable light.

14. *Hide company sponsorship*: Many physicians are starting to get the message that research conducted by drug firms may be biased in favor of the company's drugs. Numerous reviews have shown that the likelihood of an industry-sponsored study showing the superiority of the drug in question is substantially greater than in studies paid for by neutral sources.[23] It may therefore be of strategic value to hide the company sponsorship of certain trials. This is especially easy to do in large multicenter trials that are conducted simultaneously at many different medical centers. Several intermediaries can be created to administer the study, and the source of the actual funds may effectively be concealed from those reading the eventual publication.

While many studies have shown that research publications funded by industry are much more likely to favor the sponsor's product than research funded by nonprofit sources, it has not always been clear why this happens. Als-Nielsen and colleagues attempted to answer this question by carefully reviewing 370 randomized drug trials selected for inclusion in meta-analyses by the international Cochrane Collaboration. A number of measures of the general quality of the research did not distinguish between for-profit and nonprofit sponsorship, and the actual drug effect size did not differ substantially. (Equal quality is not surprising as the Cochrane Collaboration has strict guidelines for including or excluding research trials from their reviews based on the quality of the study.) The major difference they found was simply how the authors "spun" the conclusions (#11 on the list above). That is, regardless of what the data showed, the authors wrote at the end of the article that the company's drug was clearly the drug of choice for the disease in question. Als-Nielsen and colleagues concluded that the reader of journal articles could eliminate most of the bias in these studies simply by reading a paper carefully and asking whether the hard numbers actually supported the conclusions.[24] Unfortunately, that assumes two things—first, that busy medical practitioners have the time to read the literature that way, and second, that all the studies conducted by drug companies, the reprints of which are passed out to practitioners by detail people, are equal in quality to the "elite" studies selected by the Cochrane Collaboration for inclusion in their systematic reviews.

Finally, there are more subtle ways that marketing may influence research. Psychiatrist and historian David Healy claims that there is no "scientific" reason that the SSRI drugs like Prozac, Zoloft, and Paxil should be viewed as antidepressants rather than as antianxiety or tranquilizer drugs. The symptoms that they are used for treating could equally be classified as depression or as anxiety. As these drugs came into more widespread use in the United States and Britain, the number of diagnoses of anxiety disorders went way down and the number of diagnoses of depression went way up—a phenomenon not seen in other parts of the world where the sales of these drugs had never taken off. Depression is supposed to place patients at much higher risk for suicide, but there is no evidence that the suicide rate went down in response to the widespread prescription of these agents. Finally, Dr. Healy asserts that there is precious little evidence that the serotonin system has anything much to do with either anxiety or depression.

The reason these drugs are "antidepressants," Dr. Healy claims, is simple. The first drug to act primarily on the serotonin system, buspirone, was marketed in the late 1980s as a nonaddicting tranquillizer—and it flopped. Physicians had been too well programmed by the publicity over the benzodiazepines like Valium and Librium—they knew that tranquillizers could be habit-forming while antidepressants were not thought to be habit-forming. So the message to the industry was simple. Tell physicians that these new drugs are antidepressants; and then reeducate them to believe that what they used to call anxiety is now depression. It worked so well that the public became reeducated too, and now average people on the street talk with each other about whether or not they have enough serotonin activity in their brains. Dr. Healy added:

> By 1996, the World Health Organization had reported that depression was the second greatest source of disability on the planet. The response from psychiatry to this news appeared to be satisfaction that the discipline was now the second most important in medicine after cardiology. Nobody seemed to question how a society could have become so depressed so fast. Depression was now being touted as a serious illness; but the emergence of a comparable epidemic of any other serious illness on this scale would have led to serious questioning as to what had happened. There appeared to be no such questioning in the case of depression.[25]

In such a fashion an entire medical specialty meekly handed over to industry the right to define the very nature of its practice—as well as the right to decide which risks of SSRIs, such as suicidal behavior, would ever see the light of day.

GHOSTWRITING

Bero and Rennie, and Safer, argued that the process of publishing research results, and the integrity of that process, was part of the overall research endeavor. It is therefore pertinent to look at an especially egregious ethical violation—the ghostwriting of research publications.

Some Ghostwriting Stories

Dr. David Healy, the psychiatrist at the University of Wales, was invited in 1999 to speak at a medical conference in London about the drug milnacipran. The panel would be sponsored by Pierre-Fabre, the manufacturer. The plan called for the papers of the panelists later to appear in a company-sponsored supplement to the *International Journal of Psychiatry in Clinical Practice*. Healy agreed and planned to begin work on the paper. He was then surprised to receive an e-mail from Mike Briley, Pierre-Fabre's scientific director of worldwide operations, that read in part: "In order to reduced [*sic*] your workload, we have had our ghostwriters produce a first draft based on your published work. I enclose it here as an attachement [*sic*] (it is in Word 6 format and ASCII format). We would be grateful if you could read through it and make whatever corrections you consider appropriate."

Dr. Healy read through the paper and noted that the anonymous writer had indeed done a pretty good job of capturing his writing style and the general thrust of his work. Still, he took exception to the paper's glowing praise for the drug: "Newer antidepressants such as milnacipran . . . provide therapeutic benefit for a wide range of patients and may off [*sic*] advantages over selective agents." He e-mailed back to Briley that he thought that the article could be improved and set out to prepare his own draft. Briley welcomed the changes, but told Healy to hurry up as their deadline was quickly approaching.

When Dr. Healy sent in his own first draft, Briley e-mailed back, "[I]t was a pity to try to modify it since it reads so well. On the other hand we need to bring across one or two points that are not accentuated in your M/S. We have therefore decided to publish [Healy's draft] as it is in the supplement (I'm e-mailing it to the publishers today) but also to publish the other manuscript. Siegried [*sic*] Kasper has kindly offered to author this one. We would however like your talk to be more on the first [ghostwritten] manuscript . . . in order to bring out the main commercially important points."

Dr. Healy appeared at the panel and gave the paper that he had written himself. He then had the pleasure of hearing his colleague, Siegfried Kasper of the University of Vienna, get up and read the same ghostwritten draft that Briley had originally sent to Healy. The ghostwritten paper, with Dr. Kasper's name as author and no indication of any company role in the writing of the paper, eventually appeared in the journal supplement along with the paper Dr. Healy had written.[26]

Dr. Healy later wrote that he became curious about industry claims that the putative academic authors of the papers always had the right to edit a company-prepared manuscript as they saw fit. When asked to be the purported author of a paper ghostwritten for him, to be delivered at a 2001 conference, he inserted two changes, both of which revealed blemishes on the company's drug, in this case the antidepressant venlafaxine (Effexor). Dr. Healy next saw the paper when it had already been sent to the journal; both of the changes he had inserted had been omitted. He then demanded that his name be removed, which was done.[27]

Most people involved with the ghostwriting of medical-journal articles are not as eager as Dr. Healy to seek publicity for this practice. CBC News reporter Erica Johnson was able to identify several Canadian ghostwriters, as well as a number of physicians who had signed their names to the articles. None of the physicians would agree to comment on the record, and most ghostwriters refused to talk, but one writer agreed to be interviewed as long as his or her identity would remain a secret. So Johnson told us the story of "Blair Snitch," who makes $100,000 a year working for a medical writing company. He is told what studies to include in the article and knows that his job is to make the drug look good—fail at that, and cross off that company's future business. The pay is based on the quality of the journal that eventually prints the paper. Get the paper into the *New England Journal*, the *Lancet*, or similar high-visibility journals, and the fee is $20,000. The acceptance, of course, is based on tricking the journal editor into thinking that the distinguished academic physician who signs his or her name to the paper was the actual author. "Doctors don't have time to write those articles," Blair Snitch explains. "The people who have their names on those articles are very busy professionals."

Blair Snitch admitted that he was concerned about what he was doing—the patient might get a drug due to spin and not due to science. But he eventually made peace with his six-figure income: "As long as I do my job well, it's not up to me to decide how the drug is positioned. I'm just following the information I'm being given. . . . The way I look at it, if doctors . . . have their name on it, that's their responsibility, not mine."[28] Other sources have noted that the average reimbursement for the "author" who allows his name to be placed on the final article, and who has done little, if any, work on the actual writing, is about a thousand dollars.[29]

Ghostwriting Then and Now

Ghostwriting, like many problematic practices at the profession-industry interface, appears to have a venerable history. Instances have been recorded as far back as the early 1960s, and the practice is probably much older than that.[30] How extensive is ghostwriting today? For obvious reasons there are no hard data. Flanagin and colleagues surveyed articles published in three major U.S. medical journals in 1996 and detected evidence of ghostwriting in 11 percent.[31] David Healy describes in some detail the example of a firm called Current Medical Directions (CMD) of New York. In 1998, CMD, working for Pfizer, coordinated eighty-seven articles on the blockbuster antidepressant, Zoloft (sertraline). By early 2001, fifty-five of these articles had been published, in journals including the *New England Journal of Medicine*, *JAMA*, *Archives of General Psychiatry*, and the *American Journal of Psychiatry*. "Based on contact with the authors and other sources, my judgment is that in only 5 cases were the authors likely to have the raw data from the studies they reported on."[32] Most of the eighty-seven articles appeared to have originated at CMD, and authors were listed as "TBD" (to be determined). Healy

calculated that authors whose names appeared on CMD articles on average published three times as many articles as non-CMD authors, and CMD articles have a
three-times higher rate of being cited in other scientific publications.[33] "Based on
this it seems safe to say that by the turn of the century, around 50 percent of the
'scientific' literature in pharmacotherapeutics was ghost-written, originated within
companies, or was published in non-peer-reviewed supplements to journals."[34]

One might object: what is the big concern about ghostwriting? We have already
seen how the industry, simply by sponsoring the research, is generally able to secure a published paper that speaks positively about the drug under study. If the
paper written inside the company headquarters (or at a contract medical-writing
firm) by a ghostwriter, and a paper written by a scientist who has close financial
ties to the company, are equally likely to praise the drug, then who cares who actually wrote the paper?

We should worry about the basic integrity of the medical profession and what
happens when it becomes common practice for physicians to claim that they wrote
papers that they did not write. And we should worry about the integrity of medical
journals and whether we are entitled to take at face value anything we read there
(including something as basic as who wrote the paper). It should give us pause
when a former employee of a medical-writing firm describes the practices of carefully cleaning computer files to try to remove all traces of ghostwriting before the
article is sent by the reputed "author" to a medical journal.[35]

We should also worry about the impact of ghostwriting on the bias of published
papers. As a rule, the person who writes the first draft of an article exercises considerable control. A scientific paper is not simply a recitation of the facts revealed
by a particular research trial. It takes the form, "Here are the facts, and because
these facts are true, it follows that certain conclusions are probably true also."
What conclusions the facts support, and how the facts are ordered and organized
to reach the conclusion, are usually set by the writer of the first draft. A later editing job can change the choice of words and add or take away emphasis from certain conclusions. But it is very hard by a later editing to change the entire thrust of
the paper.

Let's imagine that one can do a lot to change the extent to which a paper favors
the drug, simply by editing carefully an already-prepared draft. The question still
remains—*will* the academic "author" engage in that careful editing? The same
rationalization that defends ghostwriting in the first place argues that no such careful editing is likely to occur. If the prestigious scientist is too busy to write the paper on his own, he presumably will also be too busy to do a careful job of editing.
He is likely to save time here for the same reasons he saved time before—those
nice people at the drug company always have treated him well in the past, and so
far he has never gotten into trouble over any other paper he has signed his name
to, so why not simply sign off after a cursory read and trust them to have done a
good job? David Healy puts it as follows:

> The usual company line in these instances is that, even when articles are ghost-writ-
> ten, their notional authors check them closely and sign off on them. As Bert Spilker of
> the Pharmaceutical Research and Manufacturers of America put it when the issue was

raised in the *Washington Post*, "Academic researchers participating in studies 'are given every opportunity to review, make suggestions, and sign off on manuscripts [and] except for some very, very rare exceptions . . . [the process] is working very well.'" In practice, as shown in the litigation surrounding Redux, senior figures are prepared to incorporate any changes suggested to them by companies or agencies and to sign off on articles without suggesting a single change of their own.[36]

Healy argues that the process has become so insidious that top-flight scientists now express surprise on hearing that some of their colleagues still write their own papers.[37] This sort of system leads to an unfortunate class division within medical science: the elite scientists, who enjoy all the perks of working closely with the drug industry, including having their papers ghostwritten for them by the best writers available, and the grunt scientists, who have to write their own papers and wait at the end of the line for the journal to accept or reject them. The elite status is emphasized by the other association Healy noted, that the "authors" of the ghostwritten articles tended to publish more papers and to have their articles cited more often in other scientific articles.[38] The message for the grunts is clear: if you want to become an elite scientist, you need to start emulating those of your peers who play the industry game by industry rules, and to start doing so as early as possible in your career.

Healy has pointed out a further deleterious effect of this system. As he puts it, ghostwriting tends to produce ghost scientists:

The other side of this coin is that many of the most senior figures in the field are becoming "ghost" scientists: an ever-larger part of their work is not theirs in any meaningful sense of the word. These academics become opinion leaders in a therapeutics field because they appear to have their names on a larger proportion of the literature in the most prestigious journals than do others and because they get asked to international meetings to present this data. . . . And the culmination of this change could be that the dominant figures in therapeutics will soon have comparatively little first-hand research experience and little raw data that they can share with others.[39]

Healy points to his own research on the SSRI antidepressant drugs to show why this "ghost" status matters. It is Healy's claim, well documented in his book *Let Them Eat Prozac*, that these drugs have a rare but very serious side effect called akathisia. Akathisia tends to occur very early in the treatment of depression with SSRIs and is characterized by a severe agitation and distortion of reality. It is in a state of akathisia that a number of people taking SSRIs have committed suicide or homicide. The pharmaceutical companies making SSRIs have tended to dismiss akathisia and have claimed that these patients committed suicide because of their underlying depression, and not due to any side effect of the drugs. Healy has shown that the checklist instruments used in many of the studies of SSRI side effects don't have any categories for akathisia symptoms, and so those research studies were bound to miss akathisia even if it occurred among those subjects.

Healy's argument is that if a "real" physician-scientist were conducting studies of SSRIs, she would make sure that she was personally involved in at least some of the interactions with the research subjects and would directly query them about their experiences while taking the medication. In the process she might well pick up on the fact that a few of them were experiencing a side effect not specifically coded for in the study instrument. By contrast, the "ghost" scientist, whose time is presumably too valuable for the day-to-day tasks of gathering raw data from research subjects, would delegate all contact with the patients to the research technicians, and would only see summaries of the data later on—if he even saw that much, as opposed to simply letting the statisticians at the drug company analyze the data for him.[40] This "ghost" scientist would never be in a position to notice a flaw in the instruments that were being used in the study. Healy points out that the present system of rewarding the so-called elite scientists is creating an ever-larger class of these "ghosts," and worse yet, is putting them on a pedestal as if they represent the cream of the scientific crop. The new system further ensures that the elite scientist will never have a new idea about a drug that was not directly fed to him by company employees.

Healy adds that a major problem here is the replacement of smaller trials, in which the investigator can have personal contact with most or all of the research subjects, with huge, dispersed multicenter trials in which any local investigator may see only a few of the subjects. The smaller trial setting better allows the thoughtful investigator to observe an unexpected effect of the drug, whether positive or negative. To the objection that these huge trials are needed to recruit sufficient numbers of subjects, Healy retorts that industry needs large numbers to show the superiority of their new drugs, only because the new drugs are very little better (if at all) than the older drugs. If the industry truly had new drugs that lived up to their hype, and were head and shoulders above all existing drugs, a small study would be ample to prove their benefit.[41]

At least some people within the industry itself believe that the ghostwriting problem has gotten out of hand. A proposed code of "good publication practice" for the industry, published in 2003, defends the use of paid medical writers, arguing that they can help with the timeliness and the quality of publications and help to coordinate the writing of papers for multicenter research studies where no single academic investigator has firsthand awareness of what is going on at each center at which the research is being conducted. However, the guidelines would require that the writer consult closely with the scientists before writing a first draft, be in regular touch with the other authors during each stage of editing, provide all other authors with adequate time to comment and edit, and (most importantly) be openly acknowledged in the final publication.[42] It is too early to know if these guidelines will be adopted by any pharmaceutical companies and if so, whether they will actually be enforced.[43]

In this and the previous several chapters, we have learned a number of things. We have seen that there are a number of disconnects between the rosy picture the pharmaceutical industry paints of itself as the discoverer of new medical breakthroughs and the actual amounts spent on research; the relationship between research funding and high profits; and the scientific quality, validity, and integrity of at least some of the research that is conducted. We have seen reasons to worry that the huge sums of money that hinge on the results of scientific studies create an irresistible temptation for those in power to manipulate the study results.

Moreover, we have, along the way, seen evidence to show that these problems are not new. Had anyone been interested in looking, evidence of the problems could have been found decades ago. It should not have taken Vioxx, or adolescents becoming suicidal while taking antidepressants, to suddenly cause us to wake up to these matters.

The next major area we need to explore is the marketing activity of the industry, or what, still as part of the rosy picture, the companies prefer whenever possible to call "education." Once again, if we look at the record, we can see that the patterns of today actually have a long and venerable history.

NOTES

1. L. Kowalczyk, "Drug Company Push on Doctors Disclosed," *Boston Globe*, May 19, 2002:A1. The memo was revealed as a result of lawsuits against the company for fraudulent marketing of the drug for off-label (unapproved by FDA) uses.

2. M. Silverman and P. R. Lee, *Pills, Profits and Politics* (Berkeley: University of California Press, 1974), 132.

3. P. J. Hilts, *Protecting America's Health: The FDA, Business, and One Hundred Years of Regulation* (New York: Knopf, 2003), 168.

4. J. Abraham, *Science, Politics, and the Pharmaceutical Industry: Controversy and Bias in Drug Regulation* (London: UCL Press, 1995), 93–96. Later, when Pfizer submitted evidence to the FDA to defend its NSAID, Feldene, from accusations from Public Citizen's Health Research Group, John Harter, head of the NSAID group at the FDA, summarized his impressions of the Pfizer scientists' work: "The clinical trial data submitted [by Pfizer] . . . is so poorly presented and analyzed that it is virtually worthless to assist us . . . I am disappointed that Pfizer after a year and a half of working on these studies has come up with such a pitiful effort"; Abraham, *Science, Politics and the Pharmaceutical Industry*, 200.

5. Anturane Reinfarction Trial Study Group, "Sulfinpyrazone in the Prevention of Sudden Death after Myocardial Infarction," *N Engl J Med* 1980; 302:250–56.

6. Hilts, *Protecting America's Health*, 226–27; R. J. Temple and G. W. Pledger, "The FDA's Critique of the Anturane Reinfarction Trial," *N Engl J Med* 1980; 303:1488–92; Anturane Reinfarction Trial Policy Committee, "The Anturane Reinfarction Trial: Reevaluation of Outcome," *N Engl J Med* 1982; 306:1005–8.

7. Hilts, *Protecting America's Health*, 227.

8. T. Bodenheimer, "Uneasy Alliance—Clinical Investigators and the Pharmaceutical Industry," *N Engl J Med* 2000; 342:1539–44.

9. R. Steinbrook, "Gag Clauses in Clinical-Trial Agreements," *N Engl J Med* 2005; 352:2160–62.

10. K. Morin, H. Rakatansky, F. A. Riddick Jr., et al., "Managing Conflicts of Interest in the Conduct of Clinical Trials," *JAMA* 2002; 287:78–84.

11. Bodenheimer, "Uneasy Alliance"; see also R. A. Rettig, "The Industrialization of Clinical Research," *Health Aff (Millwood)* 2000; 19:129–46.

12. Bodenheimer, "Uneasy Alliance."

13. J.-P. Bassand, J. Martin, L. Ryden, and M. Simoons, "The Need for Resources for Clinical Research: The European Society of Cardiology Calls for European, International Collaboration," *Lancet* 2002; 360:1866–69. But see also E. J. Emanuel, L. E. Schnipper, D. Y. Kamin, J. Levinson, and A. S. Lichter, "The Costs of Conducting Clinical Research," *J Clin Oncol* 2003; 21:4145–50, claiming that current industry research costs are generally justified.

14. J. A. Fisher, "Pharmaceutical Paternalism and the Privatization of Clinical Trials" (unpublished doctoral dissertation, Rensselaer Polytechnic Institute, 2005).

15. J. Braithwaite, *Corporate Crime in the Pharmaceutical Industry* (Boston: Routledge & Kegan Paul, 1984), 57.

16. K. Eichenwald and G. Kolata, "A Doctor's Drug Studies Turn into Fraud," *New York Times*, May 17, 1999:1.

17. S. Stecklow and L. Johannes, "Drug Makers Relied on Clinical Researchers Who Now Await Trial," *Wall Street Journal*, August 15, 1997:A1; "Borison, the Con Man" [editorial], *Augusta* (GA) *Chronicle*, October 10, 1998.

18. To give just one example, in a systematic review of 308 Phase II trials of cancer therapy published in 1997, 96 percent lacked a control group and 80 percent lacked any discussion of the statistical methods employed; L. Mariani and E. Marubini, "Content and Quality of Currently Published Phase II Cancer Trials," *J Clin Oncol* 2000; 18:429–36.

19. M. Petersen, "Madison Ave. Plays Growing Role in Drug Research," *New York Times*, November 22, 2002:A1.

20. L. A. Bero and D. Rennie, "Influences on the Quality of Published Drug Studies," *Int J Technol Assess Health Care* 1996; 12:209–37; D. J. Safer, "Design and Reporting Modifications in Industry-Sponsored Comparative Psychopharmacology Trials," *J Nerv Ment Dis* 2002; 190:583–92. For a shorter but somewhat similar review, see V. M. Montori, R. Jaeschke, H. J. Schunemann, et al., "Users' Guide to Detecting Misleading Claims in Clinical Research Reports," *BMJ* 2004; 329:1093–96.

21. Division of Neuropharmacological Drug Products (FDA), "Tacrine as a Treatment for Alzheimer's Disease" (Editor's note: An interim report from the FDA and a response from Summers et al.), *N Engl J Med* 1991; 324:349–52.

22. P. C. Gøtzsche, "Methodology and Overt and Hidden Bias in Reports of 196 Double-Blind Trials of Nonsteroidal Anti-Inflammatory Drugs in Rheumatoid Arthritis," *Control Clin Trials* 1989; 10:31–56.

23. While numerous studies have supported this conclusion, perhaps the most comprehensive is J. Lexchin, L. A. Bero, B. Djulbegovic, and O. Clark, "Pharmaceutical Industry Sponsorship and Research Outcome and Quality: Systematic Review," *BMJ* 2003; 326:1167–70.

24. B. Als-Nielsen, W. Chen, C. Gluud, and L. L. Kjaergard, "Association of Funding and Conclusions in Randomized Drug Trials: A Reflection of Treatment Effect or Adverse Events?" *JAMA* 2003; 290:921–28.

25. D. Healy, "Shaping the Intimate: Influences on the Experience of Everyday Nerves," *Soc Stud Sci* 2004; 34:219–45; quote p. 224. Incidentally, the notion that antidepressants as a class are not habit-forming obscures growing evidence that one SSRI at least, paroxetine (Paxil), can produce a serious withdrawal syndrome.

26. Dr. Healy obligingly posted the e-mail correspondence, the draft of the ghostwritten paper, and the two published papers on his website, www.healyprozac.com/GhostlyData/default.htm (accessed March 9, 2005). For a similar account of another ghostwritten paper, see R. Rubin, "Medical Editors: One-Sided Drug Reviews Hard to Swallow," *USA Today*, May 31, 2005:5D.

27. Healy, "Shaping the Intimate."

28. E. Johnson, "Medical Ghostwriting," *CBC News-Marketplace*, CBC News, March 25, 2003, www.cbc.ca/consumers/market/files/health/ghostwriting/ (accessed March 9, 2005).

29. Kowalczyk, "Drug Company Push."

30. Two members of the AMA's Council on Pharmacy and Chemistry wrote an article in 1929 decrying the "commercial domination of therapeutics." They mentioned the older practice of throwing drugs together in unscientific combinations and trying the results out

on unsuspecting patients in a series of uncontrolled experiments: "Perhaps the physician might be induced to publish his favorable clinical trials in some medical journal sorely pressed for copy. Such articles, reporting clinical trials, were not uncommonly published over the signature of one connected with the firm who could append the 'M.D.' to his name; such M.D.s could be hired then—and probably now—at no very high salary"; W. A. Puckner and P. Leech, "The Introduction of New Drugs," *JAMA* 1929; 93:1627–30. If this reference is indeed to the practice of ghostwriting, it would seem to have been prevalent well before 1929. N. Rasmussen, "The Drug Industry and Clinical Research in Interwar America: Three Types of Physician Collaborator," *Bull Hist Med* 2005; 79:50–80. Rasmussen went on to say of the research conducted by Philadelphia rhinologist Joseph Scarano in the mid-1930s under the sponsorship of Smith, Kline: "For Smith, Kline it was routine to outline Scarano's protocols in advance, prepare his illustrations, and submit papers to journals for him (presumably after editing by the firm). . . . In print, the only trace of Smith, Kline's hand borne by Scarano's publications . . . was acknowledgment that drugs were supplied by the firm" (67–68). One notable event during the thalidomide tragedy in the early 1960s was the effort to place a ghostwritten paper, reputedly by obstetrician Ray O. Nulsen, in the *American Journal of Obstetrics and Gynecology*; R. Brynner and T. Stephens, *Dark Remedy: The Impact of Thalidomide and Its Revival as a Vital Medicine* (Cambridge, MA: Perseus, 2001), 44–48; Insight Team of *The Sunday Times* of London, *Suffer the Children: The Story of Thalidomide* (New York: Viking, 1979), 84–85. The article insisted that the drug was perfectly safe during pregnancy. The irony is that Nulsen said that he gave premarketing samples of thalidomide to eighty pregnant women in his practice. Later record reviews suggested that he delivered five infants afflicted with phocomelia, the limb deformity caused by thalidomide, but failed to recognize the syndrome. Had he been doing real science instead of putting his name on articles written by others, he might have been the first physician in the world to report the link between thalidomide and birth defects; Hilts, *Protecting America's Health*, 157; Insight Team, *Suffer the Children*, 84–85.

31. A. Flanagin, L. A. Carey, P. B. Fontanarosa, et al., "Prevalence of Articles with Honorary Authors and Ghost Authors in Peer-Reviewed Medical Journals," *JAMA* 1998; 280:222–24.

32. D. Healy, *Let Them Eat Prozac: The Unhealthy Relationship between the Pharmaceutical Industry and Depression* (New York: New York University Press, 2004), 186.

33. D. Healy and D. Cattell, "Interface between Authorship, Industry and Science in the Domain of Therapeutics," *Br J Psychiatry* 2003; 183:22–27.

34. Healy, *Let Them Eat Prozac*: 187. In a later publication, Healy went even further: "First, up to 75% of the papers on randomized controlled trials on therapeutic agents appearing in major journals may now be ghost-written. Second, in terms of citation rates, the most cited papers in therapeutics are now likely to be ghost-written"; Healy, "Shaping the Intimate," 231. How he arrives at these figures is not explained fully. Presumably, he is speaking specifically of articles in his own specialty, psychiatry.

35. S. T. Rees, "Who Actually Wrote the Research Paper? How to Find It Out," *BMJ Rapid Response*, June 12, 2003, http://bmj.bmjjournals.com/cgi/eletters/326/7400/1202 (accessed March 9, 2005).

36. Healy, *Let Them Eat Prozac*, 183. We will discuss the case of Redux in more detail in later chapters on the FDA.

37. Healy, *Let Them Eat Prozac*, 193.

38. Healy and Cattell, "Interface between Authorship, Industry and Science."

39. Healy, *Let Them Eat Prozac*, 188.

40. A further example is provided by the Advantage study comparing Vioxx with naproxen; J. R. Lisse, M. Perlman, G. Johansson, et al., "Gastrointestinal Tolerability and

Effectiveness of Rofecoxib versus Naproxen in the Treatment of Osteoarthritis: A Randomized, Controlled Trial," *Ann Intern Med* 2003; 139:539–46. Alex Berenson wrote about this
study in 2005 after internal Merck documents were released as a result of the Vioxx lawsuits
that arose after the drug was taken off the market for safety reasons. The documents suggested that Merck senior scientists manipulated the causes of death attributed to some
subjects in the Advantage study. In the end, three patients who probably had died of heart
disease were reclassified as noncardiac deaths, just enough to make the difference between
Vioxx and naproxen not statistically significant. When Berenson queried the purported first
author, Dr. Jeffrey R. Lisse, about these possible discrepancies, Dr. Lisse was forced to admit that he had not written the manuscript and had never seen the full set of raw data.
"Merck designed the trial, paid for the trial, ran the trial. . . . Merck came to me after the
study was completed and said, 'We want your help to work on the paper.' The initial paper
was written at Merck, and then it was sent to me for editing." Berenson added that Dr. Lisse
had never heard of the cases of questioned cardiac deaths until the reporter informed him;
A. Berenson, "Evidence in Vioxx Suits Shows Intervention by Merck Officials," *New York
Times*, April 24, 2005:1.

41. Healy, *Let Them Eat Prozac*, 369, 382.

42. E. Wager, E. A. Field, and L. Grossman, "Good Publication Practice for Pharmaceutical Companies," *Current Medical Research and Opinions* 2003; 19:149–54.

43. As of late 2003, six pharmaceutical firms, mostly smaller firms, had endorsed these
guidelines, and ten medical communications firms had agreed to recommend these guidelines to their corporate clients. www.gpp-guidelines.org (accessed 12/29/03). As of March
2005, there were still only six companies that had signed on.

8

THE DRUG REP:
HISTORICAL BACKGROUND

Every medical journal, every reputable drug reference, and every authority on this drug has repeatedly cautioned against misuse of chloramphenicol. Yet, against the combined authoritative voice of the whole medical profession, drug company promotion has carried the day hardly drawing a deep breath.

—Sen. Gaylord Nelson, 1969[1]

The most critical player at the interface between the medical profession and the pharmaceutical industry is the pharmaceutical sales representative, otherwise known as the detail person, or more simply the "drug rep." It is in the persona of the drug rep that the industry has the most frequent and extended personal contact with the physician. What practicing physicians think of the drug rep will guide what they think of the industry and of their own interaction with it.

Modern drug reps arrived on the scene at an auspicious time in the twentieth century. They bore, by implication, the stamp of approval of organized medicine; and they filled a vital role that no one else at the time was able to fill. How physicians perceive reps today has been heavily conditioned by this historical backdrop.

THE AMA AND THE INDUSTRY

Around 1890–1900, the American Medical Association (AMA), which had consolidated its power as the political force speaking for mainstream medical practice, looked with particular dismay at one segment of the pharmaceutical industry. The

AMA's ire was concentrated on the manufacturers of so-called "patent medicines." There were two major reasons for dismay, one public-spirited and scientific, the other self-serving. The better reason had to do with the secrecy surrounding the formulas of these medicines.[2] The AMA had argued in its original code of ethics in 1847 that physicians could not in good conscience prescribe or recommend a medicine whose contents were unknown and whose safety and effectiveness could not be subjected to the scrutiny of the scientific community. The self-serving reason for the AMA to oppose patent medicines was that they were marketed directly to the public and usually could be obtained without prescription. The advertisement for the medicine, or the salesman who promoted them, offered both diagnosis and treatment, without the need to see a physician and pay a fee. At a time when most American physicians were barely managing to survive financially, these lost revenues were a sore subject with the AMA's members.[3]

The AMA looked for allies in its battle against the patent medicine makers, and found some among the relatively small firms that manufactured the pure drugs that were needed to make up the physician's prescriptions. In that era, most prescriptions contained two or three drugs and had to be compounded individually by the pharmacist; it would be some years before the market was dominated by tablets and capsules made by the manufacturer and merely dispensed by the pharmacist. The manufacturers of pure drugs openly labeled their products and marketed them directly to physicians and pharmacists, not to the general public. They advertised based on the purity and quality of their chemicals, not on inflated claims of miracle cures. To distinguish these scientifically respectable firms from the patent medicine makers, the AMA took to calling the former the "ethical" drug companies.[4]

While the AMA sought assistance among the "ethical" drug makers, the real turning of the tide in the battle against patent medicines came during the muckraking era at the beginning of the twentieth century. Exposés by investigative reporters revealed the unreliable and unsafe ingredients in patent medicines and grossly fraudulent advertising.[5] Slowly the public began to turn against the makers of Lydia Pinkham's pills and similar products. Probably even more important were the scientific advances in bacteriology and other branches of medicine during this era. The public's perception of the value of consulting a physician instead of picking something off the counter of the drug store finally swung in favor of the physician. As physicians gained public respect, the "ethical" drug companies rose in stature along with them. From the 1930s, when less than 10 percent of medicine sales in the United States were in the form of prescription drugs, to the 1950s, when the new wonder drugs of the postwar era were flooding the market, the drug firms grew in size and importance.[6]

One example of early pharmaceutical marketing helps us grasp the image of the "ethical" drug company of that time. A volume called *Excerpta Therapeutica* was distributed free to physicians by the U.S. branch of the London-based drug firm, Burroughs Wellcome and Company.[7] The 1916 edition of this work is about four by seven inches and half-an-inch thick, a convenient size to slip into a pocket, though it holds more than four hundred pages. Most of the volume consists of two alphabetical lists—the first of drug preparations, the second of diseases. The drug list briefly states what each drug is used for and then lists the different forms in which it is available. The second list contains a summary of the recommended drugs for treatment under the name of each disease. It appears that Burroughs Wellcome manufactured virtually every drug in the U.S. pharmacopeia, so a list of its own products was largely indistinguishable from any noncommercial list of drugs. The book does, however, point out in several places that the word "Tabloid" in the name of a drug preparation is a trademark of Burroughs Wellcome, so that if the physician wishes to be sure that a drug is of the highest quality and purity, all he has to do is begin his prescription with "Rx Tabloid . . . " followed by the usual name of the drug, such as "Rx Tabloid Hyoscine."

Excerpta Therapeutica then provides the physician with a number of tables of information on assessing pregnancy and gestation, urine analysis, recommended diets for different diseases, and other medical topics. At the end is a price list of the company's drugs, and many pages of color photos of medicine cases sold by Burroughs Wellcome. The cases are quite handsome (some covered in fine leather or silver-plated) and presumably are designed specially to fit bottles sold by Burroughs Wellcome and not to accommodate the bottles of other manufacturers. The cases reflect the various forms of transport physicians might have used in 1916—pocket cases, a saddle case, a case designed to be hung on a bicycle, and even a case designed to look like a life preserver and to be hung up in a boat.

Other items scattered through the volume describe the company's London manufacturing plant and New York offices, and a page of color photos shows fields of herbal products growing under the careful attention of Burroughs Wellcome experts.

We can imagine the impact a book like this would have had on the average physician of the day. According to the AMA nomenclature, Burroughs Wellcome was an "ethical" drug firm, and indeed at the time perhaps the largest and most important such firm. This little volume seems a solid statement of how the company proposed to work in partnership with the medical practitioner. Here was one-stop shopping brought to its limit. From one firm the physician could obtain every drug he needed to use, plus a handy little book to tell him how and when to use each one, and to top it all off, a handsome medicine case to show off his professional stature to the admiring community. The Burroughs Wellcome salesman who showed up to provide the doctor with his free copy of this year's *Excerpta Therapeutica* could hardly have expected anything other than a warm welcome.[8]

ORIGINS OF THE "DETAIL MAN"

Drug wholesalers employed salesmen as long ago as the 1850s. William Osler, professor of medicine at Johns Hopkins and the most famous American physician of his era, wrote in 1902 that "the 'drummer' of the drug house" was a "dangerous enemy to the mental virility of the general practitioner."[9] When Rufus L. McQuillan was mustered out of the Army Ambulance Corps in May 1919 and took a job with a major drug house, the jobs of salesman and detail man were intermingled.[10] Many physicians still dispensed drugs from their offices and could be expected to place an order with a salesman, but McQuillan was still expected to "detail" (provide all the details of medications to) physicians who did not order from him directly but who instead wrote prescriptions. As his territory was all of Illinois and Indiana, he would be lucky if he saw rural physicians annually.[11] In 1920 there were only an estimated 2,000 detail men in the United States, compared to 15,000 in the late 1950s.[12]

By the early 1930s, prescription products were bringing in larger profits than over-the-counter drugs. It therefore began to make economic sense for companies to invest more heavily in sales staff who had the credentials and the techniques to win over physicians.[13] In 1940, a book of instructions for detail men was published, with its author drawing upon many years of sales experience, and an article describing the modern detail man appeared in *Fortune* magazine.[14] A description of the job responsibilities of the detail person appeared for the first time in 1949 in an official government list of occupations.[15]

The 1940 article in *Fortune* explained the tradeoffs for the "ethical drug house." The company gave up lucrative patent-medicine sales and direct-to-consumer advertising as the price of developing a special relationship with the medical profession. The company trained its detail men to give physicians important, up-to-date information about its products and paid a select group of physicians research grants to perform scientific studies on new drugs. The physicians, in turn, warmly embraced the detail man, seeing him as a friend and colleague, and prescribed the drugs that he recommended. This company representative did not take any orders directly, and usually avoided any hint of having "made a deal" with the physician, creating the comforting aura that he was of a completely different breed from any vulgar "salesman."[16]

What did the "detail man" think of himself? Tom Jones, in his 1940 instructional book for his fellow reps, said forthrightly and up front, "Detailing is, in reality, sales promotion and every detail man should keep that fact constantly in mind."[17] Arthur F. Peterson, in his manual on detailing published in 1949 and reissued in 1959, seemed at first to be aiming for a higher, explicitly professional standard. He referred to detail men as "Professional Service Pharmacists," describing their work as follows:

> The well-informed "detail-man" is one of the most influential and highly respected individuals in the public-health professions. His niche is an extremely important one in the dissemination of scientific information to the medical, pharmaceutical, and allied professions. Upon him frequently depends the saving of life or relieving from suffering by virtue of his timely introduction of a therapeutic product and his intelligent discussion of it with a physician. His opportunity to render service of extraordinary value to physicians for the benefit of their patients is in itself a source of real satisfaction. He serves humanity well.[18]

But Peterson was unable to maintain this high tone for long. A few pages later, he wrote, "The Professional Service Pharmacist's job is one of scientific selling in every sense of the word. . . . He must be a *salesman* first, last, and always"; and, "It is apparent that the first qualification for a prospective Professional Service Pharmacist is sales ability, a love for selling, a 'selling heart.'"[19] Later he added, "The representative who has an idea that he is not supposed to sell but only to impart scientific information in his contacts as a service offered by his firm is very much 'off the beam.' The ultimate objective of every phase of any business is *to produce more sales at a better profit.*"[20]

Salesmen or otherwise, the pharmaceutical reps who appeared in physician's offices, saying, "I'm from Merck" or "I'm from Squibb," had the distinct advantage of the AMA's "ethical" terminology. The AMA said, in effect, "This drug firm has been on our side during our long fight with the patent-medicine crowd, forgoing any profits that might have been made by catering to the general public, and advertising their products only to you. Now, this friendly and knowledgeable person has come to add a new dimension to our relationship with this company. In an era when new drugs are appearing so fast that it's tremendously hard to keep up, this person is here to tell you about the latest pharmaceutical miracles. You owe it both to this *ethical* manufacturer and to your patients to listen carefully to what he has to say." Small wonder that in a 1959 survey American physicians indicated an overwhelming disapproval (by a ratio of 17 to 1) of any of their brethren who might refuse to talk with reps.[21]

THE MIDDLE OF THE TWENTIETH CENTURY: AN ALIGNMENT OF PLANETS

Between 1945 and 1955, three major factors came into congruence—a sort of alignment of the planets. Without this alignment it is unlikely that the drug reps would have come to play the special role within medicine that they enjoy today. The factors were:

- The explosion in new drugs
- The failure of medical education to address the drug explosion
- The retreat of the AMA from objective drug assessment

Physicians who were delighted to have diphtheria antitoxin in the 1890s had to wait until the 1920s for the advent of insulin. But starting in the mid-1930s, when the first sulfa drugs for treating infections appeared, the pace of pharmaceutical innovation increased by leaps and bounds. Penicillin was first mass-produced during World War II and was quickly followed by the first antibiotics effective against tuberculosis, the cortisone-type hormones, and an array of tranquilizers. Dr. William B. Bean, editor of the *Archives of Internal Medicine*, described the effects of the drug explosion in 1955:

A generation of physicians whose orientation fell between therapeutic nihilism and the uncritical employment of ever-changing placebos was ill prepared to handle a baffling array of really powerful compounds. The advent of sulfa drugs; the emergence of effective antibiotics; the transformation of endocrine therapy from a stage only a step in advance of mysticism to one with many hormones available for a great variety of therapeutic manipulations; the isolation of vitamins in bewildering abundance which soon outran the known vitamin-deficiency disorders; the development of drugs with potent but still not completely mapped effects on emotions—all these have made it difficult if not impossible for the most conscientious and critical physician to "keep up" with the torrent which has now become a flood.[22]

John Lear, science editor of the *Saturday Review*, noted in 1959 that new "wonder" drugs were replacing one another so quickly that pharmacists complained about regularly being stuck with hundreds of dollars' worth of obsolete, nonreturnable drugs.[23]

What preparation had the average physician to deal with this massive amount of novel information? The pharmacology course he had in medical school was rudimentary even by pre-World War II standards. Throughout medical school and internship he had heard no mention of any of these new drugs even by therapeutic class or group, let alone specifically by name. Moreover, his education had prepared him very poorly to critically assess a report of a scientific study in a medical journal. The double-blind randomized trial, today's gold standard for assessing the value of a new drug, had only been introduced into the research arena during the late 1940s, and even in the 1950s few medical schools addressed how to assess the methods and quality of a research trial in the standard curriculum.

In hindsight it appears obvious that the academic medical establishment had a crisis of sorts on its hands. Incredibly powerful drugs were being developed daily and were being prescribed by physicians who had virtually no solid grasp of how to use them. The medical schools and teaching hospitals were entering a phase of rapid growth, stimulated by massive infusions of federal funds, that turned them from the small institutions of the 1930s into the behemoth academic medical centers of today.[24] But they did not see the plight of the local practitioner as any problem of theirs.

The establishment, it seems, was hung up on the ambiguous meaning of the concept that medical education is *scientific*. Since the revolution in medical-school curriculum that was capped by the publication of the Flexner Report in 1910, medical schools had certainly taught an abundance of scientific *facts* to newly minted physicians. And at least some of those facts were imparted in teaching laboratories, where students dutifully repeated experiments under the direction of their faculty. But being made to memorize facts was a far cry from learning scientific *skills*—what the scientific investigator uses to discover new knowledge and to assess the validity and reliability of his experimental results. Still, the medical schools assumed that in training their students, they had produced a cadre of scientists. All these physicians had to do was recall what they had been taught and keep up with what was being printed in the academic journals—which the faculty fondly imagined each practitioner read religiously. No special effort on the part of the medical teaching institutions was needed to ensure that practitioners learned what they needed to know about novel drugs.

In hindsight, this was dangerous nonsense. It was not until the turn of the twenty-first century that medical school faculty became serious about teaching courses in "critical appraisal" of the literature, and "evidence-based medicine," as major components of the standard curriculum. And today most advocates of evidence-based medicine have come to agree that the average physician in practice has neither the time nor the skills to go back to the medical journals, assemble all that is known about a particular drug or disease, assess the relative quality of the various research studies, and reach a practical conclusion about how to treat an individual patient. The biggest challenge facing evidence-based medicine today is how to package the best medical information in easy-to-use nuggets that overworked practitioners can retrieve precisely when they need them and apply immediately to patient care.[25] By imagining that some combination of academic journals and occasional continuing education lectures would keep physicians up-to-date about pharmaceutical advances, academic medicine in the early 1950s basically abandoned the field to the forces of commercialism. By the time some tentative warning voices were raised in the 1960s, the victory of the commercial army was already assured.

There was only one noncommercial organization with sufficient resources and prestige to occupy the educational niche that academic medicine did not realize it had vacated. It is therefore an important part of the alignment of planets that, precisely at this critical juncture, the AMA abandoned its traditional role as an objective source of information on pharmaceuticals.

Since 1905, when the AMA was lobbying against the patent medicine makers for the creation of the FDA, the organization had had a Council on Pharmacy and Chemistry, and operated its own drug-testing laboratories. For decades there was free scientific exchange between the AMA council, the FDA, and the top medical schools, so that the council could draw on the best authorities in the field. Like most medical school teachers, the council advocated prescribing by generic rather than by brand name. The council bestowed a "Seal of Acceptance" on drug products they found worthy, and the "ethical" drug houses eagerly sought that mark of approval.[26] No drug could be advertised in the weekly *Journal of the American Medical Association* without that seal, so practitioners could rely upon the ads in their most widely read journal as an indicator of pharmaceutical quality.[27] Part of the reason the average physician of the 1940s had so much trust in the AMA is that the organization "had been a key source of information about the problems and relative value of drugs, an efficient watchdog. The AMA had published lists of fraudulent and useless drugs and often gave critical evaluations of the others. Its committees of top experts spoke always for reining in unscrupulous companies."[28]

But now the power balance shifted. The formerly small "ethical" drug firms had become huge, wealthy corporations. They could flex their financial muscle by bypassing the AMA, relying instead on direct-mail advertising and personal visits from drug reps to carry their messages directly to the doctors. The council's Seal of Acceptance was now more of a burden than a benefit to them. The AMA leadership became alarmed as revenue from drug advertising in their journal lagged in the 1940s and 1950s. A conservative clique of leaders staged a coup. Privately they assured the drug industry that they could silence the AMA's criticism if they would bring back their advertising. The Seal of Acceptance, the test laboratories, and finally the Council on Pharmacy and Chemistry itself were dismantled. No more was said about prescribing by generic name. "After the turnaround, the AMA's advertising revenues represented more than half the entire income of the association."[29]

The AMA had ceased to be an independent watchdog. But the individual practitioner, who had developed over many decades the habit of trusting the AMA to decide both what was "ethical" and what drugs to prescribe, would not quickly change. Many physicians continued to assume that the publication of an advertisement in the AMA *Journal* constituted a product endorsement by the organization. With this alignment of the planets, the drug industry found the path to the Promised Land lying open. The industry itself could virtually take over the task of informing physicians about new drugs. As the journal *Advertising Age* proclaimed in 1963:

> Most of the drugs that are prescribed today by doctors were not in existence when the doctor was in medical school. And survey after survey has shown conclusively that the medical profession's principal sources of information about these new drugs are the advertising and promotion programs of the pharmaceutical manufacturers.
>
> Medical advertising may therefore be properly called post-graduate education of the doctor. There is no question that this advertising aims to *sell* products—by brand name. A drug manufacturer naturally wants doctors to prescribe his product rather than a competitor's. Acceptance of this profit motive, however, does not take away the fact that communication between the pharmaceutical industry and the medical profession is a necessary link in our health scheme.[30]

But it would take a while for the industry to figure out how to use its new power.

THE DICHTER STUDY

A group that called itself the Pharmaceutical Advertising Club collaborated with the Institute for Motivational Research, headed by Ernest Dichter, to produce a volume called *A Research Study on Pharmaceutical Advertising* in 1955.[31] This volume, sometimes called the "Dichter Study," appears to have become a classic in pharmaceutical promotion and has since been widely cited. It marks a turning point in pharmaceutical marketing. The pharmaceutical executive who took the Dichter Study seriously would probably not view marketing in the same way afterward. It was a turning point in another way as well. After the 1950s, the pharmaceutical industry would hardly ever again allow such a document to be disseminated openly.

In 1955, most pharmaceutical promotion took the form of direct mailings to physicians, with relatively less effort going into journal advertisements and detailing. Still, the Dichter Study approached all three areas as interconnected and gave recommendations for each. For that reason the study's conclusions remained pertinent even as direct mail disappeared and detailing took on greater importance.

When Dichter's team approached drug advertising in 1955, they found many within the "ethical drug industry" viewing detailing and advertising in highly idealistic terms, as a way of transmitting accurate and current scientific information. Using then-popular projective techniques (cousins of the Rorschach ink-blot test) as well as in-depth interviews, Dichter's team showed conclusively that this was an inadequate picture of drug advertising—at least if the company wanted to sell drugs.

The physician of 1955, said the study report, was a very threatened individual. His work was becoming increasingly complex. His day was getting busier and busier. New drugs were appearing at a phenomenal rate. The physician feared being looked down upon both by colleagues and by patients if he was not among the first to prescribe some new wonder drug.

At the beginning of an interview, the physician would complain about his time being wasted by detail men, and how he hated the mountains of ads that showed up every day in his mail.[32] Once he was done going through the ritual exercise of proclaiming himself a scientific practitioner who thought independently and who could never be swayed by mere advertising, he would eventually admit that he relied heavily on the ads and the detail men to keep informed about drugs and to make sense of what he had neither the time nor the knowledge to extract from the journals.

The physician dealt with this cognitive dissonance, according to the Dichter study, by distinguishing between the run-of-the-mill drug house and the "*really* ethical drug company." Once again, the physician would at first claim that the "better" company manufactured better quality drugs. On pressing below the surface, the research showed that the distinction was almost always made on emotional grounds. The detail man from the *best* drug house, for example, was a personal friend with whom the physician had a first-name relationship for an extended period. The detail man was scientifically accomplished so that the physician could rely on his accuracy, but he never waved his knowledge in the physician's face as if he thought he knew more than the physician did. The print ads from the "ideal" company similarly walked a fine line. They were visually appealing and catchy rather than full of technical information; yet they never appeared too superficial or glitzy, as if the physician were a housewife being sold a new laundry soap. In a world where many forces seemed to be threatening the physician's self-respect, the "*really* ethical drug house" seemed to understand the physician's plight and to offer help and support. Dichter's team proclaimed that it was this aura of bonding with and supporting the ego of the beleaguered physician, refusing to treat him as a scientist while never letting on to him that you are not treating him as a scientist, that characterized successful pharmaceutical advertising.

The Dichter study broke new ground by identifying how important the process of *rationalization* was in successful pharmaceutical marketing. The company had to treat the physician in one way yet be perceived as if they were treating him in a very different way. The ideal contact with the company fed message and rationalization simultaneously. For example, a visit from the rep might *really* be a break in a busy afternoon of seeing patients, a chance to talk with an old buddy about a hobby, or an exchange of gossip about other physicians in town. But just enough scientific information had to be exchanged—even a brochure that would never be read—so that the physician could rationalize the visit as "education." The importance of rationalization hints at why the drug rep was more valuable than print advertising. It is hard for a print ad to get the mix of commercial message and rationalization just right, unlike conversation with a human being. We will see in the next chapter how many of the lessons of the Dichter Study still appear to guide pharmaceutical marketing today.

THE REP IN THE 1950S AND 1960S

The earliest studies of reps started to appear in the 1950s, though publications of that era have two distinguishing features. First, the majority of attention is paid to direct-mail and journal ads, even in studies that show that the reps are more important than ads in swaying physician opinion. Second, when reps are mentioned, virtually nothing is said about gifts to physicians, other than drug samples. It might have been the case that no gifts in fact changed hands during that period—gifts do not appear to have been a feature of the drug rep's activities in the years prior to 1950.[33] Alternatively, the gifts may have been on the order of pens and calendars, considered so innocuous and trivial as to escape mention. A 1959 paper characterized typical gifts as "pens or notebooks and various forms of entertainment."[34] By contrast, Richard Carter, in a 1958 exposé of the business side of medicine, described, "social outings, banquets, award presentations, . . . cocktail parties, duck shoots, barbecues, fishing tournaments, bowling tournaments, golf tournaments, picnics, and anything else that the authorities will stand for" as typical examples of industry-sponsored hospitality.[35]

A flaw in many of these studies was the failure to correct for social desirability bias. The Dichter group had realized that physicians feel required, on first approach, to act like people think physicians are supposed to act—to proclaim themselves objective scientists who are not swayed by advertising. Dichter's study methods allowed his group to get below the surface and eventually get at the physicians' true opinions. Many other studies took the socially acceptable answers at face value.[36]

The studies of reps published in the 1950s and 1960s portrayed a largely favorable picture. The detail men (women are not mentioned until the early 1970s) were viewed as well informed and honest, just as the physicians tended to view the large drug manufacturers in benign terms. When Ben Gaffin and Associates, surveying a national sample of physicians for the AMA in 1957–1958, asked what information sources they found personally most useful in familiarizing themselves with new drugs, reps appeared at the top of the list, mentioned by 68 percent.[37] The average physician in 1956 spent 0.91 hours every week talking with detail men.[38] Dr. Solomon Garb at the Albany Medical College became concerned about physicians' uncritical acceptance of drug advertising and developed an elective course for medical students. At one session the faculty and students met with a group of reps. While the course seemed successful at instilling in the students a good deal of skepticism regarding the information contained in printed drug ads, it did not (nor did Garb apparently intend that it should) create a similar level of skepticism about reps. Indeed, where the students discovered the reps' information to be unreliable, they gave the rep the benefit of the doubt, arguing that the company might have informed them poorly.[39]

Where physicians voiced complaints, it was about the occasional rep who was poorly trained or overly pushy, or in a few cases, about the sheer number of demands for the busy physician's time. Even in early studies a few physicians were noted to harbor very negative feelings about reps and to refuse to see most or all of them, but such naysayers were viewed as an odd minority. Such rare naysayers, for instance, included these correspondents who responded to John Lear's 1959 *Saturday Review* article about the overuse of antibiotics:

"I feel that it would be a fine thing if all doctors everywhere would refuse to accept any samples of any drugs and read only the most realistic accounts of new drugs. The savings which could result to the drug houses would reduce the cost of necessary drugs to patients, I would guess, by at least fifty percent of the present costs."—Esther B. Clark, MD, Palo Alto Medical Clinic

"It is time that we as a profession were returning to some of our old ethical standards. A doctor cannot listen to the voice of the huckster and practice honest conscientious medicine."—Edwin R. Sage, MD, Assistant Director of Public Health, San Francisco[40]

The more typical physician of that era probably resembled one who wrote a letter to the *Medical Journal*, which was in turn quoted with approval by the experienced rep, Rufus McQuillan. The physician noted that reps might see six physicians in an average day and could be kept waiting as much as an hour. The physician continued:

Since there is so much criticism these days about the high cost of prescriptions, it occurred to me that we doctors might in a modest way help to cut drug costs, if we were helpful in facilitating the visits of these men in our office. I feel that I learn something from almost all of them. I believe that if we could tell our girls not to be so protective, but to give these men one or two minutes after the next patient we are seeing, they could see many more doctors in a day. I believe that this could be a source of advertising cost savings for the drug industry.[41]

For this physician, it seemed clear that the interests of the drug industry and of medicine coincided fully, and that reps were fellow professionals deserving of every consideration—even being put into line ahead of waiting patients.

CALLING "ETHICAL" INTO QUESTION, 1961

Few in those days seemed aware of how the word "ethical" was greasing the pathway for the entry of the reps into the mainstream of medical practice, or whether the behavior of the drug companies was in conformity with that accolade. An early skeptic was Dr. Charles D. May, professor of pediatrics at Columbia and a member of the Physician's Council, "an independent group of eighteen eminent physicians who organized in 1956 'to seek means of maintaining high standards for the material on health that is disseminated through the media of mass communication.'"[42] May wrote a long paper in 1961 to take issue with a major claim of the drug industry—that its marketing efforts should be viewed as medical "education." May was quite willing to admit that the profession had fallen woefully short of its responsibilities to educate the mass of physicians about the plethora of new drugs. But this failure, to May, hardly justified the profession's handing over its "educational" task to commercially interested parties.[43]

May's critique of the industry in 1961 foreshadowed many of the themes that would be raised by similar critics over the next four decades. His first paragraph raised the ethical questions of professional integrity, conflicts of interest, and public trust:

> Is the public likely to benefit if practicing physicians and medical educators must perform their duties amidst the clamor and striving of merchants seeking to increase the sales of drugs by conscripting "education" in the service of promotion? Is it prudent for physicians to become greatly dependent upon pharmaceutical manufacturers for support of scientific journals and medical societies, for entertainment, and now also for a large part of their education? Do all concerned realize the hazard of arousing the wrath of the people by an unwholesome entanglement of doctors with the makers and sellers of drugs?[44]

May, unlike later critics, expressed evenhanded concern for the integrity of the industry, arguing that the "unwholesome" practices he opposed did as much to "degrad[e] the reputation of the pharmaceutical industry" as they did to "lower . . . the prestige of the medical profession."[45]

May started by addressing the quality of information contained in typical drug ads in medical journals. In the late 1950s the drug industry went berserk in marketing products that in retrospect were highly irrational. The companies decided that if one antibiotic was a wonder drug, two or three antibiotics mixed together in one pill were even more wondrous. If antibiotics cured infections while vitamins were essential for good nutrition, then mixing vitamins with antibiotics would be even better. Beside the problems of combination drugs that were heavily marketed to physicians without having any rational use, the industry created a smokescreen by marketing the same antibiotic under as many as ten different brand names, using their "education" to ensure that the physician remembered only the brand names and never the generic name. Hence the physician might not realize that the patient had received the same antibiotic three times rather than three different antibiotics. Thus, May had no trouble finding ads that were seriously misleading.

May then called attention to how much of the cost of drugs was due to the money spent by industry on these promotional activities and that, even in 1961, the amount spent by industry to influence physician behavior was approaching the total sum of money available to all U.S. medical schools. That same year, Kefauver's Senate Committee on Antitrust reported that the industry spent $750 million annually on promotion while the total medical school budgets of the nation amounted to $200 million.[46] Without employing the term, May showed a firm grasp of the ethical idea of conflict of interest. "There is sufficient talent and idealism in industry and the profession to formulate a wholesome partnership," he stated, as long as one could successfully "search out the principles which will bring the trade and the profession into proper alignment in fulfilling their obligations to the people."[47] May noted how laws in the nineteenth century had gradually divorced the practice of medicine from the selling of drugs, and suggested that the public would soon be up in arms again if it perceived that the industry was exerting undue influence over the profession.

May took aim at practices that seemed to violate ethical principles for managing the relationship in the public interest:

- While many physicians seemed to believe that the FDA exercised control over the content of drug ads, the FDA of that time was relatively powerless to police false or misleading ads aimed solely at physicians.
- Of all the new drugs released onto the market, about four hundred per year in the late 1950s, only a handful were genuinely novel products with new chemical makeup. The vast majority were what would later be called "me-too" drugs, offering no real advantage over drugs already on the market. A truly educational campaign would ensure that physicians understood the difference between these two categories of new drugs; marketing campaigns were based on the need to obfuscate that difference and to make physicians think that every "me-too" drug was in fact a unique therapeutic advance. A vicious cycle was created—physicians became more confused by these obfuscating marketing techniques; physicians were then in need of more "education" and were prey to new marketing efforts by industry. As Dr. Dale Console, former medical director of Squibb turned drug industry critic, told the Kefauver Senate hearings, "The basic maxim of detail men . . . was 'If you can't convince them, confuse them.'"[48]
- Like any effective advertising, drug ads and marketing are designed to bypass rational and critical thought on the part of physicians, whereas true education would simulate thought. The industry farms out this task (quite reasonably) to advertising agencies, not educators.
- May labeled as "payola" the gifts given by industry to secure the ongoing goodwill and close relationship between its reps and physicians. He singled out Eli Lilly for giving free instruments to medical students while emphasizing to the students that the deans of the medical schools approved, and Pfizer and Schering for employing needy medical students as reps. Under "payola" May included gifts and entertainment for individual physicians, money to support the activities of professional organizations and medical journals, and research grants to medical investigators. Perhaps back in the 1940s gifts had mostly been restricted to pens and calendars, but May suggested that by 1961, expensive meals and lavish entertainment had become commonplace.
- There is a major mismatch between the resources of scientific medical journals and the slick magazines that offer nothing besides drug company promotion. The legitimate journals are usually managed by a skeleton staff trained in science rather than in writing, editing, and publication, and they lack the money to hire illustrators and others who might make the publication more interesting and meaningful to the average practitioner. Meanwhile the less worthy publications can spend top dollar to deliver to the busy practitioner a well-written, fully illustrated article that conveys the message the drug company desires, mixed with just the right amount of scientific-sounding "facts."
- Even journals that contain valid scientific articles depend on drug ads for their survival and make virtually no effort to screen the ads for accuracy. They thus allow the scientific reputation of the journal to carry over onto

misleading advertising. May admitted that there were probably more "scientific" journals than the field really needed, because it was too easy to pay the publication costs of a new journal by securing enough drug ads. May noted the publication founded in 1959, the *Medical Letter*, a brief newsletter that was supported by subscription only (no drug advertising) and offered expert assessments of newly released drugs. May expressed hope that physicians would embrace the *Medical Letter* as a readable, concise, and current source of commercially unbiased drug information. His hope failed to bear fruit; at no time has more than a relatively small minority of U.S. physicians subscribed to this periodical.[49]

- May noted with particular dismay the willingness of his colleagues in academic medicine to lend their names and reputations to the drug industry's marketing, presumably for their share of "payola." (In an earlier editorial, Dr. Louis Lasagna of Johns Hopkins, despite a generally benign attitude toward the pharmaceutical industry, had decried the pressure that grants from drug companies placed on academic investigators to produce results favorable to drug sales.[50])

In passing, May became perhaps the first to call attention to the way that the industry had benefited from the AMA's label of "ethical." "Ethical," he claimed, should be reserved for how the business actually behaves, and not simply pasted on as a bit of rhetoric. May noted that as a spin-off from the too-free use of the term, the profession had developed an unscientific distaste for any open criticism of specific drug brands or firms—out of fear, it was said, that patients would be unduly distressed if they found out that the drug they were taking had been the subject of unfavorable publicity.

May might have here had in mind the experience of Congressman John A. Blatnik of Minnesota. Before the more widely publicized Kefauver hearings in the U.S. Senate, Blatnik became concerned about how the Federal Trade Commission was regulating the advertising of tranquilizers. He held four days of essentially inconclusive hearings. The lead-off witness, Dr. Nathan S. Kline of Rockland State Hospital in New York, prevailed on the committee to cite no drug or manufacturer by name. Mention of specific drugs publicly could violate the sanctity of the physician-patient relationship, he argued, causing patients to question their physicians' choice of drug. The Congress of the United States knuckled under and referred only to "Drug A," "Drug B," and so forth.[51]

May also anticipated the rejoinder that physicians are thoughtful scientists immune from the blandishments of advertising, by becoming the first in a long line of commentators to say of the large sums spent by industry on promotional activities, "Keen businessmen do not continue to lay out huge sums without results."[52]

May wrote during the time of the Kefauver Senate hearings, when Congress was actively investigating the drug industry and threatening to pass new laws. As befits a physician during an era when organized medicine opposed any governmental interference, May called for self-regulation on the part of both industry and profession. He seemed to think that a number of forces were lined up favorably for such efforts. He viewed it as only a matter of time before the industry's overbearing and expensive promotional activities aroused an angry backlash among both physicians and the general public. He also believed that within the industry itself there were more and less "ethical" elements, and that the more responsible companies might be persuaded to disown the tactics of the few companies that employed the most aggressive promotional methods. In all these predictions, May proved mistaken. Later critics of the industry would write virtually identical books and articles covering virtually the same points for the next forty-plus years.

Ironically, May may have contributed to a trend very different from what he intended. He criticized the industry and his fellow physicians who believed its pitches and accepted its "payola," from his vantage point as an elite physician attached to a prestigious New York medical school. The message taken home by the average practitioner was that the ivory-tower intellectuals simply did not understand what real medicine was like in the trenches.[53] One FDA staff physician of that era explained:

> Plenty of doctors are crazy about detail men. . . . In small towns, they not only bring doctors free samples and information but open up their bags and give them presents of all sorts—desk sets, expensive calendars, elaborate medical charts, illuminated anatomy figures, monogrammed golf balls, and so on. They're regular Santa Clauses. And they also bring news from other towns on the circuit. When you come down to it, they're very much like old-fashioned drummers, and plenty of doctors look forward to their visits. This is not to say, however, that they do anything to advance the cause of medicine.[54]

Advancing the cause or not, the rank-and-file doctors felt by then more loyalty to the reps than to academic physicians like May who criticized them.[55]

The reps had already done battle with people like Charles May over the new drugs flooding the market in the 1950s, such as the combination antibiotics. Dr. May and his academic colleagues had argued to their colleagues that these products were irrational and dangerous. The reps showed up at the office, handed out gifts, and gave examples of all the other physician on their route who were already prescribing these drugs, hinting that the physician would be thought out-of-date if he did not join the crowd. The sales figures showed that the reps won that battle, hands down. Silverman and Lee summarized that period of U.S. medical practice by remarking, "It is probable that never before in history had so many physicians— all of them supposedly trained as scientifically knowledgeable professionals—been so effectively and profitably brainwashed."[56] If the reps could win this battle with Charles May and his ilk regarding the very area of May's academic expertise, they could even more easily win the battle over accepted professional ethics.

One story that dates from the 1950s and 1960s is worth recounting in detail. Perhaps chloramphenicol, better than any other drug, illustrates the power that the drug-rep system came to have over the practice of medicine in America.

THE CHLORAMPHENICOL STORY

Chloramphenicol was one of the new "miracle" antibiotics to come into use in the years immediately after penicillin. It was the first broad-spectrum antibiotic, effective for a much wider variety of bacteria than was penicillin. When it arrived in 1949, it impressed both infectious disease experts and the average physician. Early research showed that the drug was effective in treating two longstanding epidemic threats, typhoid fever and typhus. Indeed chloramphenicol remained for years the most effective treatment available for typhoid fever. The average physician (who treated few cases of these dread diseases) was impressed for different reasons. Chloramphenicol seemed to be effective for just about any infectious condition for which it was prescribed. And the drug appeared in daily use to have almost no unpleasant side effects. Streptomycin, the first antibiotic effective against tuberculosis, had been found to be toxic to both the kidneys and the inner ear. By contrast, virtually no patients who received chloramphenicol suffered any immediate ill effects.

Chloramphenicol (brand name: Chloromycetin) was produced by the Detroit drug firm, Parke, Davis. Previously known as a maker of vitamins, Parke, Davis hoped to move into the mainstream of the larger, more prestigious drug firms. The company had a good reputation among physicians. Its sales reps in those days were almost all trained pharmacists. Physicians commonly said that receiving a visit from a Parke, Davis rep was something like having a minicourse in pharmacology walk into their offices.[57] Parke, Davis's hopes for its new drug were soon fulfilled; in 1951 the company topped the industry with $135 million in sales (equivalent to about $950 million today).[58]

Parke, Davis chemists noted that one of the components of the chloramphenicol molecule, the nitrobenzene radical, was potentially poisonous to the bone marrow that makes blood cells. Some of the same early scientific papers that praised the effectiveness of the drug also included warnings that it would have to be watched closely for marrow toxicity. Soon after the drug was introduced, reports began to appear at medical meetings and in journals that some patients seemed to have developed blood disorders after taking the drug. The worst disorder was a fatal aplastic anemia, in which the bone marrow stopped making new blood cells.

One of the first physicians to become aware of what was happening was an ordinary general practitioner, Dr. Albe Watkins, in a Los Angeles suburb. In his own practice he had been happy to use the new broad-spectrum antibiotics. In 1951, his eight-year-old son James developed problems urinating and eventually had to have minor surgery to remove a blockage in his urethra. For a while he needed to have a catheter inserted into his bladder. James received two doses of chloramphenicol—not because he had any clear evidence of an infection (and not because, even if he had had an infection, it clearly needed chloramphenicol), but simply to be on the safe side in the surgeon's judgment.

In 1952 James developed a fever of 104°. Dr. Watkins now had some doubts. He recalled how some patients had become deaf from streptomycin, after that antibiotic had been touted as being free of any serious side effects. Watkins sought reassurance from his local Parke, Davis detail man. The rep said that he had heard no reports whatever of major side effects. There had actually been several deaths linked to chloramphenicol in that sales area, and a colleague later told Dr. Watkins that the rep clearly had lied because the colleague had personally told the rep about one of the deaths.

Reassured, Dr. Watkins gave James a dose of chloramphenicol for his fever. The two earlier doses had probably sensitized his system to the drug, and the third dose now caused a catastrophic reaction. James became lethargic and pale, and bruises started to pop up all over his body. He was soon diagnosed with aplastic anemia—his bone marrow had stopped making red cells and also was producing hardly any platelets, the particles that cause the blood to clot. One of the doctors Dr. Watkins consulted on James's case said that he had already seen four cases apparently linked to chloramphenicol.

Despite more than fifty blood transfusions, James became progressively worse and died in May 1952. In retrospect, he had never needed chloramphenicol at all. The first two times, he probably needed no antibiotic of any sort. On the third occasion, several safer antibiotics would have worked just as well.

The distraught Dr. Watkins wrote to Parke, Davis. He became even more suspicious when he received a reply from its medical director, insisting that no evidence connected chloramphenicol to aplastic anemia. Unable to concentrate on his routine medical practice, Watkins decided to take his family on a cross-country auto trip. In each town where they stopped for the night, he called local physicians and asked if they had seen any cases of aplastic anemia, and warned them about his own experience. When he got to Washington, he met with the FDA's antibiotics chief, Henry Welch. Watkins brought with him reports of forty cases he had collected en route, while Welch replied that the FDA had records of fifty cases and thirty-six deaths, with new reports arriving almost daily.[59]

Parke, Davis and the FDA now each faced its own dilemma. To jump ahead in the story for a moment, the risk of developing aplastic anemia after taking chloramphenicol was later found to be somewhere between one in eight thousand and one in twenty thousand, and no test was ever developed to predict who was at greatest risk. These numbers meant that the average physician might practice for a lifetime and never personally see a case of aplastic anemia caused by the antibiotic—and also explained why no cases of aplastic anemia might have occurred among the subjects of the initial trials run by Parke, Davis. Under the circumstances it would not be surprising if the company officials were reluctant to conclude that their miracle drug, the goose that was laying their golden egg, was the cause of these deaths. Thomas S. Maeder, in his history of the drug, puts the problem this way:

> What does a pharmaceutical company do when one of its products turns out to harm people? How does one weigh the possible dangers against the therapeutic benefits and the risks of corporate liability versus the financial rewards of successful products? How can a for-profit company devoted to the development of drugs to treat illness simultaneously satisfy its legal obligations to its shareholders and its ethical duty to humanity? When the suggestion of danger is inconclusive, as medical issues so often are, how much proof ought a company to demand before taking action? These questions form the leitmotif that runs through the entire chloramphenicol story and, indeed, through the history of all pharmaceuticals.[60]

An additional factor in the case of Parke, Davis was its president. Harry Loynd (b. 1898) had managed a drug store and gotten a pharmacist's license before he went to work as a salesman for Parke, Davis' Kansas City branch at the height of the Depression. He worked his way to the top, becoming president in 1951. Loynd had been heard to say to his sales force at company meetings, "If we put horse manure in a capsule, we could sell it to 95 percent of these doctors," as well as, "Pills are to sell, not to take."[61] Loynd was not one to lie down and play dead if he sensed that his company was under threat.

From the FDA side, the dilemma looked somewhat different. The agency had the authority to order an unsafe drug off the market. But the agency also wished to defer to scientific opinion, and experts in antibiotics were quick to point out that chloramphenicol had unique advantages for typhoid fever and a few other serious infections. No group of infectious disease experts was going to recommend that this drug simply be banned from use.

In the ideal world, there was an obvious solution to the FDA's problem. Physicians simply needed to become educated and informed that the drug's use should be restricted to life-threatening infections for which no other antibiotic would work. In that select group of patients, the risk of dying from the untreated infection far outweighed the very small risk of later coming down with aplastic anemia. Moreover, the number of U.S. patients receiving chloramphenicol under these guidelines would perhaps be only in the tens of thousands per year, at most. This would in turn translate into very few cases of aplastic anemia.

The restricted-use guidelines that the FDA scientists sought to promote were quite different from the way that U.S. physicians were using the drug in the mid-1950s. This was due to the confluence of two factors—drug company marketing, and certain basic facts of daily medical practice in the real world. Dr. Dale Console described the circumstances favoring widespread use of chloramphenicol in this way:

> There are two quite different ways to practice medicine. One calls for precise, pinpoint diagnosis and the aiming of a handloaded rifle bullet at the center of the target. Unfortunately, this method is not always available; an overwhelming potentially fatal infection is an obvious exception, but this is the primary method taught in medical schools. The other method, which is not taught in medical school, seeks only some general categorization of the patient's illness, such as anemia, infection, or gastro-intestinal disorder and either letting loose a shotgun blast in the hope that one of the pellets will find the mark, or firing one or more rifle bullets in random fashion hoping, again, that one will reach the bull's eye. These are examples of irrational prescribing and unsound medical practice.
>
> The latter method of practice requires far less skill, much less time, and uses much more medication than sound medical practice. Because it is easier, it has more and more appeal as the physician becomes more hurried, more harried, and more confused. Because it uses more drugs, the drug industry encourages the practice in the "education" it gives in its advertising and promotion efforts. It is easier than you will believe to fall into the habit of thinking fever equals infection equals a prescription for chloramphenicol. Viewed in this light, the misuse of chloramphenicol becomes more understandable since chloramphenicol is one of the biggest shotguns of them all.[62]

Here Dr. Console took a position that would have been approved of by Dr. Charles May and his colleagues in academic medicine. The problem was that in several ways, this characterization was unfair to the community practitioner. The "rifle" analogy made a number of assumptions. It assumed that the physician would be able to diagnose each infectious disease precisely, by culturing the bacterium responsible for it from the appropriate body fluids. This in turn assumed that the physician either had a working bacteriological laboratory in his office, or that he could readily make use of the laboratory at his local hospital while seeing patients at their homes or in his office. It further assumed that it was feasible in this environment to postpone final treatment until the cultures were completed, often a matter of two or three days.

These assumptions generally fit well with work in an academic medical center. The university physicians typically saw relatively few patients per day and had a fully equipped laboratory just down the hall. They also had the help of residents, medical students, and technicians to do the work of gathering the culture specimens, processing the culture plates or tubes, and monitoring the patient all during the process. Most of these "ivory tower" experts had little way to realize that conditions were completely different in the world of community practice.[63]

So, in the shotgun world of everyday American medicine, chloramphenicol was prescribed to millions of patients, hardly any of whom had the dread diseases for which the drug was of real benefit. The vast majority of patients who received this drug fell into one of two categories. Either they had a bacterial infection, such as an uncomplicated bladder infection, for which several other, safer antibiotics would have worked just as well. Or, even more tragically, they had no bacterial infection of any sort. They had viral colds, which did not then and do not today respond to any available antibiotic. These cold patients had no need for any antibiotic at all, far less for one that amounted to a game of Russian roulette with a deadly blood disease.

Since millions, rather than tens of thousands of patients were annually receiving chloramphenicol, anyone could do the math and see what was going to happen. Dozens or even hundreds of cases of aplastic anemia continued to occur as a result of the use of the drug. No one appears to have calculated a reliable estimate of the total death toll.

The FDA was fully aware of all these factors and did its best to combat them. It was hampered by the fact that during most of the time that the drug was heavily marketed, the agency either lacked the legal authority to play real hardball with the company or at least had no tradition of treating companies that way. The FDA was also hampered by its own culture of secrecy, allowing Parke, Davis's public relations campaigns to put almost whatever spin on events the company wished.

The FDA convened three different scientific panels to review the chloramphenicol case. Each concluded, in essence, that the drug caused aplastic anemia in a certain number of cases, should be used with great caution, but should not be taken off the market completely. The agency then ordered Parke, Davis to send warning letters to all U.S. physicians about the drug's dangers. By the time Loynd's company was through, the warning letter sounded like yet another advertising campaign for the drug. The company stressed that three scientific panels of national experts had uniformly supported the continued marketing of the drug. The warning about aplastic anemia was phrased in such a shrouded fashion that some physicians could not even be sure why the letter was sent at all. Parke, Davis's sales figures fell off temporarily in 1952, but rebounded over the next several years and by 1958 were higher than ever.

The company relied now as it had before on the individual sales reps, who would meet with physicians one on one in private and whose conversations could never be effectively monitored by the FDA. The reps used specific pitches, provided by the company, to deal with the threat. The real problem, they would say, is that chloramphenicol had been so popular that it got the attention of the news media, and the supposed dangers were simply an example of what happens when the newspapers and magazines tried to tell doctors what to do. The reps were told by the company to say that both the FDA and the National Research Council had given their "unqualified" support to the drug, which was untrue, as both bodies had warned of the risk of blood disorders.[64] The reps were also told to mention that fifty-nine published papers, involving seventeen hundred patients taking chloramphenicol, had not turned up a single case of aplastic anemia—an irrelevant fact given the known frequency of the disorder. Even if the company had been eager to spread the true message about chloramphenicol among American physicians, as Maeder noted, "It was, of course, a difficult position in which to place a salesman, essentially sending him to peddle a product that accounted for up to 43 percent of his income but asking him to warn customers of its dangers and advise them not to use it very much."[65]

The official company statement that Harry Loynd put before the world was: "This antibiotic . . . has now successfully passed three intensive investigations, originally by Parke, Davis & Company, and more recently by the Food and Drug Administration and the . . . National Research Council. Physicians may continue to prescribe chloramphenicol for the treatment of any disease as they see fit."[66] Legally, everything Loynd said was true. If a drug is on the market, physicians can legally prescribe it for anything, no matter how unwise it would be for them to do so.

Perhaps the most disquieting evidence of how well Parke, Davis's campaign worked was discovered by Maeder in an old FDA file of a never-completed investigation. The files told of a physician in Kountze, Texas, who had graduated from medical school in 1955 and completed his internship in 1956. He had been impressed during his training with the dangers of chloramphenicol, so he used the drug sparingly in his practice. According to the later FDA field office report,

> when asked by Parke, Davis detail men how he was using the drug, he had answered that normally he used it as a "reserve." The detail men at that time suggested that the doctor go ahead and use it as a first choice drug. They further stated that Parke Davis had gone back and reinvestigated cases of blood dyscrasias that had theoretically been caused by Chloromycetin and had found that the drug was not the real cause of the anemias. One of the detail men also told Dr. ___ that research by Parke, Davis, Inc. had shown that the drug was not responsible for blood dyscrasias and the warning on the Chloromycetin and literature was there only because the FDA required such on that type of drug.[67]

Compare the case of this Texas physician with his California colleague, Dr. Watkins. Dr. Watkins, when he went through his training, was never told that a drug such as chloramphenicol existed. He had no academic understanding of the pros and cons of this drug; any information provided to him by the drug reps from

Parke, Davis therefore had no effective counterbalance in his existing medical knowledge. The Texas physician was from a newer generation. He had been taught specifically about this drug in both medical school and internship.

In one tragic way, however, this Texas physician was just like Dr. Watkins. Faced with the disconnect between what he had been taught and what the rep told him, he elected to believe the rep and dismiss what he had been taught. The physician's own seven-year-old son developed an ear and throat infection, and the local rep advised him to treat it with chloramphenicol. He did, and the child later died of aplastic anemia.[68] FDA was able to track down one other death in the immediate area in which doctor had been told same thing by Parke, Davis reps.

In 1965, James Goddard became the FDA commissioner. He was armed with new legal authority as a result of the Kefauver-Harris amendments passed in the wake of thalidomide, and was willing to do battle with the industry. Nonetheless, Goddard was reduced to saying in 1968, "Despite the risks associated with the use of chloramphenicol, if one may judge from the sales figures, use of the drug continues to be excessive. Where have the FDA, the manufacturer, and the medical profession failed? Is the general medical community unaware of, or unconcerned about, the risks associated with this drug? . . . The 'box warning' in the labeling is strongly worded and tells the physician quite bluntly the dangers of the drug, yet it has not accomplished its intended purpose."[69]

Through the mid-1960s, physicians continued to prescribe chloramphenicol in the same promiscuous fashion. Then, in 1966, the patent expired and the drug was available in generic form. It was no longer worthwhile for Parke, Davis reps to push the drug. Virtually overnight, use of the antibiotic plummeted. The average physician, asked now why he did not use the drug more often, would say something like, "Are you kidding? That drug kills people!" Once the voice of the drug rep had been stilled, the voice of medical science suddenly could be heard clearly. But before that, while the voice of the drug rep remained loud and persistent, there was, as Senator Nelson noted, no contest. As with the unfortunate physician in Texas, the rep's voice easily won the day.

Thus affairs stood in the 1960s. In the next chapters we will bring this portrayal up to date and look at some more recent data on physician-pharmaceutical representative interactions.

NOTES

1. Quoted in T. Maeder, *Adverse Reactions* (New York: William Morrow and Company, 1994), 9.

2. For that reason the name "patent medicine" is a misnomer; if the medicine were patented the formula would have to be on file with the government and would be publicly accessible. In actuality these firms sought copyright and not patent protection. P. Starr, *The Social Transformation of American Medicine* (New York: Basic Books, 1982), 128.

3. Starr, *Social Transformation*.

4. The specific term "ethical drug company" appeared around the turn of the twentieth century. I have been unable to identify its exact origins. According to AMA *Journal* editor George H. Simmons, writing in 1907, the first resolution attacking proprietary (copy-

righted) medicines as specifically contrary to the AMA Code of Ethics was passed in 1879, but it did not specifically mention "ethical drugs" or "ethical drug houses," and those terms appear to have come into use somewhat later; G. H. Simmons, "The Commercial Domination of Therapeutics and the Movement for Reform," *JAMA* 1907; 48:1645–53.

5. On the Progressive Era and the battle against patent medicines, see Starr, *Social Transformation*, 127–31; P. J. Hilts, *Protecting America's Health: The FDA, Business, and One Hundred Years of Regulation* (New York: Alfred A. Knopf, 2003), 35–55. Two of the more important muckraking articles exposing the patent medicine makers were Samuel Hopkins Adams's "The Great American Fraud," published in *Collier's Magazine* in 1905–1906, and Mark Sullivan's accounts of the Lydia Pinkham company, summarized by editor E. Bok, "The Patent Medicine Curse," *Ladies' Home Journal*, September, 1905, 15.

6. On the data for prescription drugs in the 1930s, see N. Hawkins, "Detailmen and Preference Behavior," *Southwestern Social Science Quarterly* 1959; 40:213–34.

7. *Wellcome's Excerpta Therapeutica*, U.S.A. 1916 ed. (New York: Burroughs Wellcome and Company, 1916).

8. I am grateful to Declan O'Reilly for drawing this volume to my attention.

9. M. Smith, *Principles of Pharmaceutical Marketing* (Philadelphia: Lea & Febiger, 1975), 314.

10. A 1907 address by George H. Simmons of the AMA quotes a resolution to the AMA House of Delegates from three years before that refers to drug company salesmen as "drummers," but then goes on to mention "detail men" twice, suggesting that at least by that date the latter term was in common usage; Simmons, "Commercial Domination of Therapeutics."

11. R. L. McQuillan, *Is the Doctor In? The Story of a Drug Detail Man's Fifty Years of Public Relations with Doctors and Druggists* (New York: Exposition Press, 1963). McQuillan did not name the company he worked for. He recounted receiving only a few hours of informal training before being turned loose.

12. J. A. Greene, "Attention to 'Details': Etiquette and the Pharmaceutical Salesman in Postwar American" [*sic*]. *Soc Stud Sci* 2004; 34:271–92.

13. S. M. Rothman and D. J. Rothman, *The Pursuit of Perfection: The Promise and Perils of Medical Enhancement* (New York: Vintage, 2004), 49, in turn citing a study by the Committee on the Cost of Medical Care (1932). By contrast, another source claimed that in the 1930s, only about 3 to 8 percent of drug sales were accounted for by prescription drugs; Hawkins, "Detailmen and Preference Behavior." On the date at which the "drummer" or old-fashioned drug salesman could have been said to have been transformed into the modern "detail man," Puckner and Leech wrote in 1929, "In the past, when medical schools taught much about drugs and little that was scientific about the actions of drugs, physicians were inclined to look to the pharmaceutic 'detail man' for instruction in the use of medicines"; W. A. Puckner and P. Leech, "The Introduction of New Drugs," *JAMA* 1929; 93:1627–30, quote p. 1627; quoted in N. Rasmussen, "The Drug Industry and Clinical Research in Interwar America: Three Types of Physician Collaborator," *Bull Hist Med* 2005; 79:50–80. The notion of the "detail man" therefore appears to have predated 1929 by a goodly margin.

14. Rothman and Rothman, *The Pursuit of Perfection*, 54–55.

15. Hawkins, "Detailmen and Preference Behavior."

16. Rothman and Rothman, *The Pursuit of Perfection*, 55, citing in turn "Abbott Laboratories," *Fortune* 22 (August 1940): 63–66.

17. T. Jones, *Detailing the Physician: Sales Promotion by Personal Contact with the Medical and Allied Professions* (New York: Romaine Pierson Publishers, 1940), 17.

18. A. F. Peterson, *Pharmaceutical Selling, "Detailing," and Sales Training,* 2nd ed. (Scarsdale, NY: Heathcote-Woodbridge, Inc., 1959), 2. Jeremy Greene uses this passage (which appeared in both the 1949 and 1959 editions of Peterson) as evidence that a fundamental shift had occurred in the self-perception and professional aspirations of reps since Jones wrote in 1940; Greene, "Attention to 'Details,'" 274. As I will argue shortly, I believe that this interpretation takes the single quotation from Peterson out of context.

19. Peterson, *Pharmaceutical Selling,* 5.

20. Peterson, *Pharmaceutical Selling,* 227.

21. The 17:1 ratio is from Ben Gaffin and Associates, *Attitudes of U.S. Physicians toward the American Pharmaceutical Industry,* Chicago, 1959; I have been unable to obtain a copy of this document. The statistic is quoted in R. Bauer and L. Wortzel, "Doctor's Choice: The Physician and His Sources of Information about Drugs," *Journal of Marketing Research* 1966; 3:40–47. Caplow reported in 1952 that a sample of 129 practitioners in the Midwest characterized drug reps as follows: would prefer not to see them at all—14 percent; generally favorable but there are too many of them and/or they are not well informed—17 percent; generally favorable—47 percent; enthusiastic—22 percent; T. Caplow, "Marketing Attitudes: A Research Report from the Medical Field," *Harvard Bus Rev* 1952; 30:105–12. Rufus McQuillan, who was a detail man from roughly 1919 to 1959, could conceive of no legitimate reason why a physician would refuse to see him, unless the physician was either extremely quirky, unutterably rude, or an incurable snob; McQuillan, *Is the Doctor In?* Peterson wrote in his 1959 manual, "But in fact the erudite [representative] will meet with so few physicians who do not receive him cordially that discourtesy is hardly worth a mention"; Peterson, *Pharmaceutical Selling,* 129.

22. W. Bean, "Vitamania, Polypharmacy and Witchcraft," *AMA Archives of Internal Medicine* 1955; 96:137–41.

23. J. Lear, "The Certification of Antibiotics," *Saturday Review,* February 7, 1959: 43–48; quote p. 45.

24. K. M. Ludmerer, *Time to Heal: American Medical Education from the Turn of the Century to the Era of Managed Care* (New York: Oxford University Press, 1999).

25. See, for example, J. W. Ely, J. A. Osheroff, M. L. Chambliss, et al., "Answering Physicians' Clinical Questions: Obstacles and Potential Solutions," *J Am Med Inform Assoc* 2005; 12:217–24.

26. Before 1938, when the FDA gained new powers to demand evidence of drug safety prior to marketing, companies routinely devoted more effort to gaining AMA council acceptance than to getting FDA approval; Rasmussen, "Drug Industry and Clinical Research in Interwar America."

27. A survey conducted in 1939 reported that 81 percent of physicians in Chicago read the *Journal of the American Medical Association* regularly and 79 percent noticed the ads in it; J. E. Jeuck, "Direct-Mail Advertising to Doctors," *J Bus* 1940; 13:17–38. A follow-up survey of physicians in smaller towns across the nation showed an even higher readership of 85 percent; R. B. Rand, "Pharmaceutical Advertising to Doctors," *J Bus* 1941; 14:150–68.

28. Hilts, *Protecting America's Health,* 126.

29. Hilts, *Protecting America's Health,* 127; for a less critical account see H. F. Dowling, *Medicines for Man: The Development, Regulation, and Use of Prescription Drugs* (New York: Alfred A. Knopf, 1970), 153–77.

30. "Medical Advertising—Sales Tool, Postgraduate Course for M.D.," *Advertising Age* 1963; 34(1): 216–19.

31. Pharmaceutical Advertising Club, *A Research Study on Pharmaceutical Advertising* (Croton-on-Hudson, NY: Pharmaceutical Advertising Club), 1955.

32. Testimony before the Kefauver Senate hearings on the drug industry in the early 1960s showed how persistent the firms could be in flooding physicians' mailboxes. One doctor testified that he had ordered his staff to throw away all ads that arrived as bulk mail. The ads began to arrive in his office as first-class mailings with no company name on the envelope and giving the name of the medical director of the company as the return address. When he caught onto this ploy, the companies started to send him ads airmail. Finally the firms resorted to mailing the advertising material from foreign countries. Apparently detail people in the area tipped off the companies to what was or was not working. R. Harris, *The Real Voice* (New York: Macmillan, 1964), 90: "Any device, regardless of expense, will be used to overcome the physician's resistance." Caplow reported in 1952 that the volume of mail ads had roughly doubled between 1940 and 1950, and physicians were five times as likely to report that they resented direct-mail ads in the latter year; Caplow, "Marketing Attitudes."

33. Neither Tom Jones nor Arthur Peterson makes any mention of gifts of any sort, besides drug samples, in manuals for detail men; Jones, *Detailing the Physician*; Peterson, *Pharmaceutical Selling*. Peterson, in fact, specifically advises against giving small gifts and trinkets to the receptionist as a way to gain admission to the physician, and argues for a miserly policy with regard to giving free samples of medications. Similarly, though McQuillen, in his reminiscences of forty years as a detail man starting in 1919, several times describes in detail the contents of a typical traveling bag, it is full of samples and literature but never of other giveaway items; McQuillan, *Is the Doctor In?* 87.

34. M. Nickerson, "Doctors, Drugs and Drug Promotion," *Can Med Assoc J* 1959; 80:520–24, quote p. 520; this paper was one of the few of its era to take a generally negative slant toward the commercial bias of industry marketing: "[I]f one does not have the time, the facilities or the inclination personally to evaluate [the] wares [pushed by drug advertising and detailers], less harm will be done if they are ignored completely. Remember that advertising is advertising"(p. 524).

35. R. Carter, *The Doctor Business* (Garden City, NY: Doubleday, 1958), 140. Dr. Dale Console, former medical director of Squibb, testified before a Senate committee in the early 1960s about "the free cocktail party and the golf outing complete with three golf balls stamped with the name of the doctor and the company in contrasting colors." P. R. Garai, "Advertising and Promotion of Drugs," in *Drugs in Our Society*, ed. P. Talalay and J. H. Murnaghan (Baltimore: Johns Hopkins University Press, 1964), 189–202; quote p. 192.

36. Studies demonstrating social desirability bias include Caplow, "Marketing Attitudes"; C. Rabe, "The Doctor Measures Detailmen," *Med Economics* 1952; 11:19–25; T. Caplow and J. Raymond, "Factors Influencing the Selection of Pharmaceutical Products," *Journal of Marketing* 1954; 19:18–23; H. Menzel and E. Katz, "Social Relations and Innovation in the Medical Profession: The Epidemiology of a New Drug," *Public Opinion Quarterly* 1955–56; 19:337–52; J. Coleman, E. Katz, and H. Menzel, "The Diffusion of an Innovation among Physicians," *Sociometry* 1957; 20:253–70; R. Ferber and H. G. Wales, *The Effectiveness of Pharmaceutical Promotion* (Urbana: University of Illinois College of Commerce and Business Administration, 1958); J. Coleman, E. Menzel, and E. Katz, "Social Processes in Physicians' Adoption of a New Drug," *J Chron Dis* 1959; 9:1–19; Hawkins, "Detailmen and Preference Behavior"; R. Bauer, "Risk Handling in Drug Adoption: Role of Company Preferences," *Public Opinion Quarterly* 1961; 25:546–59; D. Burkholder, "Role of the Pharmaceutical Detailmen in a Large Teaching Hospital," *Am J Hosp Pharm* 1963; 20:274–85; C. Wilson, "Influence of Different Sources of Therapeutic Information on Prescribing by General Practitioners," *Br Med J* 1963; 2:599–604; C. Wilson, "Therapeutic Sources for Prescribing in Great Britain," *Journal of New Drugs* 1963; 3:276–86; Bauer and Wortzel,

"Doctor's Choice"; R. W. Fassold and C. W. Gowdey, "A Survey of Physicians' Reactions to Drug Promotion," *Can Med Assoc J* 1968; 98:701–5. A review of much of this literature is D. B. Worthen, "Prescribing Influences: An Overview," *Br J Med Educ* 1973; 7:109–17. A rare study in which interactions between physicians and reps were directly observed, as opposed to relying on self-reporting, was R. R. Rehder, "Communication and Opinion Formation in a Medical Community: The Significance of the Detail Man," *Academy of Management Journal* 1965; 8:282–91.

37. Bauer and Wortzel, "Doctor's Choice." Gaffin tried to correct for social desirability bias by asking physicians also what sources the physicians thought *other doctors* relied on, and received roughly the same answers.

38. Bauer and Wortzel, "Doctor's Choice," quoting D. Noyes, "Your Share of Disposable Professional Time," *Modern Medicine Topics* 17 (June 1956): 5–7. This figure was actually down from a reported 1.3 hours in 1952.

39. S. Garb, "The Reaction of Medical Students to Drug Advertising," *N Engl J Med* 1958; 259:121–23; S. Garb, "Teaching Medical Students to Evaluate Drug Advertising," *J Med Educ* 1960; 35:729–39.

40. Lear, "Certification of Antibiotics," 44–45.

41. McQuillan, *Is the Doctor In?* McQuillan failed to specify the physician's name or the year of publication, and left unclear whether "Medical Journal" is the full name or only an abbreviation for the publication.

42. C. D. May, "Selling Drugs by 'Educating' Physicians," *J Med Educ* 1961; 36:1–23; quote p. 1.

43. As we will see in more detail later, when we review the history of the FDA, many things were happening around the time May wrote this article. Senator Estes Kefauver was holding a series of hearings in the U.S. Senate that mostly attacked the pharmaceutical industry but that also indirectly embarrassed medicine. John Lear, science editor of the *Saturday Review*, had written a series of articles that exposed the silliness of combination antibiotics, the shameless methods used by the industry to promote them, and the ease with which physicians had been swayed by that marketing. It seems to be a general truth that medicine belatedly wakes up to its own professional obligations when the outside world starts to peer in and comment.

44. May, "Selling Drugs," 1.

45. May, "Selling Drugs," 1.

46. Cited by Garai, "Advertising and Promotion of Drugs." *Advertising Age* estimated in 1963 that the industry spent one thousand dollars per U.S. physician annually on promotion, at that time with the largest proportion of the money being spent on print ads; "Medical Advertising—Sales Tool, Postgraduate Course for M.D." Adjusting for inflation, this would represent approximately six thousand dollars in 2003 dollars. This suggests, according to modern estimates, that the per-physician promotional spending by industry has roughly doubled in that interval; S. Wolfe, "Why Do American Drug Companies Spend More Than $12 Billion a Year Pushing Drugs? Is It Education or Promotion?" *J Gen Intern Med* 1996; 11:637–39.

47. May, "Selling Drugs," 7.

48. Harris, *The Real Voice*, 91.

49. Pierre Garai reported in 1964 that no more than 25,000 out of the 180,000 physicians in North America had subscribed to this inexpensive, "indispensable adjunct to conscientious practice"; Garai, "Advertising and Promotion of Drugs." Currently the *Medical Letter* website claims a total circulation of 120,000 but does not state how many of these are U.S. physicians; www.medletter.com/html/who.htm (accessed March 6, 2005).

50. L. Lasagna, "The Drug Industry and American Medicine," *J Chronic Dis* 1958; 7:440–43.

51. Harris, *The Real Voice*, 15–16.

52. May, "Selling Drugs," 16.

53. This response of the pharmaceutical industry to academic critics had been tried, with apparent success, well before 1961. Dr. Henry Harrower was the founder of Harrower Laboratory, Inc. in California, manufacturer of Henry Harrower's Gonad Tablets (an "ethical" product since it was marketed directly to physicians and druggists only). Harrower had at first been a legitimate investigator but broke with his fellow endocrinologists over the profligate use of hormones. He then began to edit his own journal, *The Endocrine Survey*, aimed at the general practitioner. The *Survey* was full of editorials deriding the academic physicians for their prejudices and narrow-mindedness and urging physicians to prescribe drugs based rather on their own common sense and personal testimonials from grateful patients; Rothman and Rothman, *The Pursuit of Perfection*, 144–45.

54. Harris, *The Real Voice*, 92.

55. A more ominous rebuttal to critiques of drug marketing came from George R. Cain, president of Abbott Laboratories, writing in the *Bulletin of the New York Academy of Medicine* in 1962: "Critics have claimed that the detail man is of little value in the total health picture, and yet surveys show that 96 per cent of all doctors who see detail men value their services and the information they supply. . . . [I]t is clear that various critics are trying to accomplish certain objectives leading toward socialized medicine." G. R. Cain, "The Detail Man—What the Pharmaceutical Industry Expects of Him," *Bull NY Acad Med* 1962; 38:126–34, quote pp. 133–34.

56. M. Silverman and P. R. Lee, *Pills, Profits and Politics* (Berkeley: University of California Press, 1974), 110.

57. T. S. Maeder, *Adverse Reactions* (New York: William Morrow and Company, 1994), 207. Maeder's book as a whole is a comprehensive analysis of chloramphenicol.

58. Hilts, *Protecting America's Health*, 108–16, provides a concise history of chloramphenicol.

59. Later, in our chapter on the FDA, we will see that Welch became involved in the first major conflict-of-interest scandal at that agency. There is no evidence, however, that he dealt with the chloramphenicol case with anything less than complete integrity.

60. Maeder, *Adverse Reactions*, 152.

61. Maeder, *Adverse Reactions*, 160.

62. *Competitive Problems in the Drug Industry*, Part 11, 91st Congress, 1st session, 1969, 4484–85; quoted in Maeder, *Adverse Reactions*, 191–92.

63. The "ivory tower" view implicitly made yet another assumption—that bacteriological cultures yielded 100 percent accurate results. This is not the place for a discourse on clinical epidemiology, quantitative decision analysis, and evidence-based medicine. Suffice it to say that by the 1990s, it had become more clear among thoughtful primary care physicians that the strategy most spurned by the "experts" of Dr. Console's day—treating a disease "empirically" without first making a precise bacteriological or tissue diagnosis—was in some instances the *most rational* strategy, statistically shown to produce the largest number of good outcomes. The old community GP who treated his patients according to "what happened to be going around town" at any given time turned out in hindsight to be, unwittingly, practicing the most rational medicine.

64. Hilts, *Protecting America's Health*, 112.

65. Maeder, *Adverse Reactions*, 212.

66. Hilts, *Protecting America's Health*, 112.

67. Quoted in Maeder, *Adverse Reactions*, 222.

68. Maeder, *Adverse Reactions*, 222. The FDA was able to track down one other death in the immediate area in which the doctor had reportedly been told essentially the same thing by Parke, Davis reps. Apparently the evidence in the two cases was in the end insufficient to take any formal action.

69. M. C. Smith, "Drug Product Advertising and Prescribing: A Review of the Evidence," *Am J Hosp Pharm* 1977; 34:1208–24, quote p. 1220.

9

THE DRUG REP TODAY

Few doctors accept that they themselves have been corrupted. Most doctors believe that they are quite untouched by the seductive ways of industry marketing men; that they are uninfluenced by the promotional propaganda they receive; that they can enjoy a company's "generosity" in the form of gifts and hospitality without prescribing its products. The degree to which the profession, mainly composed of honourable and decent people, can practice such self deceit is quite extraordinary. No drug company gives away its shareholders' money in an act of disinterested generosity.

—Dr. M. D. Rawlins, 1984[1]

INTO THE TWENTY-FIRST CENTURY

In chapter 8, we saw how Dr. Charles May in 1961 had included expensive meals and lavish entertainment in his list of typical gifts received by practitioners from drug reps.[2] And an FDA staff physician explained the popularity of reps among rural physicians, during the same time period, by noting, "In small towns, they not only bring doctors free samples and information but open up their bags and give them presents of all sorts—desk sets, expensive calendars, elaborate medical charts, illuminated anatomy figures, monogrammed golf balls, and so on."[3] May's remarks about gifts, and the FDA physician's allusion to desk sets and monogrammed golf balls, suggest that between the 1940s and the 1960s the spigot of largesse gradually opened wider and wider.

One of the few serious efforts to quantify the value of these gifts, on a per-physician-per-year basis, came with the hearings held by Senator Edward Kennedy (D-Mass.) in 1991.[4] These hearings set the estimated value at about $125; but this figure could easily be a serious underestimate, and could also mask the fact that a small minority of physicians received unusually lavish gifts. In 2004, the first annual report was issued by the attorney general of Vermont, under a new law that required the companies to report gifts worth more than $25. According to that report, the average Vermont prescriber (not all of whom are physicians) was the recipient of $228.[5] Again there are many reasons to regard this figure as a serious underestimate, especially since we can imagine that the Vermont reps made special efforts to package their gifts in ways that brought many exchanges under the $25 reporting limit.

In 1991, Jared Haft Goldstein, a family physician in Randleman, North Carolina, decided to come clean on "the following noninclusive list of material influences received from drug companies since my freshman year in medical school":

> Breakfasts, lunches, dinners, candy, popcorn, tea, herbs, sherry, doughnuts, pizza, wassail mix, books, free journals subsidized by advertising, subscription journals kept to a low price because of advertising subsidies, stethoscope, reflex hammer, black bag, pencils, pens, eraser, EKG caliper, tape measure, various anatomic models, diaphragm fitting set, various wall charts, calendars, *Physicians' Desk References*, date-due calculation wheel, mugs, magnifying glass, penlights, refrigerator magnets, umbrella, cassette holder, various tape cassettes (medical and nonmedical), gym bag, towel, cooler, antique medicine bottle, Moebius strip, sandglasses, facial tissues, picture frames, clocks, paperclip holders, penholders, desk set, paperweights, chart holders, drug samples for personal and family use, notepads, parenteral drug samples for office administration, prescription pads, calculator, pocket diaries, electronic diary, appointment book, paperclips, "honoraria," two children's worth of formula, sun visor, waterproof keyholder, Thermos, maps, coaster, slide viewer, wallet, drug-dosage card, nailclippers, pocketknife, teddy bear pin, letter opener, tongue depressors, bookends, toothbrush, Chapstick, keyring, sunscreen, adhesive bandage dispenser, kilt pin, candy jar, novelty pens, and, my personal favorite, a lighted night-table paper-and-pen holder.[6]

As the gifts increased in number and value, the ethical antennae of the physicians were slow to recalibrate. Once the habit of seeing the reps, listening to their advice, and accepting their trinkets became part and parcel of everyday medical practice, physicians were unlikely to notice that the stakes gradually got larger and larger from one year to the next—except, as we shall see later, for a small number of greedy physicians who appear willing to milk the system for whatever they can get. Among most physicians, the greater value of gifts received would simply trigger more creative rationalizations—rationalizations that the reps themselves, always eager to further cement their friendly relationships with the practitioner and to bypass his critical faculties, were happy to suggest and supply. That made it much easier for the medical rank and file to reject the Charles Mays of the profession as ivory-tower intellectuals totally removed from "real" medicine.

THE CAREER OF A TYPICAL DRUG REP

Drug reps increased from 56,000 in 1990 to almost 88,000 in 2000—a 57 percent increase as compared with a 10 percent increase in research and development staff during the same period.[7] By 2001 it was reported that there were 90,000 reps, 1 for every 4.7 office-based physicians.[8] "A St. Louis, Missouri, opening for a salesperson with a college degree and at least a year of experience seems fairly typical: It offers base pay of $45,000 to $60,000 a year, plus commission, 5,000 shares of stock options, medical and dental coverage, a 401(k) and a company car."[9]

It's very hard to locate, in the published literature on the pharmaceutical industry, a candid interview with a pharmaceutical sales representative who is willing to speak on the record. An extended confession of a former drug rep, published on the Healthy Skepticism website, apparently saw print because the author concealed not only his name and the name of the companies he had worked for, but even the country in which he lived.[10]

I had the good fortune to be able to interview several former drug reps who later ended up in medical school. What follows is based on a compilation of their recollections.[11] I'll call the "typical" drug rep depicted in this story "Stan," and the company that employed him "Pinkham."

Finding a Job

Stan was a biology major in college and then taught high school biology. He found this boring and thought about going to medical school, but he was turned down the first year he applied. He then got a job working in a medical office to be closer to the world he hoped to enter. He started to meet the drug reps who came to visit the office and realized that they had much better paying jobs than he did. He recalled that a college friend had contacts in the industry, and through that friend he landed an interview with a Pinkham sales recruiter.

The interview went well. Stan wondered if his lack of sales experience would count against him, but it seemed that Pinkham was looking for a likeable person who could get along well with physicians and office staff, not a "pushy" sales-type person. "They don't hire car salesmen," was how Stan put it. When Stan started his training two months later, he also discovered that a college science background was not required. He found himself among lawyers and literature majors as well as many other types.[12]

Pinkham had assigned Stan to the sales force for its anti-ulcer drugs. Stan read up on the scientific mechanisms by which these drugs worked and the clinical trial studies that reported how the drugs performed in human subjects. He also learned about all the competitor drugs on the market and how each company was positioning its drug for potential sales. His fellow reps with poorer science backgrounds got extra tutoring. Pinkham did not generally flunk reps out of the initial training program, but there were regular pop quizzes and "it was pretty intense."[13]

Stan was given a thick book of materials—he remembers how excited he was when the huge carton from Pinkham first arrived at his home. He was instructed never to show this to a physician as it was not formally FDA approved. For the same reason, reps were told never to work up their own materials. Stan was asked to sign a form to keep everything in his training manual confidential. "Most of us didn't read it all the way through and just signed."

The training program focused both on sales and on building relationships with physicians. For instance, Stan learned that the best way to sell was to stress how the drug helps *the physician* as well as the patient. He might say, for instance, that because the drug caused fewer side effects, the physician would be bothered by fewer irate phone calls. Other sessions focused less on relationship building and more on sales techniques. Stan was told never to settle for vague agreement, but always to "close," to get the physician to commit to prescribing the drug. Role play activities honed these skills: "They told us that the relationship is important but you've got to sell your drug."

Training then turned to the gifts reps would be giving to physicians. Stan was told that on average, one hundred dollars was the upper limit for the value of a gift. It was considered out of line to drop a bottle of alcohol at the physician's office; but it was all right to buy a bottle if Stan was with the physician at an entertainment venue where it was sold. When the reps asked questions, they were often told "use your judgment" and that they would find a lot of variation from one territory to another.

During his training, Stan came to feel proud that he worked for Pinkham, which was viewed as having high standards, as opposed to Company X, whose "reps who would run over their own grandmother to make a sale." Stan heard accounts of Pinkham reps going to offices and hospitals where they saw flyers left by other company reps for things they knew were out of line—"Come to dinner and we'll fill up your gas," or even travel on a cruise ship. He also heard stories of how Company X reps had trashed the Pinkham samples or educational handouts when they were allowed unattended into the physicians' back offices.

One incident during training was a less pleasant reminder of how much loyalty was demanded by the company. During one session, Stan and another rep trainee asked a few rather pointed, technical questions about the side effects of one of the drugs they would be detailing. Stan was remembering his biology training and that he still hoped some day to get into medical school. After that session the two of them were pulled aside by one of the supervisors. Why were they asking these questions? In what way did they imagine this would help them do a better job in company sales? Nothing of a threatening nature was said out loud. But Stan came away knowing that asking more questions along those lines in the future would pretty clearly mark him as lacking an essential quality that Pinkham would be looking for when it came time to pass out bonuses and promotions.

In the Field

Stan trained at headquarters for a month and then was sent to his first assignment, knowing that every four to six months he'd be called back for some brief refresher training. He felt very fortunate to be assigned to a territory in Metropolis, covering a portion of the inner city and some of the adjoining suburbs, because he would have a partner who already knew the region well. Stan spent his first week setting up his home office, getting all his supplies and stocks of samples organized. Two pieces of equipment were essential—a thick binder that his partner showed him, and his personal laptop. The binder listed the food and entertainment sources in the territory, about fifty restaurants and caterers. Stan was told that they would occasionally use all of them but that they'd concentrate on about fifteen that had proven themselves highly reliable and would deliver. Stan knew that his main job was to keep the laptop up-to-date. Each week he'd receive a company data download, giving Pinkham's total sales in his territory, and what anti-ulcer drugs each of his assigned physicians had prescribed, both Pinkham's and the competitors'. (There was about a three- to six-week lag from the week when the prescriptions were written to the week Stan received the data on his laptop.) Stan would use this same laptop to enter a log of each contact with a physician: did you see the doctor or only office staff; did you leave samples; any details about what worked or what didn't that would help a later rep. In Stan's case he did not have to rely so much on the laptop database, as his partner filled him in on what worked for each of the one hundred physicians in their territory, and whom to talk to in the office to get access.

After his get-acquainted week, Stan started out in earnest. He and his partner split the territory in half, the inner city and the suburbs, each taking one part for a week at a time. Their goal was ideally that each doctor would be visited by one of the two partners each week; actually they managed more like two visits per month.

"I still remember my first detail," Stan said. "I saw a family doc who was an important guy in the community, and he was a big user of our product. The community was about to throw a party in his honor after twenty-five years in practice. He asked me for a donation of four to five hundred dollars for this party. I wasn't ready for that request. I said I'd see about it and went back to my district manager. She said, 'Is the guy important for sales in your region? Okay, then if he's really important, we'll go ahead.' I gave him four hundred dollars. I later realized that was why he agreed to see me in the first place, with me being the new rep and all—because he wanted that money."

Just where did that four hundred dollars come from? Stan described how the books were kept at Pinkham, so far as he was allowed to see. First, he had his salary—at the time the standard starting salary was around fifty thousand dollars. To that would be added bonuses, which we'll get to later. Stan also enjoyed a very generous set of fringe benefits, and full-time use of a company car. Then he had an "immediate-needs account" which covered phone bills, gas, and similar expenses. Two kinds of supplies were simply ordered in quantity; Stan never paid for them and was never told what they cost. These were the "branding items" (the pens, notepads, coffee mugs, and whatever had the Pinkham logo on it) and the drug samples.

Then there was the "entertainment account." This would pay for all food and entertainment expenses for both Stan and the physician, as long as the physician was present at the time of the expense. These items all had to be recorded and submitted to the district manager for reimbursement. Presumably the four hundred dollars for the family physician's twenty-five-year party came out of this fund. How much was in the "entertainment account" seemed to be a secret at the managerial level. Stan got the impression that the limit on this account was "over six figures." He knew from his own accounting that during one year he exceeded a hundred thousand dollars in entertainment plus his own office supplies, and no one complained. Whenever he asked the manager about spending limits, he was told that things were all right because sales were good in that territory, or else that if he was spending too much, the district manager would tell him. "I never felt money was an issue."[14]

Stan got to witness two different bonus systems during his time at Pinkham. The company, at the time he was hired on, was a high-salary, low-bonus firm. At first Stan got only about a five-thousand-dollar annual bonus, based on Pinkham's over-all sales performance that year. But soon Pinkham found itself losing some of its best reps to competitors with more generous bonus plans. A new plan was insti-tuted with a bonus paid quarterly, pegged to Stan's individual sales performance. Last year's sales set the benchmark, and he could earn a bonus depending on how far he exceeded them each quarter. On this new system Stan found that he could sometimes earn an extra seven thousand dollars per quarter.

The Physicians Respond

Stan soon got to know the daily routine of his territory. He found the inner-city physicians generally much easier to visit. They needed his free samples for their indigent patients and came to depend on the notepads and pens, so they always seemed happy to see him. Stan had been trained to try to discourage the doctors from using samples to treat a patient long term, but those with a heavy indigent population felt they had no choice. It was better if Stan could persuade them to use a starter coupon, good for a free prescription; that at least got the physician started writing a prescription for the drug. Stan soon discovered how much red tape was involved with samples. He had to fill out forms for all samples and was told to keep copies of those forms for five years after he left the company.

The suburban doctors were a harder sell. To Stan, they seemed to view them-selves as more elite. He felt he had to fight harder to get any of the coveted "face time" with them, and they always seemed less appreciative for whatever they re-ceived. But even here, Stan gradually came to find out what worked. His laptop gradually logged in all the weaknesses of each doctor—their favorite foods, their favorite drinks, their birthdays. "I could go to their offices on the right day and say 'Happy Birthday' and it meant a lot. If all else failed I could use the medical school ploy—tell them I planned to reapply to medical school and I was seeking their advice."

And golf, of course. Stan took golf lessons and considered it a good investment for his career. "I loved those golf games because I had so much time with the docs. You could do the sales part in a couple of holes and all the rest of the time was just getting to know them personally. When we had a game, the physician would never pay for anything. I paid all the fees, bought lunch and drinks, sometimes cigars. I'd buy them golf balls sometimes, but usually not right there at the club; that was get-ting near the limit of what we were allowed." The district manager had an extra pot of money that Stan knew little about, but she used that to buy three or four of their highest-prescribing physicians memberships in upscale golf clubs, costing about ten thousand dollars each, Stan guessed. At the district rep meetings Stan ob-served that some of the women reps who did not play golf, or who played badly, seemed to suffer as a result.

Stan looked back at his experiences and made estimates about the total popula-tion of physicians he dealt with. Maybe 5 to 7 percent of the physicians refused any contact with the reps. He was supposed to hand out reprints of the scientific studies of the performance of his drugs, but a relatively small percentage seemed very interested in getting these. About 60 to 70 percent seemed eager to push for better and bigger gifts. At various times he was asked for a dress, a hundred-dollar gift certificate, and dinner out at plush restaurant without a sales talk. Stan thought his most extreme request was a physician who wanted a weekend trip to a local amusement park for her child's birthday. Stan said no to the amusement park and the dress. In both cases he really felt used by the physician, but he also ran it by the district manager, who agreed these were out of line and supported him. Both doctors who were denied the gifts were angry, and they showed it by writing fewer prescriptions for Stan's drugs. By contrast, Stan discovered that the high-prescribing physicians were usually not the ones making the more outrageous requests. Indeed they were often so busy that it was hard to get them to come out to any free events.

Lest one think that Stan is exaggerating about the extent to which physicians tried to shake him down for expensive gifts, let's turn briefly to some published anecdotes. Fran Hawthorne, for her book on Merck, interviewed a drug rep who recalled taking an internist to a New York Jets pregame show. The physician brought along his six-year-old daughter, who during the show leaned over to the rep and asked if he could buy her a T-shirt. Hawthorne commented, "Even for a drug sales rep who doles out $10,000 worth of freebies a year, getting hit up by a 6-year-old is a bit much."[15] *Chicago Tribune* reporter Bruce Japsen combed the documents released in the TAP-Lupron fraud trial for examples of extreme extortion by physicians. A Cleveland urologist, who had prescribed a million dollars' worth of Lupron, threatened to switch to the competitor drug Zoladex unless he was given airline tickets and all-expense-paid trips to resorts. The same urologist also charged more than seven thousand dollars to a rep's credit card for dinners for himself and his colleagues. A Pittsburgh urologist demanded a family vacation in Italy when he could not make a scheduled trip offered to reward high-volume Lupron prescribers. Even the TAP reps refused that particular request.[16]

"You have your good days and bad days," Stan summarized. "A good day is real face-to-face interaction with a doc, maybe five minutes in the office, or if you have a lunch appointment you might have thirty minutes. You get in a groove and learn what works for different docs. In my case, I felt good about the quality of Pinkham's drug. The docs seemed to recognize that drug as quality, so it was relatively easy to sell. It felt good to push the product." Asked to describe his "ideal" practice, Stan recalled a clinic he had in his territory. "It was a private practice, they scheduled reps fifteen minutes at a time, they asked for samples but did not demand food." Bringing food for the physician and office staff, Stan said, "got to the point where it definitely demeans your character. It was a tough battle every night to have to ask did you compromise your ethics." But in many offices, feeding the staff was the magic ticket to get them to arrange the coveted face time with the physician.

Fooling the "Consultant"

Stan described an event that occurred several times during his career as a drug rep. He and perhaps twenty or twenty-five of his fellow reps in the area would rotate through a hotel meeting room at a central location in their district. Each would do his standard "detail" presentation on a single Pinkham drug. Sitting in the room, listening to each rep in turn, was a local physician. "The physician was hired for the day to be a consultant to the firm," Stan explained. "He was told that his job was to rate all these reps' presentations. He had a one-page evaluation form to fill out on each of us after he had heard us. The company explained that they wanted to fine-tune the marketing campaign, and wanted to know what worked and what didn't in the standard detail. Because he was thought of as a leading physician in the area, his views were very important to us. The company paid him five hundred or seven hundred fifty dollars for the day, plus a fancy lunch at the hotel."

"As we went in and out of the room where he sat, all us reps were laughing at the guy behind his back. What we knew, and what he didn't know, was that no one paid any attention to the papers he was filling out and that he wasn't in fact a consultant at all. Rather, he'd been selected because our data showed that he was a relatively low prescriber of our drug, but he had a very busy practice and had been targeted as a potentially much higher prescriber. Basically, the company was willing to bet five hundred or seven hundred fifty dollars that if he heard the same drug pitch all day, by the end of the day he'd be so brainwashed that he could not possibly prescribe any other drug but ours."

"A bunch of us reps did this one day where they had several of these docs in different rooms in the hotel and we shuffled among them. The district managers were running around trying to make sure that none of the docs got wind of the others being there at the same time."

Changing Times

Even in the relatively few years that Stan worked for Pinkham, he saw some changes occurring. After a while a new district manager was appointed, whom Stan found harder to work with. "I took one of the physicians to a Major League baseball game and while we were there I bought him a T-shirt. I put it down that way on my expense report and the DM refused to pay for it. It came out of my pocket. That guy was a stickler; the old DM would have had no problem. As far as that went, I was often told to buy the thing anyway, just don't write it down that way, say it was a big dinner event. I did that once when a physician said she'd start using our drug if I paid for her winter skiing weekend. I thought at first that she was joking, so I sort of backed into that one without realizing what I had promised. I did get it paid for but I couldn't write down 'ski weekend.'"

Stan also ran up against another obstacle. "The new PhRMA guidelines came into effect my last year in the field.[17] Our Pinkham CEO was on the committee to write the code so it was presented to us that this was important, we should be a leader within the industry. It was not just a charade, we meant it. I wish it had been a charade, because it hurt sales. I did a lot more lunches because now the golf and the golf balls were out. If we did a dinner now we always had to have a speaker. Our finicky DM watched the expense accounts closer. I don't know how closely the guidelines were followed in later years. For that matter, I know in other regions there was a great variability. So in the end I am not sure how much of that was my own DM as opposed to the company policy; the DM really sets the tone for what is allowed or not allowed in your area."

What about those laptop files that included virtually every prescription written by each physician in the territory? "We were told not to tell the docs we had this information, that they didn't want to know and it would just upset them. Also they said don't tell the pharmacists we would occasionally visit. I would ask a doc how much of my product he was writing, he'd say 'a lot,' and I'd know he was lying but would never say so." Stan guessed that maybe five out of his one hundred physicians knew that he had these data.[18]

WRITING THE BOOK ON INFLUENCE

I have suggested that today's drug rep uses many techniques that would suggest that the spirit, if not the letter, of the 1955 Dichter study still animates the industry's marketing. Lest one think that the industry has fallen behind the times, it is worth taking a look at a more recent review of marketing success, to ask how well reps follow that advice.

Influence: The Psychology of Persuasion is the title of a popular book by Arizona State University psychologist Robert B. Cialdini.[19] Cialdini's goal is to arm average consumers against the wiles of influence peddlers, by reviewing the best recent psychological research on what persuasion techniques work and why. He breaks the armamentarium of influence into six basic categories.[20]

One of Cialdini's categories, "scarcity," derives from the fact that many of us will buy something we don't really want, if we are told it will be available at this price for only a short time, or that there are only a handful of them left. Drug reps can hardly use this marketing tool in any systematic way, because the person they seek to influence, the physician, is not the purchaser or user of the product. The physician cannot write the prescription for the magic cure for erectile dysfunction until the drooping patient shows up in the office. He wants to know that this drug will be available when needed, not to hear that it is in incredibly short supply.

But all the rest of Cialdini's categories for highly effective persuasion seem directly applicable to the rep's daily routine. Cialdini notes that every one of his categories represents a natural human psychological reaction that is, in most instances, genuinely helpful (and time- and effort-saving). That means that we are conditioned at very early ages to react in these ways. The marketer need not invent a new behavior pattern. She must simply push the right button to trigger an existing, largely automatic response.

- *Reciprocation*: The salesperson who gives us a small gift or who does us a small favor is much more likely later to make a sale. Cialdini stresses how much social survival depends on reciprocity, and how important it is for the social system that the person who initiates a gift exchange can be confident that his cooperative gesture will be replied to with a similarly cooperative gesture; therefore, the sense of obligation that we owe to one who does us a favor or gives us a gift is programmed both early and deeply. Psychologists have shown that "free samples" work especially well in triggering a sense of obligation—even if they are described explicitly not as gifts but in utilitarian terms as merely "a chance to try out the product for yourself."

- *Commitment and Consistency*: Sales increase when the customer can be made to feel that *not* buying the product is at odds with a commitment he previously made or a position he previously took. Reps are trained to try to get physicians to make verbal commitments to take specific actions regarding the drug. Knowing the doctors in their territory as well as they do, they are in an excellent position to say, "You have always told me that avoiding side effects was one of your highest priorities. So when I tell you that our new pill for hypertension has the lowest side-effect profile of the ten top-selling drugs, you'll naturally want to prescribe it frequently."

- *Social Proof*: We are programmed to do what all of those around us seem to be doing. The rep is a one-person network among the local physicians, always able to tell Dr. A that Drs. B, C, D, and E are prescribing the company's new drug for all of their patients with that disease.

- *Liking*: The sales person who is attractive and likeable can sell the proverbial refrigerators to Inuits. Stan, as we saw, found a mix of people from many different backgrounds in his training course, some of whom needed considerable tutoring before they could master the scientific information. What we can assume that they all had in common was being reasonably attractive and likeable—as most who have seen groups of drug reps can readily attest. Cialdini adds that research dating back to the 1930s shows that we like people better, and are more likely to be influenced by them, when we associate them with events at which food is served.[21]

- *Authority*: We have a strong tendency—the strength of which we repeatedly underestimate—to obey and defer to those in authority or accompanied by the trappings of authority. Reps are always ready to tell us that the major "opinion-leader" physicians within our community prescribe their drugs, or to hand us reprints showing that "experts" at Harvard or Hopkins have given their drug the seal of approval.

In short, one wishing to write a book on successful marketing could use the activities of today's drug reps as virtually the centerpiece for the work.

ANOTHER PERSPECTIVE ON TODAY'S REP

Michael J. Oldani of Princeton has a unique perspective on the drug rep. He spent nine years as a rep himself before going to graduate school in anthropology.[22] Now he combines his expertise in anthropology with his own past experiences, supplemented by testimony from other personal contacts. Oldani offers the following observations that supplement our account of Stan's career.[23]

- The rep's training focuses heavily on spin. For example, one goal is to find a way to turn every objection the physician offers against the drug into a point in the drug's favor. The objection, in the first place, may have simply been a gambit on the physician's part—testing the rep to see if he knew his facts; or for that matter, just putting in a word so as not to appear too easily to be swayed by the sales pitch. The objection, for instance, that an antibiotic fails to cover the *Pseudomonas* bacteria is turned on its head by the reply (following the requisite display of empathy, "I can certainly understand, Doctor, why that would concern you") that pseudomonas is seldom acquired in the community where most infections of the type being discussed occur. The spin leads immediately to the "close" of, "Now, can I count on you to write a script for antibiotic X the next time you need to treat this infection?"[24] As always, the goal is the sale, not a dispassionate sharing of scientific information.

- Reps were also trained to take full advantage of any indebtedness the physician felt toward them. For example, a physician might call a rep to come over quickly with new information on a drug that had recently been advertised to the public. The rep was taught, in that case, to lead off with sales pitches about several older products the physician had *not* asked about, before providing the requested information on the new pill. The physician, having asked the rep to do her a favor, had no choice but to listen to the entire spiel.

- "The actual everyday pharmaceutical economy is based on social relationships that are forged and strengthened through repetitive and *calculated* acts of giving." It is important, notes Oldani, that, "Actual 'business' transactions are never conducted."[25] The physician and the rep construct a complex relationship over time, based on a variety of material exchanges—the rep giving the physician a succession of gifts, the physician showing gratitude by writing more prescriptions, which translate eventually into the rep's bonus—and yet manage all along to maintain the illusion that this is all some combination of friendship and science, that no *money* is changing hands. Oldani would be the first to chuckle at the standard physician's rationalization, "Do you think I am so pliable or unscientific that I could be bought by a pen or a sandwich?" The single pen or the sandwich is meaningless in itself; it is important only insofar as it plays a role in this complex network of exchanges and relationships.

- In further commentary on how these relationships are structured, Oldani notes, "[T]he everyday function of the pharmaceutical gift economy . . . works by 'limiting and disguising the play of economic interest and calculation' that exists at every level of pharmaceutical product promotion. The industry works very hard to maintain a *feel-good economy* for doctors and reps to coexist, where decisions for prescriptions can be based on other criteria. Thus, a paradoxical health-care economy has been created, one that is all about the patient, while simultaneously not about the patient at all."[26] Oldani adds that the first and foremost goal of the rep system is what was called at his company "moving drug," and the fact that "these drugs move in a particular direction: through patient bodies" could easily be lost sight of.[27]

- The reps learn the importance of giving first-hand. Pharmaceuticals build employee loyalty partly by the intensive training program in which reps learn basic medical language and information, and partly by showering the reps themselves with "gifts large and small: clothes, luggage, crystal bowls, social events, fine dining, company parties, increases in salary, and so on. Future sales reps *learned* the value of giving almost immediately (consciously or unconsciously) and, in return, sold products by performing these same acts with doctors. We were indoctrinated almost immediately into a corporate culture of giving."[28] Oldani's company (which he does not identify) did not pay out end-of-year cash bonuses only; it also provided points that could be redeemed in a merchandise catalogue for items ranging from TV sets to family vacations.

- As many have commented, food is the reps' "weapon of choice," causing some older reps, lugging supplies to their tenth food event of the week, to complain that they were nothing but "meals on wheels."[29]
- Stan became a rep only after the pharmaceutical industry had outsourced the task of gathering data on physicians' prescribing practices, paying independent companies to gather these data which were then downloaded weekly into the reps' laptops. When Oldani began his career in 1989, it was still the job of the rep to gather much of his information personally from local pharmacies and nursing staffs at clinics. Oldani believes that the shift to computerized data, which occurred during his sales career, substantially changed the nature and tempo of the rep-physician relationship. The rep no longer had to develop the extensive network of relationships with nonphysicians and could concentrate in seeking "face time" with the prescription writer—meaning of course that more and more reps were now competing for the coveted face time. Moreover, the data now showed much more clearly exactly who were the highest-prescribing physicians, and the reps competed even more fiercely for face time with that select group. The gift-giving wars escalated even beyond anything he had seen previously.

LAUNCHING A NEW DRUG

One of Stan's retraining weeks took him to Las Vegas, where Pinkham paid all his expenses for an entire week. The reason for this special treatment was a launch, or "roll-out," of one of the company's newest drugs. Some serious work was done, such as role-playing exercises in which reps tried out sales strategies for the new drug. But in other ways Stan reported that the week was more or less a "big party." The goal was as much to get the entire sales force excited about the new drug as to get some work done.

The highlight of the week, Stan recalled, was a musical review, put on especially for the company staff. Rather than rely on one rep's recollections of what such an event was like, I turn instead to a published account, which Stan vouched for as being completely realistic based on his own experience.

AN ANTIDEPRESSANT LAUNCH STORY

Writer Andrew Solomon has compiled one of the most comprehensive and well-researched recent books on depression.[30] Solomon is generally a defender of the pharmaceutical industry, for two reasons—first, his father works for a drug company; and second, he is extremely grateful for the industry's products that aided his own struggle with serious, recurrent depression. Solomon writes, "I tremble to think where I would be if industry had not developed the medications that have saved my life."[31]

But Solomon admitted to being somewhat uncomfortable when, presumably as a result of his father's contacts, he became one of the few outside the industry to attend the launch of a new antidepressant medication.[32] Solomon kept mum about where this was held as well as the name of the drug and the company. Solomon reported upwards of two thousand people in attendance at the launch he witnessed. The overall goal of the launch events was to prepare the company sales force to go out and aggressively market the new medication and to work them up to a fever pitch of excitement and motivation.

Solomon described the keynote event of his launch taking place in a cavernous conference center. The first thing the audience saw was an entire orchestra rising out of the stage, the way the actors first appear in the musical *Cats*. After "Forget Your Troubles, C'mon Get Happy," the orchestra swung into Tears for Fears's "Everybody Wants to Rule the World." Photos of the Grand Canyon and of a woodland brook appeared on huge screens while the booming voice of a hidden speaker, as in *The Wizard of Oz*, welcomed everyone and began to extol the new product. The lights went up on a set designed as a construction site. From the back of the stage slowly rose a wall of gigantic bricks, each emblazoned with the name of a competitor antidepressant drug. A scaffold appeared and became the moving stage on which a chorus of dancers in boots and hard hats and carrying pickaxes began to gyrate athletically and kick-dance. The names of the other antidepressants were now obscured by beams of laser light, shot out from a spacecraft hovering at the back of the auditorium and forming the new drug's logo. This became the cue for the kick-dancers to attack the wall of bricks with their pickaxes. The bricks, made of stage plaster, crashed down in huge clouds of dust. A visible speaker now appeared for the first time. The company's head of sales strode over the ruins of the competition, enthusing over the profit figures that were now being projected onto the big screen.

With the crowd now as excited as Super Bowl fans at half-time, the program suddenly switched emotional gears and started to play to the humanitarian theme. A short film depicted patients who had taken the new antidepressant during Phase III trials extolling the relief they had found from serious depression that in some cases had ruined their lives for years. The blurry focus at the edges of the screen added machine-made sentimentality, but Solomon saw the sales reps around him becoming visibly moved by the real-life stories they heard.

Solomon attended several more gatherings in the few days after the main launch event, all bouncing between the poles of hype and humanism. "In the end, however, everyone was showered with products: I came home with a T-shirt, a polo shirt, a windbreaker, a notepad, a baseball cap, an airplane carry-on, twenty pens, and a range of other goods that had the product's logo displayed as boldly as a Gucci label."[33]

NOTES

1. M. D. Rawlins, "Doctors and the Drug Makers," *Lancet* 1984; 2:814.

2. C. D. May, "Selling Drugs by 'Educating' Physicians," *J Med Educ* 1961; 36:1–23.

3. R. Harris, *The Real Voice* (New York: Macmillan, 1964), 92.

4. Senate Committee on Labor and Human Resources, *U.S. Senate Examining Practices of U.S. Pharmaceutical Companies and How Drug Prices and Prescriptions are Affected* (Washington, D.C.: U.S. Government Printing Office, 1991).

5. W. T. Sorrell, "Pharmaceutical Marketing Disclosures: Report of Vermont Attorney General," Montpelier, VT, 2004. www.atg.state.vt.us/upload/1077728093_Pharmaceutical_Marketing_Disclosures_Report.pdf (accessed March 6, 2005).

6. J. H. Goldstein, "Of Mugs and Marketing," *JAMA* 1991; 265:2391–92, quote p. 2391.

7. K. Greider, *The Big Fix: How the Pharmaceutical Industry Rips Off American Consumers.* (New York: PublicAffairs, 2003), 66

8. D. Blumenthal, "Doctors and Drug Companies," *N Engl J Med* 2004; 351:1885–90.

9. Greider, *The Big Fix*, 56; the further commission stated to be, "13K at quota, uncapped" (p. 67).

10. "Memoirs of Methods Used to Sell Drugs," MaLAM, February–March, 1999; www.healthyskepticism.org (accessed November 9, 2002).

11. An older published account that tends to confirm the general content of these interviews is M. Waldholz, "How a 'Detail Man' Promotes New Drugs to Tennessee Doctors," *Wall Street Journal*, November 8, 1982. Further general support for the details obtained in these interviews is provided by a recent drug rep memoir, J. Reidy, *Hard Sell: The Evolution of a Viagra Salesman* (Kansas City, MO: Andrews McMeel, 2005)—although Reidy's entertaining book is perhaps less about the typical drug rep and more about the rep who is devoted primarily to doing as little work as possible while covering his tracks. Another good recent source on drug rep activities is D. D. Kirkpatrick, "Inside the Happiness Business," *New York*, May 15, 2000, 37–43 (an in-depth study of the marketing of the antidepressant Celexa).

12. After this manuscript was largely completed, Stephanie Saul reported in the *New York Times* that college cheerleaders were a hot item in pharmaceutical company recruitment for future reps, so much so that a special firm had been set up to match graduating cheerleaders with companies seeking them; S. Saul, "Gimme an Rx! Cheerleaders Pep Up Drug Sales," *New York Times*, November 28, 2005:1.

13. Drug firms spent approximately $40,000 on selecting and training each rep, as of 1994; R. Levy, "The Role and Value of Pharmaceutical Marketing," *Arch Fam Med* 1994; 3:327–32, quote p. 330.

14. By contrast, Jamie Reidy reported that as a new rep for Pfizer in the mid-1990s, he was given an account for "Travel and Entertainment" that was capped at $20,000 annually; Reidy, *Hard Sell*, 74.

15. F. Hawthorne, *The Merck Druggernaut: The Inside Story of a Pharmaceutical Giant* (Hoboken, NJ: John Wiley & Sons, 2003), 136; as we have seen from Stan's account, the $10,000 figure is probably a low estimate.

16. B. Japsen, "Medicine's Gift Culture Put in an Uncomfortable Light," *Chicago Tribune*, May 16, 2004:1. For more on expensive gifts, see K. Moore and J. Harvey, "Drug Companies Push Pills to Doctors," *Cleveland Morning Journal*, August 7, 2002; S. Murphy, "Gifts Seen Effective by Drug Company Reps," *Boston Globe*, November 17, 2002; on companies' use of gifts disguised as consultant fees to evade regulations, see M. Petersen, "Merck Is Said to Limit Perks in Marketing to Physicians," *New York Times*, January 18, 2002:C1.

17. S. Hensley, "Drug Group Sets Guidelines to Curb Hard-sell Tactics," *Wall Street Journal*, April 19, 2002:A2; the code can be viewed at www.phrma.org/publications/policy// 2004-01-19.391.pdf (accessed January 31, 2005).

18. A 2001 Kaiser Family Foundation nationwide survey concluded that this practice was more widely known, with 60 percent of physicians stating that they were aware of drug reps having detailed information about their prescribing; "National Survey of Physicians, Part II: Doctors and Prescription Drugs," Kaiser Family Foundation, March 2002, www.kff.org/rxdrugs/loader.cfm?url=/commonspot/security/getfile.cfm&PageID=13965 (accessed February 2, 2005). Nevertheless, Brownlee and Lenzer, writing in 2005, still apparently felt that most physicians were unaware of these practices; S. Brownlee and J. Lenzer, "Spin Doctored: How Drug Companies Keep Tabs on Physicians," *Slate Medical Examiner*, May 31, 2005, http://slate.msn.com/id/2119712/ (accessed June 1, 2005).

19. R. B. Cialdini, *Influence: The Psychology of Persuasion* (New York: Quill/William Morrow, 1993). I am grateful to Brian Winters for suggesting this volume.

20. For a similar analysis, applied directly to pharmaceutical reps in an empirical study, see E. E. Roughead, K. J. Harvey, and A. L. Gilbert, "Commercial Detailing Techniques Used by Pharmaceutical Representatives to Influence Prescribing," *Aust N Z J Med* 1998; 28:306–10.

21. Cialdini, *Influence*, 193.

22. On his career as a drug rep, and how he came to be demoted and eventually forced out of the field, see M. J. Oldani, "Tales from the 'Script': An Insider/Outside View of Pharmaceutical Sales Practices," *Kroeber Anthropological Society Papers* 2002; 87:147–76.

23. M. J. Oldani, "Thick Prescriptions: Toward an Interpretation of Pharmaceutical Sales Practices," *Med Anthropol Q* 2004; 18:325–56.

24. Oldani, "Thick Prescriptions," 328.

25. Oldani, "Thick Prescriptions," 332.

26. Oldani, "Thick Prescriptions," 343.

27. Oldani, "Thick Prescriptions," 345.

28. Oldani, "Thick Prescriptions," 333.

29. Oldani, "Thick Prescriptions," 334.

30. A. Solomon, *The Noonday Demon: An Atlas of Depression*, New York: Scribner, 2001.

31. Solomon, *The Noonday Demon*, 395.

32. Solomon is quite reticent about the exact role that his father occupies within the industry or the firm he works for. It is therefore of interest to learn that his father is Howard Solomon, CEO of Forest Laboratories. When Forest launched its own antidepressant, Celexa (a drug the company had licensed for U.S. sale from its European manufacturer), Howard Solomon tried to inspire the sales force by reading passages from Andrew's book manuscript; Kirkpatrick, "Inside the Happiness Business," 37–43. It is not clear whether the antidepressant launch event described by Andrew Solomon is the Celexa launch or that of a different drug; the few details reported by Kirkpatrick for the Celexa launch do not fit the description given by Solomon, except for the total number in attendance.

33. Solomon, *The Noonday Demon*, 396.

⑩

THE INFLUENCE OF DRUG REPS: WHAT THE DATA SHOW

Medical training should not include acquiring a sense of entitlement to the largesse of drug companies.

—David J. Rothman[1]

Now that we have seen the activities that typical reps engage in, what do we know about the impact of this activity on medical practice? The industry position is that the activity is a benign educational service that supplies physicians with important information about pharmaceuticals in a timely way. It is also self-policing, since if any company distributed false or biased information to physicians, reps from competing companies would quickly point this out and use the fact to the first firm's detriment. How well do the facts jibe with this picture?

One of the most important resources for the facts about detailing is a website, "Drug Promotion Database," maintained by Joel Lexchin of York University, Toronto, in collaboration with the World Health Organization Department of Essential Drugs and Medicines.[2] The database includes some systematic reviews of the research literature, following an evidence-based format in which the quality of the research methods of each study is analyzed. At the time of this writing, the systematic reviews had been updated through mid-2003.

THE RESEARCH ON DRUG REP INFLUENCE

A number of conclusions appear justified in light of the available research. One way to review these conclusions is to select representative research studies to look at in some detail. The studies I have selected have either been replicated by a number of similar studies, or else have employed especially reliable research methods. The studies have been conducted in several different countries. I know of no evidence that suggests that the relationship between physicians and drug reps is substantially different in one part of the world compared to another. With some caution, it seems permissible to use studies from all regions as indicative of a global pattern.

How Extensive Is the Interaction Between Physicians and Reps?

Dr. Robert P. Ferguson headed a team from the University of Maryland that conducted a mail survey in 1997 of internal medicine specialists affiliated with the medical school hospital and two community hospitals in Baltimore. The study was hampered by a relatively low response rate of 40 percent, or 346 physicians.[3]

Of the sample, 83 percent had met with reps during the previous year, and 86 percent had received drug samples. Those who had trained in residency programs that adhered to a policy of limited contacts with drug reps were no less likely than their peers to have seen reps. Ferguson and colleagues found that there was a direct relationship between how busy the physicians reported themselves to be and how likely they were to see reps in their practices. It seems interesting that physicians with presumably the least amount of extra time available chose to spend it in this fashion.

Perhaps the best general data on the attitudes of U.S. physicians generally comes from the Kaiser Family Foundation national survey of physicians, conducted during 2001 with a sample size of about twenty-six hundred.[4] Fifteen percent rated information from drug reps as "very useful" and 59 percent rated it as "somewhat useful." Only 9 percent thought the information from that source was "very accurate," but 72 percent rated it as "somewhat accurate." Free drug samples had been accepted by 92 percent of respondents, and 61 percent admitted to receiving meals, free travel, or tickets to entertainment events. Only 13 percent stated they had received "financial or other in-kind benefits" and 12 percent had received "financial incentives to participate in drug trials." Asked what they thought about reps receiving information "about how often you prescribe certain drugs," 31 percent said that this was unacceptable; 43 percent said they were bothered by this but understood the reasons why it is done; and 22 percent indicated that they had no problem with the practice.

How Do Residents View the Appropriateness and Influence of Promotional Gifts?

Drs. Michael A. Steinman, Michael G. Shlipak, and Stephen McPhee, of the Division of General Internal Medicine at the University of California, San Francisco, surveyed 117 residents in their first and second years of training at an unnamed "large university-based internal medicine residency program" (we can presume it was their own) in the spring of 1999.[5] An excellent 90 percent of the residents responded. The residents were first asked about the appropriateness of nine different drug company promotional items. More than 80 percent of the residents viewed as appropriate a pocket antibiotic guide, a lunch conference, a dinner with an accompanying lecture, an article reprinted from a journal, and a pen with a company logo. Only 15 percent viewed a gift of luggage as appropriate. Generally, residents were more likely to think of a gift as appropriate if it was both inexpensive and somehow had educational value or content. Of the residents who viewed particular promotions as inappropriate, many nonetheless had still either accepted such items in the past or planned to do so in the future. None of the residents had refused to accept pens or free lunches at conferences.

One of the key findings of the study was the perception by the residents of the influence that contact with reps had on physicians. More than 60 percent described reps as having "no influence" over their prescribing and only about 2 percent thought reps exerted a moderate amount or a lot of influence over their prescribing practices. By contrast, only about 15 percent thought that reps had no influence over the prescribing practices of other physicians, compared to about a third of residents who thought that reps had moderate or a lot of influence over other physicians' prescribing. There was a striking (and statistically highly significant) disparity between the residents' views of themselves as immune from influence, and their views of others as relatively open to influence.[6]

Dr. Abigail Zuger, an AIDS specialist and writer in New York, commented on this phenomenon in an amusing anecdote. She described a colleague who happily scarfed up every gift and free dinner offered him by the drug reps. He was certain that he prescribed only the scientifically justified drugs, and that if they wished to throw their money away in vain attempts to influence his practice, that was their business. Then an AIDS drug that was released with much fanfare from the reps (but with precious little scientific proof of its value) was shown some months later to be potentially dangerous. Zuger's colleague was quite sure that he would have only a tiny number of patients taking that overhyped drug, but he dutifully checked his records so that all could be notified of the newfound risks. Zuger wrote that when she next saw him, he was a much chastened man. "It turns out I had a lot of people on that silly drug," he admitted. "I really can't understand how that happened."[7]

How Do Residents View Their Role in Drug Company Advertising?

Drs. Stephen K. Sigworth and Mary D. Nettleman, internists, and Gail M. Cohen, a pediatrician, decided to frisk their residents in May and June of 2000. Actually they did a survey of 181 primary care residents at their school, Virginia Commonwealth University in Richmond. First the residents were asked to complete a questionnaire, and then to empty the pockets of their white coats. The study had a highly respectable response rate of 91 percent.[8]

Virtually all the residents had eaten a meal paid for by a drug firm in the past year; unlike the residents at UCSF surveyed by Steinman and colleagues, 91 percent thought that they had been at least partially influenced by these events.

On emptying their pockets, 97 percent of the residents were found to be carrying at least one item with a drug company insignia on it; the average number was four. The items in highest use were pocket reference books, calipers (used for reading electrocardiograms), and pens. Fifty-five percent were carrying stethoscope tags with a drug company logo (an item of no practical use, purely for decoration). Fifty percent of all the items found in the residents' pockets had drug logos.

Sigworth and colleagues asked the residents if they would consider wearing a small advertising patch on their white coats if the drug company paid them to do so. Only 13 percent said they would, and on average they would demand payment of $100 annually. The investigators noted that the residents seemed quite willing to carry around a pocketful of drug company advertising for free when they saw their patients. There appeared to be a disconnect between the resident's refusal to wear a patch—presumably because of the bad impression this would make on their patients—and their indifference to carrying about with them numerous other items of an equally commercial nature. Sigworth and colleagues noted that the most likely explanation lay in the convenience of picking up the freebies offered by drug reps, compared to the need to go out of one's way to acquire "unbranded" equipment.

What Role Does Industry Promotion Play in the Dissemination of a New Drug?

Two Australian social scientists, Marilyn Y. Peay and Edmund R. Peay, studied the introduction of a new drug—temazepam, a benzodiazepine used primarily for inducing sleep (U.S. trade name, Restoril).[9] The point of view stressed by advocates for the drug was that the drug is eliminated from the body relatively quickly and so could be expected to be less likely to cause a morning hangover, or other side effects, compared to longer-acting benzodiazepines. Critics might reply that there were already a number of sleeping pills on the market, and that all benzodiazepines are potentially addictive, so that this drug really had no marked advantage over its rivals.

The Peays interviewed 124 private practitioners in Australia, both general practitioners and various specialists, about 13 months after temazepam was introduced into the market in 1980. Of the 124 doctors, 88 (71 percent) were familiar with temazepam, and reported that on average, they had found out about it about four months after its introduction. None of the 88 classed temazepam as a major therapeutic advance, but 59 (67 percent) of them had prescribed it, doing so on average about five weeks after they had first heard of it. About 61 percent stated they were now prescribing it routinely for suitable patients.

Of the 88 familiar with the drug, 68 percent first heard of it through commercial sources; 40 percent specifically identified the drug rep as their first source. Only 28 percent cited sources such as medical journals or professional meetings. Only about 28 percent of these physicians reported discussing the drug with other doctors.

The Peays then applied statistical analyses to their findings and discovered that the strongest predictor of temazepam awareness and use was both first having heard of it from a drug rep, and frequency with which that doctor visited with drug reps. In either case the physician was more likely to have heard of the drug earlier, to use it earlier, to view it as a more significant therapeutic advance, and now to be prescribing it regularly. By contrast, the physicians relying mostly on journals for their information were slower to learn about and to use the drug and tended now to prescribe other drugs rather than temazepam.

How Does Commercial Information Affect the Rationality of Physicians' Prescribing?

Drs. Adolfo Figueiras, Francisco Caamaño, and Juan Jesus Gestal-Otero, of Santiago, Spain, had an opportunity to do the sort of research in their region of Galicia that ordinarily only drug reps would be able to carry out in the United States.[10] All prescriptions in their region go into a central databank. The three researchers were therefore able to send a questionnaire to physicians in Galicia and compare the questionnaire results to the physicians' actual prescribing behavior—a more reliable method than asking physicians for a self-report of their prescribing, as was done by Peay and Peay in Australia.

They surveyed 311 physicians and got a reasonable response rate of 75 percent. They also developed several scales to measure the quality of each physician's prescribing. For example, they looked at how well the physician's prescriptions matched drugs that had been included in the formulary of the Spanish National Health Service, which experts had selected as the most suitable drugs for use in primary care clinics. They also looked at how many drugs had been prescribed for which there were no controlled clinical trials to show that the drug worked. From these various quality indicators they derived an overall score to rate the physician's quality of prescribing.

Figueiras and colleagues discovered that physicians who rated very highly the quality of information that they received from industry ads or sales reps tended to have lower quality-of-prescribing scores than physicians who rated more highly scientific, unbiased sources of information.[11]

How Aware Are Physicians of Commercial Influence on Prescribing?

Dr. Jerry Avorn, Milton Chen, and Dr. Robert Hartley of Harvard Medical School developed a clever "gotcha!" for practitioners, which they published in 1982.[12] They selected two drugs for which there was a clear disconnect between what the medical journals reported as the scientific findings and what was claimed for the drugs in commercial marketing. Propoxyphene (Darvon) was widely touted for relief of moderate pain, when the evidence showed it was no better than acetaminophin or aspirin. Several drugs, cerebral vasodilators, were argued to improve the symptoms of dementia by improving blood flow to the brain, but no published studies had shown them to have any useful effect.

The authors did telephone interviews with one hundred internists and general practitioners in Boston. (Fifteen refused to participate for an 85 percent response rate.) Of those answering, 68 percent described drug advertising as of "minimal importance" in their prescribing habits; 28 percent called it "moderately important"; and only 3 percent viewed advertising as "very important." Detail reps were considered somewhat more important, with respective figures of 54 percent, 26 percent, and 20 percent. By contrast, 62 percent claimed that scientific papers were "very important" in influencing which drugs they used.

Avorn and colleagues then asked about their target drugs. The physicians agreed by a 71 percent majority that "impaired cerebral blood flow is a major cause of senile dementia," and 32 percent said that they found cerebral vasodilating drugs useful in managing confused geriatric patients. Forty-nine percent stated that Darvon was more potent than aspirin; only 31 percent thought them equivalent.

In sum, these physicians seemed to believe that they were minimally influenced by drug ads and drug reps and instead used only scientific sources of information; yet they believed things that could never be found in medical journals and that could only be heard from company sources. And their own assessment of where they got their information (journal articles vs. drug reps or ads) was unrelated to what they believed to be true.[13]

Dr. James Orlowski and Leon Wateska, a pediatrician and pharmacist respectively at the Cleveland Clinic, performed a study at their medical center which has since been widely quoted. Leading physicians at the Cleveland Clinic were invited to attend a conference at a tropical beach resort, all expenses paid, to hear presentations from the company about each of the two drugs. Each drug was administered intravenously in a particular specialty unit, so that a relatively small number of physicians could greatly influence the rate at which the drug was prescribed.

Orlowski and Wateska looked at prescriptions for each drug in the twenty-two months prior to and the seventeen months after the resort trips. They found that the first drug was used at about three times the previous rate after the trip, and the second drug was used at more than twice the previous rate. Orlowski and Wateska then looked at utilization data for these drugs in all large U.S. hospitals during the same time period and found no comparable increases. They concluded that the increased prescribing could therefore not be due to any national trend.

The authors interviewed twenty physicians (ten from each resort trip group) and asked them if they thought they could possibly have been influenced in their drug prescribing behavior by these junkets. Seventeen of the twenty denied flatly that a resort trip could have any such influence. Three were less certain, but none of them felt it likely that they would be influenced.[14]

Finally, a third paper (not strictly a research paper) provides some further clues as to how aware physicians are of the way in which they are influenced. A group based at the University of Toronto, headed by Dr. Neil H. Shear, set out to design an instructional intervention for physicians. They reasoned that the vast majority of physicians see drug reps, and so it made no sense to tell them not to. Instead they decided to see if they could train physicians how to use the visit with the rep to get their own educational and informational needs better met.

Dr. Shear and his colleagues made use of a video made in Australia that depicted a physician being detailed on a fictitious antidepressant. The audience agreed that the video was very authentic, matching closely their own experiences with drug reps. Shear and colleagues reported their surprise that when they pointed out the fairly obvious and typical selling techniques used by the rep in the video to control and steer the interview, most physicians reacted as if becoming aware of these for the first time. Also, when they designed a checklist that allowed the physician to take charge of the interview and to get information on things that doctors needed to know about the medication, the direction the interview would take differed dramatically from the "normal" rep visit—showing again the error in the widely held claim by the industry that drug detailing is primarily an educational "service."[15]

Do Physicians View Drug Company Gifts as Conflicts of Interest?

Dr. Paul Palmisano of the University of Alabama in Birmingham and Joan Edelstein of Stanford Children's Hospital in Palo Alto, California, teamed up in another clever little study.[16] Both were involved in teaching health care practitioners about drug promotion and conflicts of interest and developed their questionnaire as an attitude pretest to introduce the topic to the students. While the students thought they were all getting the same questionnaire, in fact two different ones were distributed. One asked about the propriety of an elected official who awards contracts accepting a fifty-dollar gift from a prospective bidder. The other asked about a medical student accepting a fifty-dollar gift from a drug company.

Medical students disapproved of the public official's receiving the gift by an 85 percent margin, but only 46 percent thought it improper for the medical student to accept the gift. A group of nurse practitioners (who also prescribe drugs) was administered different questionnaires, asking about a fifty-dollar gift to the public official, a medical resident, and a nurse practitioner, respectively. The number of nurses who thought each gift improper was 97 percent for the public official, 64 percent for the resident, and 30 percent for the nurse.

Beside leading to very lively discussion in the teaching seminars, Palmisano and Edelstein thought the questionnaire results showed a marked double (or triple) standard of professional ethics. Both physicians and nurses were unwilling to apply to physicians the stringent standard of avoiding conflicts of interest by which they unhesitatingly judged a public official. The nurses were willing to give the physicians a relative pass on an ethical duty to avoid a conflict of interest, but were even more willing to let their fellow nurses off the hook. It seemed as if the very idea of "conflict of interest" is something one attributes to others and very seldom to oneself—at least if one works in health care.

What Do Patients Think about Pharmaceutical Gifts to Physicians?

Fewer studies look at patients' awareness of and attitudes toward the gifts physicians receive from reps. Dr. Robert L. Blake, Jr. and Elizabeth Early of the University of Missouri at Columbia surveyed 486 adults (an 83 percent response rate) in the waiting rooms of two family practice centers operated by their Department of Family and Community Medicine in the summer of 1994.[17] Patients were asked if they were aware that physicians might receive certain gifts from drug companies, and whether or not they approved. Table 10.1 summarizes the responses.

Table 10.1. Patient Awareness of and Attitude toward Commercial Gifts (adapted from Blake and Early)

Gift	Percent Aware of Gift	Percent Who Do Not Approve	Percent Who Approve	Percent with No Opinion
Dinner	22.4	48.4	34.6	14.6
Baby formula for family use	28.6	44.2	41.4	10.9
Cocktail party at conference	Not asked	43.4	40.5	13.0
Golf tournament at conference	Not asked	41.6	40.3	14.6
Coffee maker	13.8	40.7	39.1	17.3
Conference expenses	Not asked	32.5	52.7	11.5
Ice cream social at conferences	Not asked	28.0	55.6	12.8
Ballpoint pens	55.3	17.5	67.3	13.0
Medical books	34.6	16.9	70.0	9.9
Drug samples for office use	87.0	7.6	82.1	9.3

Patients generally disapproved of those items that were for personal rather than professional use. Like physicians, patients seemed to be more accepting of items that were lower in cost, or that had a clear educational value. In general, however, patient approval levels of all gifts was considerably below physician levels of acceptance in other studies looking at physicians' attitudes. There was also a fairly high rate of "no opinion" responses, suggesting that patients might be thinking about these issues for the first time; this was reflected in the relatively low level of awareness of many of these gifts—with scarcely half of patients admitting awareness of ballpoint pens. A possible bias that cannot be discounted is that these patients were waiting for appointments with their family physicians, so that negative answers might seem to be direct criticism of that physician. This could have placed pressure on patients to report lack of awareness or to express less disapproval.

In one way, patient responses exactly mirrored physician responses. Patients were quite accepting of free drug samples—the one item on the list of gifts that might benefit them personally. It seems that if there is something in it for us, our ethical compunctions immediately decrease, whether we are physicians or patients.

How Do Physicians View the Ethics of Accepting Gifts?

Many surveys ask physicians or others whether they approve or disapprove of certain gifts or practices, but few explicitly refer to the language of "ethics." Drs. Allan S. Brett, Wayne Burr, and Jamaluddin Moloo of the Department of Medicine, University of South Carolina in Columbia, specifically asked about "ethics" in their survey of the residents and faculty in their department.[18] They received completed questionnaires from thirty-nine residents (93 percent) and thirty-seven faculty physicians (73 percent). They did not specify the date of their survey; their results were published in October 2003.

The authors described eighteen scenarios, ranging from pens and note pads to an all-expenses-paid weekend at a luxury resort in exchange for attending several hours of seminars about a drug. Residents' and faculty members' responses were similar, though for the most part the faculty expressed slightly more ethical concern about a gift than the residents did. As in other surveys, gifts of lesser cost and of greater educational use were seen as less ethically problematic. The most striking finding of this survey was the relatively low level of ethical concern expressed across the board. The scenario arousing the highest level of ethical concern—the resort junket—received a mean response of 1.79 from residents and 1.72 from faculty, on a four-point scale. A score of two indicated "moderately problematic." Only about 60 percent of either residents or faculty classified the resort trip as "moderately problematic" or "very problematic." The vast majority of scenarios were ranked by the vast majority of respondents as "not problematic" or "mildly problematic."

A SUMMARY OF THE RESEARCH DATA

If we add up all the research studies, and sift through them to try to pick out the studies that use the most reliable methods, what conclusions can be drawn? We can go back to the Drug Promotion Database evidence-based review for some suggestions, beside the conclusions we have already seen:

- Physicians tend to view gifts from drug reps positively when they are of small monetary value and can be seen as directly connected to patient care. More concerns are shown as gifts increase in value and are clearly intended for personal use and enjoyment.[19]
- One study looked at the practice of drug companies paying physicians fees for enrolling patients in postmarketing research. (These so-called research studies are often called "seeding trials" because the quality of the "research" may be poor and the true underlying reason might be to "bribe" physicians to prescribe the drug.) Fifty-four percent of physicians thought such fees ethically acceptable; 56 percent of patients viewed them as ethically unacceptable.[20]
- Studies characterizing physicians who tend to rely more on industry sources of information often fail to replicate each other's findings. Among the better-supported conclusions are that such doctors are older, less conservative, lack peer contact and support, are in generalist rather than specialty fields, see more patients, and have more positive attitudes toward the use of drugs. Not surprisingly, academic physicians rely less on industry sources than do private practitioners.[21]
- Promotional activities influence physicians' attitudes toward drugs even where the physician cannot recall the promotional activity later on.[22]
- Several studies have looked at one subset of physicians—those who serve on committees that decide which drugs should be listed on a formulary for a hospital or similar institution. Increased contact with drug companies leads to increased requests by those physicians that the firm's drugs be added to the formulary.[23]
- Direct-to-consumer advertising works—patients who see drug advertising are more likely to request those medicines from their physicians. Physicians

tend to grant these requests even when they have doubts about the value of the advertised medicine.[24]

THE REASONING OF PHYSICIANS

Most of the studies we have reviewed so far are questionnaire surveys. These typically show what physicians think, but not why they think that. In order to study the reasoning process that underlies physician behavior and attitudes, one has to use more qualitative research methods, such as the in-depth, semi-structured interviews the Dichter group employed back in 1955.[25] One recent study from the United Kingdom is notable for using this sort of approach.

Helen Prosser and Tom Walley, a social scientist-pharmacologist team in Liverpool, interviewed 107 British general practitioners (GPs) in their area.[26] The sample was chosen to represent a wide range of practice size, practice location, and physician gender, as well as to include practices that had both high and low prescribing costs. The GPs were asked why they did or did not see reps and what advantages and disadvantages they perceived.

The GPs generally regarded the reps as a very efficient and indeed indispensable way of keeping informed, especially about new drugs:

> I think the answer is it's user friendly, it's very user friendly and it's easy listening, you know, with your coffee listening to what they've got to say.
>
> I'm sure you could manage if you didn't see another drug rep and I'm sure you could get the information if you wanted to, it's just that it's not that accessible, and it's also whether you would have the time to actually sit and read it.
>
> If it wasn't for the reps, all we'd have about Vioxx is two or three letters from the rheumatologist saying, "By the way, this new anti-inflammatory is OK for people with upset stomachs." That would be all we'd know . . . because there isn't any other mechanism, so if it wasn't for the drug reps we'd be left high and dry.[27]

These responses raise the possibility that the "accessibility" of rep-provided information becomes a form of self-fulfilling prophecy. If the physician (as the second interviewee hinted) were to stop seeing reps and would seek the information elsewhere, she might become both proficient and efficient in using those alternative information sources. As long as she continues to rely on the reps, whatever skills might be needed to make effective use of alternatives remain undeveloped.

Physicians are aware that it makes little sense to use an accessible source of information if it's also unreliable. So the next part of the rationale for rep-friendly behavior is to insist that reliability can be ensured. Usually this takes the form of "I can tell the difference" despite the empirical research suggesting that physicians cannot tell when they are being influenced or when they are getting inaccurate information. One form of this rejoinder is, "I can tell based on the information itself." The following quote deftly turns the knowledge that reps are often biased in their presentations into a defense of the physician who knows this and so can (presumably) be on guard:

I see reps as a useful information source. I mean, I'm hopefully streetwise enough to be quite selective.

Another version is, "I can tell based on the source." The idea that there are good and bad drug reps and that the good ones are trustworthy was observed as long ago as the 1955 Dichter study as part of the psychological processing of drug promotion by physicians, and it appears still to be going strong today:

I think if you see a rep who you know well . . . it's the same rep who you've seen for several years, they don't try and pull the wool over your eyes. They know that if they tell you lies you'll be seeing them again in six months and you'll find them out.

GPs defend the patronage and gift giving of reps in various ways. This GP appears to view his interactions with reps as a sort of charity:

I see it as their job, poor things, so the least I can do is to give them five minutes as a matter of courtesy.

The next two speakers are quite blunt in defending gifts:

I don't mind a nice hotel for a weekend. You don't get many perks unfortunately as a GP, and I don't see a problem with that.
    They entertain you, take you out to Christmas dinner and that sort of thing. You try to return their hospitality, after all they are the people producing the drugs.

A relative minority of the GPs value social and intellectual exchange. The final quote suggests that one GP has effectively turned the visits with the reps into a personally rewarding form of debate club.

Rep activity is just part of the social structure of the doctor's day. It's a break from patients, to talk to someone different.
    Some reps I've known for donkey's years and they know all about my life and I know all about their life and you have a chat about things which are totally unrelated to why they came, but it does make life more interesting and you're probably more likely to actually retain what they came in to tell you if you've had a pleasant time talking to them about your kids or something.
    It's a good discipline to sit down and look through whether something new is better and whether it is justifiable. They have to argue their corner and we argue it back.

Finally, some GPs mention the fact that seeing reps is simply part of the social landscape and they cannot imagine it being otherwise.

I think probably because we always did. With my old senior partners it was the done thing.

In sum, the interview data gathered by Prosser and Walley depict physicians who are generally very comfortable with their relationship with drug reps and who would be resistant to any "rational" arguments, based on the empirical data, to curtail those relationships. How do physicians come to have these attitudes following many years of training and practice?

THE "CULTURE OF ENTITLEMENT" HYPOTHESIS

Jerome Kassirer, former editor of the *New England Journal of Medicine*, calls the environment within medical education that promotes acceptance of reps and their gifts a "culture of entitlement."[28] I am aware of no firm empirical evidence to document that the culture develops and is reinforced in the way that Kassirer suggests, so I will state this developmental account as a hypothesis that requires further research. Nevertheless I believe it to be the most plausible account of how physicians "come of age" to be so accepting and unquestioning of drug reps and the largesse that they bestow. According to the editors of the *Lancet*,

> It begins on the first day of medical school and lasts through to retirement. . . . It starts slowly and insidiously, like an addiction, and can end up influencing the very nature of medical decision-making and practice. It first appears harmless enough: a textbook here, a penlight there, and progresses to stethoscopes and black bags, until eventually come nights "on the town" at academic conventions and all-expenses paid "educational symposia" in lovely locales.[29]

The culture-of-entitlement hypothesis is especially important because physician-investigators commonly complete medical school and residency alongside physicians whose future careers lie in practice. Their specific training in research usually occurs only later. If the "culture" operates as described, these physician-investigators have already been persuaded *before they become committed to a career in scientific research* that they are entitled to whatever goodies they can obtain from the pharmaceutical industry, and that accepting these gifts poses no threat to their professional integrity or values. This would go a good way toward explaining how supposedly scientific investigators can act in ways so at odds with basic scientific values, once they begin to receive large grants and speaking and consulting fees from the industry.

Most medical students begin their education with a sense of duty and commitment, which slowly fades and is replaced by cynicism.[30] By the time the student has become a resident, idealism has often been replaced by self-pity: we work so hard, we're underpaid, we're unappreciated, lawyers are the enemy, even patients are the enemy (by making more work for us to do at all hours of day and night). In exchange for having to put up with all this, we deserve some love, and we deserve some rewards. Perhaps even more important, the average medical graduate today may be in debt for as much as $120,000 or more after completing medical school.[31]

To take full advantage of the descent from idealism into cynicism, the pharmaceutical industry must supply physicians with an army of nice, physically attractive people who seem to appreciate them when no one else does, and who shower them with rewards. But this practice has to fly under the ethical radar of the more sensitive and idealistic students, setting off no warning bells. The industry has to carefully pace its gift giving to fit the psychological stages of the physician's progress through education into practice. In the process, industry has carefully attended to the old adage that the descent into Hades is a gradual slope.

For the idealistic first-year (or first-day) medical students, the gifts must appear noble. Nothing crass or self-serving will do. The object must be education and service to the patient.[32] So a textbook or a medical instrument will start off the relationship on the right foot. Later, something that obviously appeals to self-interest will be acceptable as long as it is of low monetary value. So medical students and residents happily line up for pizza or sandwiches at lunch. When students reach their clinical rotations, they tend to follow the lead of residents in deciding what is acceptable or not.[33] So, gradually, more and more expensive meals, and more and more trinkets and paraphernalia become "acceptable."

Once the message has been received that the drug industry is the students' friend, and wishes above all else to see them succeed in the arduous process of medical education, the industry is then free to up the ante by imperceptible degrees. At each step of the way, the messages transmitted are:

- how much the industry appreciates how hard the student has to work,
- how relatively innocent and benign is the gift, and
- how much (as a result of the first two elements) the student should feel *entitled* to the gift.

Moreover, the industry is well aware of the social psychology of gifts. We are brought up from infancy to feel a debt toward those who give us gifts, and this occurs no matter what the gift's monetary value.[34]

The end result of this slow process of acculturation is a practitioner who eagerly seeks contacts with pharmaceutical sales reps, eagerly accepts their gifts, never feels ethical unease about this state of affairs, and feels fully entitled to whatever is received.[35]

Evidence to support the culture-of-entitlement hypothesis comes from distressing instances in which physicians have moved from a role of willing recipients of drug industry largesse, into the role of shakedown artist. Dr. Richard Smith, editor of the *British Medical Journal* (now *BMJ*), described some instances two decades ago that parallel some of the worst cases Stan encountered: "Many doctors, it seems, write to drug companies asking for funds to pay for foreign trips, and 'one doctor even stated that unless his request was granted he would stop prescribing the company's products.' Another group of doctors refused to attend a film unless it was 'shown with a meal organised at a restaurant of their choice.'"[36]

More recently, the readiness of the FDA to grant exemptions to its conflict-of-interest policies for "experts" who sit on its advisory committees seems to have had some unintended consequences as FDA advisors try to cash in on their status. "Members of FDA advisory committees are said to command unusually high consulting fees from drug companies. . . . According to the *Washington Times* reporter August Gribbin, 'One drug company executive who asked not to be identified referred to the advisory committee members' approaches for obtaining [consulting] work as "shakedowns" because a company that refused to yield to such requests could doom products that cost tens of millions of dollars to develop."[37]

Recent moves by some physician groups to charge reps for "face time" provides a further illustration of the pervasive culture of entitlement. As the number of reps has recently escalated and demands on the physicians' time increase, charging a fee is ostensibly a tool to allocate limited time. To the horror even of the AMA, some of these physician groups announced that they would levy fees up to one hundred dollars for each rep who wished to speak with them.[38]

The fact that these physicians somehow felt *entitled* to this money speaks to the pervasive nature of this aspect of the medical culture. The physicians apparently never stopped to consider that they could simply have refused to see the reps because they did not wish to be subjected to unscientific bias in their prescribing. The obvious rejoinder, "But am I not entitled to be paid for my time?" misses the point about what counts as *professional* time. If I sit at home watching the Super Bowl and watch a Budweiser spot, what would make me think that I can call up Budweiser and shake them down for payment for watching their commercial?

Perhaps the most extreme illustration of a culture of entitlement is the recent revelation that as many as 10 percent of U.S. physicians might be involved in selling information to various Wall Street investment firms, including hedge funds. With approximately one trillion dollars' worth of assets now invested in hedge funds, there is a huge financial incentive to seize upon any snippet of information coming out of new drug trials. When a company's stock can drop 20 percent in value overnight at the news that a once-promising drug has gone belly-up in its latest trial, any firm to whom the news is leaked a few days early can make a tremendous profit selling the stock short. Entire firms are now devoted to recruiting physicians to be interviewed by investment firms and hedge funds, for payments ranging from $300 to $1,000 per hour.[39]

Luke Timmerman and David Heath, investigating this phenomenon for the *Seattle Times*, stated that they had found "at least 26 cases in which doctors have leaked confidential and critical details of their ongoing drug research to Wall Street firms."[40] These practices were denounced as "a moral cesspool" by Arthur Caplan, of the Center for Bioethics at the University of Pennsylvania, and as "outrageous and completely unethical" by Dr. Drummond Rennie, deputy editor of *JAMA*.[41] Perhaps the most intriguing aspect of the *Seattle Times's* coverage was the ability of the physicians interviewed to convince themselves that they had not, after all, divulged any important or key data. "They'll ask what I can't answer," said one physician. "I just answer from my personal experience in how patients seem to respond to certain therapies."[42] Somehow these physicians can imagine savvy investment firms paying them $300 to $500 per hour for vague, nonessential impressions.

These physicians have signed confidentiality agreements that limit disclosures while the trial is ongoing. Pharmaceutical companies are in a bind. They rely on these physicians to conduct their trials and to enroll subjects in the speediest possible fashion; they dare not antagonize them. But the company then may suffer the consequences if its stock plummets on Wall Street due to leaks of pessimistic information from an ongoing trial—in an extreme case, information that might perhaps be in error if the trial were allowed to run its course. If the behavior of the pharmaceutical industry was what primarily created the culture of entitlement to begin with, it is ironic that the culture has now turned to bite the hand that fed it. Industry critics might take perverse satisfaction in this development, were it not for the fact that physicians selling research secrets to Wall Street firms for personal gain marks an abysmal new low in professional ethics.

The culture-of-entitlement hypothesis is important for suggesting the source and the dynamics of the rationalizations employed by physicians to defend their current practices with regard to the pharmaceutical industry. We have seen in this chapter that there is a fairly extensive, accumulated database tending to show that the cozy relationships that have grown up between physicians and drug reps in the past sixty years have deleterious consequences. Physicians who ought to be more attentive to their professional responsibilities to serve the interests of their patients put themselves in a compromised position by maintaining these forms of relationships. The data reveal both the way that physicians are willing to compromise their core ethical responsibilities, and also the way that physicians go on believing that no ethical violation has occurred. We have previously seen what historical factors were at work during the period of the 1940s and 1950s to make this new social role of drug rep both acceptable and indeed essential to practitioners. The culture-of-entitlement hypothesis adds a personal-developmental understanding to this historical account, explaining how the history of the physician-drug rep relationship recapitulates itself (as it were) within the lifetime career history of each physician-in-training.

Ethical analysis must take a particular sort of turn in the face of deep-seated rationalization. Ordinarily we rely a good deal on personal testimony when we assess an ethical issue or dilemma. People describe what they propose to do, and assess which actions are ethical and which unethical, and give reasons to justify their ethical reasoning. We usually accept these statements as honest and trustworthy accounts of the moral issues and of an individual's moral position. We cannot grant first-person testimony the same degree of privilege when we have reason to believe that an individual's assessment of her own behaviors and motives have become systematically obscured by a pervasive set of rationalizations. It will therefore become necessary to discount a good deal of what physicians say about themselves and their reasoning when we come to assess the ethical goals of the profession-industry relationship, and especially when we come to weigh proposals for reform.

NOTES

1. D. J. Rothman, "Medical Professionalism—Focusing on the Real Issues," *N Engl J Med* 2000; 342:1283–86.

2. www.drugpromo.info (accessed December 21, 2004).

3. R. P. Ferguson, E. Rhim, W. Belizaire, L. Egede, K. Carter, and T. Lansdale, "Encounters with Pharmaceutical Sales Representatives among Practicing Internists," *Am J Med* 1999; 107:149–52.

4. Kaiser Family Foundation, "National Survey of Physicians, Part II: Doctors and Prescription Drugs," Kaiser Family Foundation, 2002, www.kff.org/rxdrugs/loader.cfm?url=/commonspot/security/getfile.cfm&PageID=13965 (accessed April 14, 2005).

5. M. A. Steinman, M. G. Shlipak, and S. J. McPhee, "Of Principles and Pens: Attitudes and Practices of Medicine Housestaff toward Pharmaceutical Industry Promotions," *Am J Med* 2001; 110:551–57.

6. Similar data were obtained in a survey of radiation oncologists; E. C. Halperin, P. Hutchison, and R. C. Barrier Jr., "A Population-Based Study of the Prevalence and Influence of Gifts to Radiation Oncologists from Pharmaceutical Companies and Medical Equipment Manufacturers," *Int J Radiat Oncol Biol Phys* 2004; 59:1477–83.

7. A. Zuger, "When Your Doctor Goes to the Beach, You May Get Burned," *New York Times*, February 24, 2004:5.

8. S. K. Sigworth, M. D. Nettleman, and G. M. Cohen, "Pharmaceutical Branding of Resident Physicians," *JAMA* 2001; 286:1024–25.

9. M. Y. Peay, and E. R. Peay, "The Role of Commercial Sources in the Adoption of a New Drug," *Soc Sci Med* 1988; 26:1183–89.

10. A. Figueiras, F. Caamano, and J. J. Gestal-Otero, "Influence of Physician's Education, Drug Information and Medical-Care Settings on the Quality of Drugs Prescribed," *Eur J Clin Pharmacol* 2000; 56:747–53.

11. Similar findings have been reported in the following studies: R. Mapes, "Aspects of British General Practitioners' Prescribing," *Med Care* 1977; 15:371–81; A. D. Bower and G. L. Burkett, "Family Physicians and Generic Drugs: A Study of Recognition, Information Sources, Prescribing Attitudes, and Practices," *J Fam Pract* 1987; 24:612–16; T. S. Caudill, M. S. Johnson, E. C. Rich, and W. P. McKinney, "Physicians, Pharmaceutical Sales Representatives, and the Cost of Prescribing," *Arch Fam Med* 1996; 5:201–6; M. H. Becker, P. D. Stolley, L. Lasagna, J. D. McEvilla, and L. M. Sloane, "Differential Education Concerning Therapeutics and Resultant Physician Prescribing Patterns," *J Med Educ* 1972; 47:118–27; D. Berings, L. Blondeel, and H. Habraken, "The Effect of Industry-Independent Drug Information on the Prescribing of Benzodiazepines in General Practice," *Eur J Clin Pharmacol* 1994; 46:501–5; F. Haayer, "Rational Prescribing and Sources of Information," *Soc Sci Med* 1982; 16:2017–23; and J. K. Stross, "Information Sources and Clinical Decisions," *J Gen Intern Med* 1987; 2:155–59.

A rare negative study of this sort is E. Hemminki, "The Effect of a Doctor's Personal Characteristics and Working Circumstances on the Prescribing of Psychotropic Drugs," *Med Care* 1974; 12:351–57.

12. J. Avorn, M. Chen, and R. Hartley, "Scientific versus Commercial Sources of Influence on the Prescribing Behavior of Physicians," *Am J Med* 1982; 73:4–8.

13. Lexchin and his colleagues on the Drug Promotion Database website (www.drugpromo.info) mention a number of methodological weaknesses of the Avorn study but then note that the general conclusions have since been replicated by later studies using better methods. See, for instance, M. G. Ziegler, P. Lew, and B. C. Singer, "The Accuracy of Drug Information from Pharmaceutical Sales Representatives," *JAMA* 1995; 273:1296–98; J. Greenwood, "Pharmaceutical Representatives and the Prescribing of Drugs by Family Doctors," (thesis, Department of Administrative and Social Studies, University of Nottingham, 1989); and M. E. Ferry, P. P. Lamy, and L. A. Becker, "Physicians' Knowledge of Prescribing for the Elderly: A Study of Primary Care Physicians in Pennsylvania," *J Am Geriatr Soc* 1985; 33:616–25.

14. J. P. Orlowski and L. Wateska, "The Effects of Pharmaceutical Firm Enticements on Physician Prescribing Patterns: There's No Such Thing as a Free Lunch," *Chest* 1992; 102:270–73.

15. N. H. Shear, F. Black, and J. Lexchin, "Examining the Physician-Detailer Interaction," *Can J Clin Pharmacol* 1996; 3:175–79.

16. P. Palmisano and J. Edelstein, "Teaching Drug Promotion Abuses to Health Profession Students," *J Med Educ* 1980; 55:453–55.

17. R. L. Blake Jr., and E. K. Early, "Patients' Attitudes about Gifts to Physicians from Pharmaceutical Companies," *J Am Board Fam Pract* 1995; 8:457–64.

18. A. S. Brett, W. Burr, and J. Moloo, "Are Gifts from Pharmaceutical Companies Ethically Problematic? A Survey of Physicians," *Arch Intern Med* 2003; 163:2213–18.

19. M. D. Sergeant, P. G. Hodgetts, M. Godwin, D. M. Walker, and P. McHenry, "Interactions with the Pharmaceutical Industry: A Survey of Family Medicine Residents in Ontario," *CMAJ* 1996; 155:1243–48; R. E. Aldir, D. Jarjoura, M. Phinney, et al., "Practicing and Resident Physicians' Views on Pharmaceutical Companies," *J Contin Educ Health Prof* 1996; 16:25–32; D. Strang, M. Gagnon, W. Molloy, et al., "National Survey on the Attitudes of Canadian Physicians towards Drug-Detailing by Pharmaceutical Representatives," *Ann R Coll Physicians Surg Can* 1996; 29:474–78; S. M. Keim, A. B. Sanders, D. B. Witzke, P. Dyne, and J. W. Fulginiti, "Beliefs and Practices of Emergency Medicine Faculty and Residents Regarding Professional Interactions with the Biomedical Industry," *Ann Emerg Med* 1993; 22:1576–81.

20. J. La Puma, C. B. Stocking, W. D. Rhoades, et al., "Financial Ties as Part of Informed Consent to Postmarketing Research: Attitudes of American Doctors and Patients," *BMJ* 1995; 310:1660–63.

21. Peay and Peay, "Role of Commercial Sources"; C. Gaither, R. P. Bagozzi, D. M. Kirking, and F. J. Ascione, "Factors Related to Physicians' Attitudes and Beliefs toward Drug Information Sources," *Drug Information Journal* 1994; 28:817–27; J. D. McCue, C. J. Hansen, and P. Gal, "Physicians' Opinions of the Accuracy, Accessibility, and Frequency of Use of Ten Sources of New Drug Information," *South Med J* 1986; 79:441–43.

22. R. L. Engle, "The Impact of a Single-Advertiser Publication on Physicians' Perceptions and Expected Prescribing Behavior," *Journal of Pharmaceutical Marketing and Management* 1994; 8:37–54; R. W. Spingarn, J. A. Berlin, and B. L. Strom, "When Pharmaceutical Manufacturers' Employees Present Grand Rounds, What Do Residents Remember?" *Acad Med* 1996; 71:86–88; W. S. Sandberg, R. Carlos, E. H. Sandberg, and M. F. Roizen, "The Effect of Educational Gifts from Pharmaceutical Firms on Medical Students' Recall of Company Names or Products," *Acad Med* 1997; 72:916–18.

23. N. Lurie, E. C. Rich, D. E. Simpson, et al., "Pharmaceutical Representatives in Academic Medical Centers: Interaction with Faculty and Housestaff," *J Gen Intern Med* 1990; 5:240–43; M. M. Chren and C. S. Landefeld, "Physicians' Behavior and Their Interactions with Drug Companies: A Controlled Study of Physicians Who Requested Additions to a Hospital Drug Formulary," *JAMA* 1994; 271:684–89.

24. M. Perri and W. M. Dickson, "Direct to Consumer Prescription Drug Advertising: Consumer Attitudes and Physician Reaction," *Journal of Pharmaceutical Marketing and Management* 1987; 2:3–23; B. Mintzes, M. L. Barer, R. L. Kravitz, et al., "How Does Direct-to-Consumer Advertising (DTCA) Affect Prescribing? A Survey in Primary Care Environments with and without Legal DTCA," *CMAJ* 2003; 169:405–12.

25. Pharmaceutical Advertising Club, *A Research Study on Pharmaceutical Advertising* (Croton-on-Hudson, New York: Institute for Motivational Research, Inc., 1955).

26. H. Prosser and T. Walley, "Understanding Why GPs See Pharmaceutical Representatives: A Qualitative Interview Study," *Br J Gen Pract* 2003; 53:305–11.

27. The irony of this interview segment is obvious today, after Vioxx has been withdrawn from the market due to excessive toxicity.

28. J. P. Kassirer, "A Piece of My Mind: Financial Indigestion," *JAMA* 2000; 284:2156–57; see also S. Brownlee, "Doctors without Borders: Why You Can't Trust Medical Journals Anymore," *Washington Monthly* April 2004, 38–43.

29. "Drug-Company Influence on Medical Education in USA" [editorial], *Lancet* 2000; 356:781.

30. See, for example, W. Woloschuk, P. H. Harasym, and W. Temple, "Attitude Change During Medical School: A Cohort Study," *Med Educ* 2004; 38:522–34; P. Haidet, J. E. Dains, D. A. Paterniti, et al., "Medical Student Attitudes toward the Doctor-Patient Relationship," *Med Educ* 2002; 36:568–74. For an argument that cynicism might be reduced through certain curricular reforms, see W. P. Roche, A. P. Scheetz, F. C. Dane, et al., "Medical Students' Attitudes in a PBL Curriculum: Trust, Altruism, and Cynicism," *Acad Med* 2003; 78:398–402.

31. Dr. Drummond Rennie, who had blown the whistle on the "Thyroid Storm"–Betty Dong case, cited the indebtedness of young physicians as one factor leading to their susceptibility to unethical solicitations of information from investment funds; D. Heath and L. Timmerman, "Some Doctors See Ethical Pitfall in Actions That Others Defend," *Seattle Times*, August 7 2005:A8.

32. Historically, one way the industry could provide an "educational" experience for medical students, while subtly creating a sense of indebtedness for the industry's largesse, was to invite the students for a tour of a pharmaceutical plant, all expenses paid. This practice appears to have a venerable history. For example, on March 22, 1900, forty students from the Rush Medical College in Chicago, accompanied by one of their professors and an equal number of pharmacy students, boarded a specially chartered Michigan Central train for the trip to Detroit, where they were all put up at the Russell House. The next day was spent in a guided tour of the Parke, Davis and Company laboratories, where, among other things, the students observed the technique for creating diphtheria antitoxin from horse serum. The day ended with a banquet with a musical quartet at the Russell House before the students took a night train back to Chicago. The company paid all the expenses; "Excursion to Parke, Davis & Co., by Chicago College of Pharmacy and Rush Medical College," *Western Druggist* 1900; 22:234. I have been informed by physicians that these tours remained common at least into the 1950s and 1960s.

33. Oldani agrees that "training" the physician in the normal and expected nature of what he calls the pharmaceutical gift economy begins with medical students and residents, and usually with a shower of low-cost gifts at the beginning. He mentions that as a rep, he often held lunches for residents and students in which he would generate extra interest by raffling off an expensive textbook (the "raffle tickets," true to form, were signed "pretend" scripts for the medication being detailed). "On more than one occasion, I was quite shocked to find that during my presentation the textbook had been taken. Residents would reassure me that somebody probably just thought it was a free give-away." M. J. Oldani, "Thick Prescriptions: Toward an Interpretation of Pharmaceutical Sales Practices," *Med Anthropol Q* 2004; 18:325–56, quote p. 349. Apparently in these cases the indoctrination into the "culture of entitlement" had worked a little too well.

34. M. M. Chren, C. S. Landefeld, and T. H. Murray, "Doctors, Drug Companies, and Gifts," *JAMA* 1989; 262:3448–51; J. Dana and G. Loewenstein, "A Social Science Perspective on Gifts to Physicians from Industry," *JAMA* 2003; 290:252–55; D. Katz, A. L. Caplan, and J. F. Merz, "All Gifts Large and Small," *Am J Bioeth* 2003; 3(3): 39–46.

35. For an especially detailed discussion of the ethics of pharmaceutical gifts from the medical trainee's point of view, see W. A. Rogers, P. R. Mansfield, A. J. Braunack-Mayer, and J. N. Jureidini, "The Ethics of Pharmaceutical Industry Relationships with Medical Students," *Med J Aust* 2004; 180:411–14. Rogers et al. point out an interesting catch-22. If medical students accept gifts from the drug companies and *do* learn that such gifts entail a debt to the giver, then they become subject to commercial bias in their prescribing at an especially formative time. If they accept such gifts and *do not* associate the gift with any sense of reciprocal indebtedness, then they learn the culture of entitlement—that they are worthy of being given lavish freebies not bestowed upon the average person, simply because they are physicians-to-be.

36. R. Smith, "Doctors and the Drug Industry: Too Close for Comfort," *Br Med J* (Clin Res Ed) 1986; 293:905–6 (quoting the 1986 report from the U.K. Royal College of Physicians, *The Relationship between Physicians and the Pharmaceutical Industry*).

37. M. Angell, *The Truth about the Drug Companies: How They Deceive Us and What to Do about It* (New York: Random House, 2004), 211; citing August Gribbin, "House Investigates Panels Involved with Drug Safety," *Washington Times*, June 18, 2001.

38. H. Jung, "Some Physicians Now Charging Drug Reps to Hear Sales Pitch," *Nando Times*, June 14, 2002, www.nandotimes.com/healthscience/v-text/story/433828p-3469159c. html (accessed June 18, 2002); C. McCanse, "Gifts-to-Physicians Issue Once Again Moves to Front Burner," *FP Report* (American Academy of Family Physicians) August, 2002; 8(8): 5–6; T. Albert, "Is It Ethical to Bill Drug Reps for Office Visit?" *American Medical News*, November 26, 2001; T. Chin, "Drug Firms Score by Paying Doctors for Time," *American Medical News*, May 6, 2002. In July 2003, Scott Hensley of the *Wall Street Journal* reported that many of these early efforts to charge reps for "face time" had collapsed; S. Hensley, "Doctors Advise Sales Reps to Do More Listening," *Wall Street Journal Online*, July 14, 2003, online.wsj.com/article/0.,SB105795444221548500.00.html.

39. E. J. Topol and D. Blumenthal, "Physicians and the Investment Industry," *JAMA* 2005; 293:2654–57.

40. L. Timmerman and D. Heath, "Drug Researchers Leak Secrets to Wall St.," *Seattle Times*, August 7, 2005:A1.

41. Timmerman and Heath, "Drug Researchers Leak Secrets," (Caplan); Heath and Timmerman, "Some Doctors See Ethical Pitfall," (Rennie).

42. Timmerman and Heath, "Drug Researchers Leak Secrets."

⓫

CONTINUING MEDICAL EDUCATION

[The pharmaceutical industry is] unique in that it can make exploitation appear a noble purpose.

—Dr. Dale Console, former medical director of Squibb, commenting how drug promotion masquerades as a system of postgraduate education at the Kefauver Senate hearings, c. 1960[1]

THE STORY OF THE BERLIN CONGRESS

E. Fuller Torrey is a distinguished senior psychiatrist, now president of the Treatment Advocacy Center in Arlington, Virginia. In the summer of 2001 he attended the Seventh World Congress of Biological Psychiatry, held in Berlin. He sent back a postcard of sorts, which was published in *The American Prospect*.[2] Similar postcards could be sent nowadays from attendees at most major medical conventions, although by most accounts the problem Torrey describes is more severe in psychiatry than in other specialties.

Torrey writes—perhaps a bit naively—about how good the old days were:

Until about a decade ago, pharmaceutical companies passed out pens or notepads with their companies' logos at such events, and most speakers presented data and opinions based upon their true scientific beliefs.

That all changed when Big Pharma took over. At the congress, I counted 15 major displays on the way to the lunch area, including an artificial garden (Janssen-Cilag), a brook running over stones (Lundbeck), and a 40-foot rotating tower (Novartis). Almost all offered free food and drink, T-shirts, or other inducements designed to get psychiatrists to pause so that an army of smiling sales representatives could give their sales pitch.[3]

Torrey found himself especially fascinated by the Organon display, advertising the antidepressant drug Remeron. Psychiatrists were lined up for a twenty-minute wait outside a colorful tent with a picture of a genie. Inside, "a red-robed young woman with sprinkles in her hair" was taking Polaroid photos of the visitors' auras. The brochure touted the "advanced biofeedback equipment" used to take the photos, which showed red, orange, yellow, or blue clouds around one's head. A yellow-robed woman, named Amber, with even more sprinkles, then offered the interpretation of the aura—Torrey, she explained, showed "intelligence and good judgment, although some hints of skepticism."[4] Torrey was indeed skeptical, and asked the sales staff "if they thought it wise to associate their product with auras, magic, New Age thinking, and anti-science."[5] As an answer, the staff simply pointed to the long line of waiting psychiatrists, like sitting ducks waiting for the obligatory sales pitch.

Still skeptical, Torrey asked about the price tags of all that he surveyed. There were, of course, formal lectures and panels; it was not all gardens, brooks and auras. Most were company-sponsored, though in some cases the sponsorship was not openly revealed. The typical reimbursement for the speaker was a $2,000–$3,000 honorarium, business class air fare, and four-star hotel accommodations. If the expert himself organized the symposium, the honorarium might go up to $5,000, or even higher if the spiel was extremely favorable to the company's product. "One American expert was paid $10,000 last year to fly to Europe to give a single lecture."[6] Many of these experts, Torrey added, own company stock and so have a direct interest in the drug's success.

There were a few sessions on topics that were unrelated to drugs. These attracted little if any industry support and were lightly attended. The speaker at one of those talks ruefully surveyed the empty seats and told Torrey that he "felt like the legitimate act at a burlesque show, included only to keep the cops out."[7]

One might wonder how all these psychiatrists found the money to fly to Berlin for this congress. Meeting officials admitted to Torrey that about half of the roughly four thousand who attended were sponsored by the drug companies. Unlike the speakers, the attendees had to settle mostly for coach-class air tickets. But they got to stay at the same hotel and had their registration fees paid, and were also invited to parties, "some literally with dancing girls."[8] Torrey observed that with the precise data each company obtains on all the prescriptions written by each physician, it was easy to monitor whether these psychiatrists showed a proper regard for the company who sent them to Berlin, and to dole out invitations to attend next summer's international congress accordingly.

As best as Torrey could determine, the total cost of the Big Pharma presence at the Berlin congress—which, of course, is passed along to all who purchase these drugs—was at least ten million dollars.

Torrey urged some serious changes to protect the interests of patients. Sadly, he wrote, "most of the profession's organizations, such as the American Psychiatric Association, are themselves so indebted to drug companies that they are unlikely to lead reform."[9]

CONTINUING MEDICAL EDUCATION

We have already learned that American medicine might not have developed such close relationships between detail persons and practicing physicians had highly effective continuing medical education (CME) programs existed in the 1940s and 1950s. New drugs were exploding onto the market in ever-increasing numbers, and physicians had only the drug rep to turn to for up-to-date information and guidance. The drug rep and related developments—printed drug ads, drug company house newsletters, throw-away medical journals—filled a gap that had been left by the medical education establishment.

Today CME is big business—amounting to an annual revenue of $ 1.77 billion in 2003.[10] But this growth in CME has occurred during an era when the drug industry has exerted considerable power and influence. Hence CME has developed in a direction that is highly congenial to the desires of the industry.

One ironic perspective on CME is that if it were to listen to itself, it would put itself out of business. Much of today's CME focuses on "evidence-based medicine." Physicians are urged to do what the evidence proves is effective, not what they always used to do out of habit or inertia. That raises the question of whether CME itself can be shown to be effective, and the answer is that very little such evidence exists. Does attending CME sessions alter the behavior of physicians in the direction of providing better quality patient care? We have little proof that this is the case.[11]

But there may be reasons why CME appears not to alter physicians' behavior. Most studies of CME tend to assume that the alternative is no education or information transfer at all—or else that physicians would simply read journals to stay informed. The pharmaceutical industry, as we have seen, has devoted huge efforts and sums over more than a half-century to developing a highly effective system of informing and influencing practitioners. We would expect that where the formal CME apparatus gives out the same message as that promoted by drug marketing and detailing—say, that proton-pump inhibitors like Prilosec and Nexium are excellent drugs for gastroesophageal reflux disease—the CME and the detailing process would work in tandem and be mutually reinforcing, making it hard to distinguish an effect due to CME alone. On the other hand, where CME gives out one message—for instance, that cheap diuretics and beta blockers are much better first-line drugs for hypertension than expensive calcium channel blockers and angiotensin receptor blockers—and detail reps give out a different message, we would expect that the reps will win. Studies of physician compliance with official guidelines for hypertension treatment show that this tends to be the case.[12] It is therefore not surprising that industry sponsorship of CME conferences has drawn criticism from some physicians for decades.[13]

CME AND THE DRUG INDUSTRY

CME has a precise scope and meaning because physicians are granted credit for each hour's worth of programs or other activities in which they participate. To give out such credits, a program must be officially recognized and approved by the Accreditation Council for Continuing Medical Education (ACCME) or one of its delegate organizations. A drug company wishing to send a message to physicians by having them attend a meeting with a speaker can proceed in two different ways. The company can simply invite the physicians to come to a dinner at which a speaker will do a presentation. Today, given the competition for the attention of busy physicians, almost all such meetings will offer a dinner with wine at a fine restaurant; and the higher-prescribing physicians will be paid additional fees (up to several hundred dollars) for attending such meetings as "consultants" (and will justify that designation, perhaps, by filling out a one-page evaluation sheet giving their judgments as to the effectiveness of the presentation). In this informal setting, no CME credit will be given, and the company speaker is free to say essentially whatever she wishes.

The other route requires the drug company to interact with another organization that has been accredited by the ACCME. That organization might be a medical school or hospital that will sponsor a CME conference after receiving funding to support the conference from the drug company. Or the organization may be a "medical communications company" whose exclusive role is putting on CME programs with drug-industry financing. The upside is that physicians now have an extra incentive to attend the meeting—they will get CME credit, which many need for licensure or for maintaining their specialty certification (often around fifty hours per year). The downside is that the company must now satisfy the regulations of the ACCME, and that places limits on what the speaker can say and how much of a commercial appeal will be allowed within the so-called "scientific" presentation.

The consequence of this two-track option is that we have a great deal of data about the drug companies' involvement in the formal CME type of program. All such programs submit annual data to the ACCME, and aggregate data are publicly available on the ACCME website. By contrast, the informal speaker-over-dinner goes under the company's budget for gifts and marketing, and those figures are among the most closely guarded secrets within the industry. So we know a great deal about the industry's relationship with formal CME activity, more than we know about most other forms of drug marketing.

Larger CME programs receive funding from industry in two ways. Industry may pay directly into the budget for the CME program costs (which typically include honoraria to pay the guest speakers, rental of meeting rooms, coffee and food served at breaks and meals, printed handouts, and planning and administrative costs such as advertising). Or the meeting may feature a hallway or an exhibit room in which a firm can set up a display or booth, paying a rental fee for the use of the space. Some think that the latter method is "cleaner" because the industry presence is kept at arm's length and presumably exercises less influence on the content of the educational program. However, a CME-sponsoring organization calculates exhibit fees as part of its predicted budget for any conference, and it is not clear that the method of industry funding makes any large difference in the influence, or the lack of influence, that the industry is able to exert. If the percentage of the total conference budget paid by industry is small, the sponsoring organization may exercise considerable freedom in choosing what information to present. If the industry pays a large percentage of the conference costs, the sponsors may think twice about presenting information that would antagonize industry and lead to less money for future conferences.

Beside the pharmaceutical companies, other companies are involved in sponsoring CME. These include mostly the makers of medical devices such as diagnostic equipment, pacemakers, operating room instruments, and so on. Table 11.1 summarizes the extent to which industry supported CME programs in the U.S. in 2003.

Table 11.1. Industry Support for All CME Activity, 2003[14]

Total income, all ACCME accredited providers	$1,774,516,395
Total commercial support	$971,100,096
Support from pharmaceutical companies	$943,608,302
Percentage of all commercial support from pharmaceutical companies	97%
Percentage of total income from pharmaceutical support	53%

Averages can be misleading. A closer inspection of ACCME figures shows that the sponsoring organizations of CME programs can be broken down into three rough categories. One group includes the commercial communications companies and similar organizations, who rely almost wholly on industry funding. A second group includes organizations like the Veterans Administration and some managed care organizations, who receive virtually no industry funding for CME. That leaves the organizations that sponsor most CME programs, notably hospitals, professional societies, and medical schools, in the middle. I have labeled those three groups of CME organizers high, middle, and low depending on the relative proportion of funding received from industry. Table 11.2 breaks down the percentage of CME revenues received from industry sources for the three types of organizations, along with the percentage of total CME programs and CME credit hours accounted for by each type (using 2002 figures).

Table 11.2. Categories of CME Organizations with Percentage of Revenue from Industry (2002 figures)

Category of sponsoring organization	Total revenues (thousands of dollars)	Revenues from pharmaceutical industry (thousands of dollars)	% of revenues from pharmaceutical industry	% of total CME activities	% of total CME hours
High	377,306	316,563	84	13	6
Middle	604,301	280,286	46	65	72
Low	614,590	123,323	20	22	22

There are a number of lessons to be drawn from table 11.2. First, several types of organizations that we might think of as relatively independent, such as hospitals and medical schools, derive quite sizeable portions of their CME budgets from industry.

Second, the "high" subcategory appears virtually to be a tool of industry, depending on the drug companies for almost their entire CME budgets—though the total amount of CME hours granted by these organizations is in the minority. Even here we should beware of average figures. Because overall, medical schools derive 59 percent of their CME budget from industry does not mean that that percentage applies to each CME program. At my own medical school, which I assume is fairly typical, CME activities vary all the way from no industry funding at all to more than 60 percent industry funding.

Scott Hensley, writing in the *Wall Street Journal* in 2002, noted that only 17 percent of a typical medical school's CME funding came from commercial sources in 1994, while by 2000 the figure had risen to more than 40 percent. CME program organizers told him that a decade before, physicians had been content to pay fees for CME that more or less covered the cost of the program. Then, as "free" CME subsidized by the industry became common, physicians demanded lower registration costs, forcing the medical schools to turn more and more to industry for CME support.[15] The "culture of entitlement" we discussed in relation to gifts from drug reps appears to have extended its reach into CME.

Table 11.2 suggests that industry funding is a mainstay of CME in the United States and that a good deal of the present CME activity would simply cease were this funding to disappear. We must now ask what effect this has on the content of CME.

REGULATING CME CONTENT

The ACCME has for some time been concerned about undue commercial bias in CME programs. While the available research is patchy, it tends to confirm the presence of procompany bias correlated with commercial sponsorship of CME.[16] Hensley, in the *Wall Street Journal*, described a lecture given in June 2002 at the Astor Ballroom in the Marriott Marquis in Times Square, New York City. Nearly four hundred physicians feasted on filet mignon and red snapper while a psychiatrist, Dr. Jay Fawyer of Fort Wayne, Indiana, discussed drug therapy for depression. Early in the talk, Dr. Fawyer highlighted the problems of patients who relapse after treatment with existing antidepressants. Later he spent time discussing a new drug, duloxetine, suggesting that this might be the answer for these otherwise refractory patients. The new drug was scheduled to be on the market about a year later under the brand name Cymbalta, manufactured by Eli Lilly.

The conference was organized by Optima Educational Solutions, a small company near Chicago. Lilly paid Optima two million dollars to offer the same "course" in a number of cities across the country, with a dozen physicians taking turns as speakers, attracting a total of 5,400 attendees. The physicians who attended received two hours of CME credit each.

Lilly and Optima both insisted to Hensley that the course was aimed at conveying scientific information about the causes and treatment of depression and that multiple products were mentioned. Optima, not Lilly, designed the slide show and the content. Optima would not say what it paid its speakers, but Dr. Fawyer said he was paid roughly one to five thousand dollars for such a presentation. He described it as a financial "break-even" situation because of the lost revenue from his practice while he was away speaking.[17]

Hensley characterized the dinner at the Astor Ballroom as typical of what happened in the wake of PhRMA's new 2001 guidelines limiting the gifts drug reps could give to physicians. The guidelines were (as our drug rep Stan reported) supposed to rein in such lavish entertainments as golf outings and sports events. Optima and other "education" firms told Hensley that they had received a substantial increase in their CME contracts as companies shifted marketing funds away from those now banned activities into CME.

Hensley also reviewed the history of efforts to regulate CME so that the sessions were truly education and not infomercials. The last round of public scrutiny of drug company excesses had occurred with the U.S. Senate hearings chaired by Senator Edward Kennedy in 1990–1991. This in turn led to calls for reform, and new ethical guidelines to (supposedly) govern reps' behavior were promulgated both by PhRMA and the AMA. The ACCME followed suit in 1991 to better regulate CME activities.[18] The relative effectiveness of those regulations can be gauged by the fact that the ACCME, in the spring of 2003, promulgated proposals for newer and tougher regulations and posted these for public comment.

According to Hensley, the FDA was also expected to enforce the separation of marketing and education, especially in one key area—the so-called "off label" use of drugs for medical problems other than those the FDA had specifically listed when the drug was approved. An industry- and manufacturer-funded free market advocacy group, the Washington Legal Foundation, successfully attacked several FDA initiatives on the grounds that they curtailed First Amendment free-speech rights to the physicians giving the lectures. The FDA then largely stopped enforcing its guidelines.

One of the major litigations against the industry in recent years was a whistleblower suit against Warner-Lambert (now part of Pfizer), charging that the Medicaid system was defrauded of hundreds of millions of dollars when physicians were persuaded to write prescriptions for inappropriate uses of the drug gabapentin (Neurontin). The company was charged with employing CME presentations as a major form of marketing for off-label uses of Neurontin. Warner-Lambert was said to have selected speakers and signed off on their presentation content specifically to ensure that physicians would hear about off-label uses, despite the law by which a company is prohibited from marketing any drug for off-label use.[19] Pfizer (on Warner-Lambert's behalf) pleaded guilty and paid a fine of $430 million, the second largest on record.[20]

There are several ways a CME presentation could be biased in favor of the sponsoring company. The most blatant is when a particular drug is touted as the best treatment. Hensley reported the unease experienced by Dr. Diana Koziupa, a psychiatrist from Sellersville, Pennsylvania, during a lecture series she presented in 1999–2000 with funding from Glaxo Wellcome. The slides the company provided for her included a series of cases, designed to test the audience's knowledge of which drug would be the best one for each patient described. Dr. Koziupa reported that the audiences always laughed when it turned out that Wellbutrin, a Glaxo product, turned out to be the "correct answer" in every one of the case studies.[21]

But bias need not be this blatant. Many companies calculate that they will earn a certain amount of money whenever physicians can be persuaded to use any of a class of drugs, such as inhaled corticosteroids for asthma. The CME speaker need never mention any drug by name at all, merely urge the use of the class, and the company profits. More generally, physicians may come away from CME programs with the message that a particular medical problem is best treated always by medications, and never by diet, exercise, or lifestyle changes. For instance, we may doubt whether Drs. Fawyer and Koziupa found any slides in the set they were provided with showing studies that documented the beneficial effects of daily walking for patients with depression.[22]

THE EVIDENCE

What evidence exists that CME programs have a demonstrable industry bias or that attending company-sponsored CME impacts physician behavior? The CME issue is less well-studied than some other aspects of pharmaceutical industry influence. An early study by Dr. Marjorie Bowman showed that the content of two CME programs was notably tilted in support of the companies' products.[23] She went on to demonstrate by a survey of physician attendees that later prescribing practices were likely to favor the products of the sponsor.[24]

Spingarn and colleagues compared residents who had attended a company-sponsored grand rounds on Lyme disease with residents who had not attended, assessing their knowledge of treatment with a survey three months later. They found the attendees more likely to use an expensive intravenous antibiotic sold by the company. The residents were prone to use that antibiotic both when it was appropriate and when it was not, and even when cheaper oral antibiotics would have done as well.[25]

Elina Hemminki and her colleagues in Finland took advantage of Estonia's shift from former Soviet republic to free-market economy during the 1990s, comparing the rate of prescriptions for female hormone replacement therapy with survey data obtained from family physicians and gynecologists. Estonia had a low rate of prescription for hormone replacement in the early 1990s but the rate rose rapidly later in the decade. Gynecologists, compared to family physicians, were more likely to view hormone replacement favorably, to believe that they had had sufficient continuing education on the topic, and to report that their last continuing education conference was partly paid for by a drug company.[26]

While their evidence is merely anecdotal, Dieperink and Drogemuller reported an experience that has been replicated numerous times at many institutions. They were surprised to find the number of prescriptions written in their Veterans Administration hospital for an unusual antipsychotic drug to have tripled within a very short period of time. The drug's appropriate uses were limited and they thought it very unlikely that suddenly their patients needed this drug three times as often. Investigating, they found that a CME conference had been funded at the hospital by the company manufacturing the drug in question, immediately before the spike in prescriptions.[27]

Since the quantitative evidence is rather lacking, indirect evidence of the effectiveness of CME can be gained from observations of industry behavior. As we will see shortly, the pharmaceutical industry has responded to threats of tightening regulations for CME with a major push-back—suggesting very strongly that the industry finds the present state of CME suitable for its goals. Lauren Walker, writing in the periodical *Medical Meetings*, may well be biased, but offered the calculation that the industry received sales revenues of $3.56 for every $1.00 spent on CME programs and other meetings.[28]

Dr. Peter Tugwell, chairman of medicine at the Ottawa Hospital, Canada, wrote a letter soliciting funds for CME conferences on behalf of an organization called OMERACT. The letter was sent to several major companies, including Bristol-Myers: "We think that support for such a meeting would be very profitable for a company with a worldwide interest in drugs targeted in these fields. The impact of sponsorship will be high as the individuals invited for this workshop, being opinion leaders in their field, are influential with the regulatory agencies. Currently we are seeking major sponsors to pledge support of U.S. $5,000 and $10,000. These major sponsors will be given the opportunity to nominate participants to represent industry's interest and to participate actively in the conference."[29] Clearly, Tugwell assumed that drug companies would not find it odd to be told that investing in CME was a profitable use of their funds, or to be promised that the amount of control over the content of the program, and how favorable it would be from their company's point of view, would be proportional to the amount of money paid in.

EARLIER EFFORTS AT CME REGULATION

The 1991 guidelines promulgated by the ACCME dealt with both disclosure and firewalls. Mandatory disclosure is the principal way that institutions in American medicine have sought to handle conflicts of interest. But, if the evidence is any indication, simple disclosure has not been successful at eliminating bias from CME.

The ACCME regulations have therefore not been content solely with disclosure of conflicts of interest. They have also been concerned with so-called "firewalls" by means of which drug company money can be kept separate from decisions about what speakers to invite and what those speakers should say. For example, no firewall exists when drug companies are allowed to contribute to a CME conference by hand-picking their own preferred speakers and supplying them with slides prepared by the firm's marketing division. With the ideal firewall, several different drug firms might pay into a budget to support a CME program and receive credit for doing so in the program announcement but all decisions about which speakers to invite and what to ask them to talk about are made by an independent expert committee. For example, slides supplied to a speaker by a drug company might be prohibited.

The earlier ACCME regulations came under fire from Dr. Arnold Relman, former editor of the *New England Journal of Medicine* and one of the most outspoken critics of the pharmaceutical industry. Relman asserted that fully half of the members of the ACCME task force responsible for its guidelines were "representatives of the pharmaceutical industry or . . . consultants for businesses that work with the industry in preparing educational programs."[30] Relman thought it outrageous that so many for-profit Medical Education and Communications Companies (MECCs), who openly advertised their wares to the drug industry by promising to design CME programs guaranteed to increase sales of their products, had been accredited by the ACCME as able to decide which programs were deserving of CME credit. Relman did not spare criticism of his own colleagues in academic medical centers. He noted that a resolution had been presented to the Society for Academic Continuing Medical Education, representing forty-eight medical schools, that would have prevented pharmaceutical companies and MECCs from awarding CME credit on their own say-so. The society tabled the resolution, allegedly because of fears of losing industry support for their own CME programs, as well as threats of a lawsuit from the MECCs.[31]

In response to Relman's and other criticisms, the ACCME proposed new guidelines in 2003 that leaned far more heavily to firewalls rather than to the mere disclosure of conflict.

One might imagine that the industry would be content with its informal apparatus for influencing physicians, and would not much care what happened in the formal CME sector. It appears, however, that the industry prefers to carry out many of its activities under the rubric of CME, perhaps wishing to make use both of the attraction to practitioners of offering them CME credits to attend an event, as well as the "halo" suggestion that if CME credits are given out, the presentation must be reasonably scientific and unbiased. Consultants to the industry (notably, those with financial stakes in the MECCs) spread tales of doom if the tighter CME guidelines were to take effect. Relman characterized the objections of the Washington Legal Foundation as alleging that virtually all well-trained and well-informed physicians already consult with the drug industry, so excluding such individuals from speaking would lead to a serious deterioration in the quality of CME.[32] As one might expect, the response of the industry to the ACCME proposed guidelines was almost completely negative.

CME AND THE INSPECTOR GENERAL'S REPORT

Early in 2004, the industry appeared well dug-in on the CME front. The threat of losing up to nearly half their existing CME funds seemed sufficient (according to Relman's accusations) to force academic medical centers into a compliant attitude when stronger CME regulations came up for a vote before the ACCME and other bodies. The Washington Legal Foundation stood poised to bring suit, claiming that such regulations violated First Amendment rights to "free commercial speech."[33] If business as usual prevailed, the ACCME would announce tough new regulations in draft form, then await an extended period for public comment. Strings would be pulled behind the scenes, and after the comment period, the ACCME would approve a set of regulations that had been considerably watered down from the draft form, in a direction favorable to industry.

But this scenario did not play out during 2004, and indeed by year's end it appeared from the outside as if the industry was in something of a retreat mode on the

CME issue. In September 2004, the ACCME announced a more stringent set of guidelines for CME funding, demanding more effective firewalls across the board.[34] Disclosure remains mandatory but would no longer be sufficient; speakers with industry ties are expected not to do presentations on those therapeutic areas.[35] Greater emphasis is placed on basing material presented on the best scientific evidence, and on eliminating commercial influence over conference planning and content. Clearer lines of demarcation are demanded between advertising and product promotion and the scientific content of CME.

Little objection was heard from industry in reply. The difference between the expected and the actual scenario was accounted for, perhaps, by the entrance of a new player into the game.

In April 2003, the Office of the Inspector General (OIG), Department of Health and Human Services, issued a report on the implications of a federal anti-kickback law for pharmaceutical manufacturers. The OIG report shocked many readers by noting that some commonly accepted business practices in the industry were potentially a violation of the federal anti-kickback law.[36] Violations could occur whenever:

- The industry gives payments or anything of any value
- The payment or gift is in return for ordering or recommending a purchase
- The purchase is reimbursable in whole or in part by a federal health care program
- The above is true even if the payment or gift has other legitimate purposes

It seems obvious from this definition that a physician taking a company pen or coffee mug from a rep would be a violation of the statute, as long as the physician had any portion of her practice covered by Medicare or Medicaid. The OIG went on to make clear that there was no intention of arresting physicians who accepted gifts from drug reps. They were after bigger fish—the pharmacy benefit managers (PBMs) and any sweetheart deals they had concluded with manufacturers. The overall goal of the OIG report was apparently to encourage the industry to create and then monitor in-house compliance systems, and much of the report explains what sort of compliance system the OIG would look for if a firm were ever audited.[37]

The OIG report discussed the industry's CME programs as well. The report recommended that companies separate the operations that give grants to fund CME from their sales and marketing functions. The anti-kickback statute would be implicated, said the OIG, if the company exerted any control over the content or the selection of speakers at a CME event.[38]

If at least one article in a pharmaceutical-friendly journal is to be believed, the industry took the OIG report seriously. In the summer of 2004, *Pharma Voice* interviewed a number of insiders among commercial CME firms, and reported that many had put their CME programs on hold while awaiting the new, tougher AC-CME guidelines.[39]

The general tone of the industry response to the new ACCME guidelines was notably meek. According to the new attitude described by *Pharma Voice*, companies were working to separate CME programming from marketing, as suggested by the

OIG report, and were in turn putting pressure on commercial suppliers of CME and conference events (the MECCs) to create separate business operations to handle CME and openly commercial activities. Indeed the "buzz" among those interviewed was that even measuring "return on investment" might bring down the wrath of the OIG in case of an audit, by showing that the company intended a close connection between CME funding and drug sales. Stop measuring return on investment and find novel ways to monitor "return on education," several sources suggested.

At this writing it is too soon to tell if anything substantive will change.[40] Will the stringent new guidelines adopted by ACCME be enforced in the trenches? If the guidelines work as intended, will the industry pull funding out of CME support, in favor of non-CME dinners and other events it can control better?[41] Will DHHS perform any audits, to reinforce the big stick represented by the OIG report? All that can be said at present is that the threat of legal action under federal anti-kickback statutes seems to have gained the industry's attention.

CONCLUSION

It is difficult to write a book about the problems of corporate influence over science and academics. The early chapters of the book have to explain how terrible the problem is—otherwise why bother to read the book? Then the last few chapters have to provide solutions—otherwise why bother to read the book? So the author spends most of the volume saying how unfixable the problems are, then pulls fixes, like a rabbit out of a hat, at the end.

Derek Bok, former president of Harvard, manages this balancing act very well in his book, *Universities in the Marketplace*.[42] He waxes pessimistic for most of the book, then discovers optimism at the end. In only one area does pessimism win out completely. He believes that universities can develop aggressive new policies to ward off the worst dangers of commercial influence before it is too late; but that funding for CME is already a lost cause: "The dependence on corporate support has reached such a point that it will be difficult for medical schools to free themselves of industry influence."[43]

CME ought to be the ultimate test of medicine's professionalism. What, after all, could be more central to its mission, than physicians assisting other physicians to keep informed of the latest scientific information so as to improve the quality of care provided to all patients? According to Bok, we have allowed what should have been a pillar of professionalism to deteriorate into a massive eBay—with the users hoping to obtain something of value without paying the full price for it; and a variety of commercial predators taking full advantage of these hopes to line their own pockets.

NOTES

1. R. Harris, *The Real Voice* (New York: Macmillan, 1964), 85.

2. E. F. Torrey, "The Going Rate on Shrinks: Big Pharma and the Buying of Psychiatry," *The American Prospect*, July 15, 2002, 15–16.

3. Torrey, "The Going Rate on Shrinks," 15.

4. Torrey, "The Going Rate on Shrinks," 15.

5. Torrey, "The Going Rate on Shrinks," 15.

6. Torrey, "The Going Rate on Shrinks," 16.

7. Torrey, "The Going Rate on Shrinks," 16.

8. Torrey, "The Going Rate on Shrinks," 16.

9. Torrey, "The Going Rate on Shrinks," 16. It would seem that the professional medical societies are willing to go to considerable length to preserve the environment in their exhibit halls that will be most congenial to the industry representatives who pay for such a large portion of the meeting budget. The *BMJ* reported (April 16, 2005), "The American College of Physicians has refused to allow the non-profit US organization No Free Lunch, a group devoted to reducing competing interests in medicine, to rent a booth at its annual meeting. The college said the presence of the group would inhibit dialogue between industry exhibitors and doctors"; "US Doctors Rebuff Drug Watchdog Group" [news in brief], *BMJ* 2005; 330:862. The press release from No Free Lunch pointed out that the College's own ethics manual warns physicians against accepting gifts, even of low value, from drug reps; www.nofreelunch.org/news.htm (accessed April 15, 2005).

10. www.accme.org/incoming/179_2003_ACCME_Annual_Report_Data.pdf (accessed August 4, 2004).

11. W. Sohn, A. I. Ismail, and M. Tellez, "Efficacy of Educational Interventions Targeting Primary Care Providers' Practice Behaviors: An Overview of Published Systematic Reviews," *J Public Health Dent* 2004; 64:164–72. These authors asked what it might take to get primary medical care providers to do a better job of screening children for oral health. They reviewed all systematic reviews of high-quality trials of various educational interventions. They decided that some interventions change provider behavior—small group discussion, outreach visits, reminders—notably, the techniques already widely used in pharmaceutical promotion. But formal CME programs could not be shown to be on the list of effective interventions.

12. D. Siegel and J. Lopez, "Trends in Antihypertensive Drug Use in the United States: Do the JNC V Recommendations Affect Prescribing?" *JAMA* 1997; 278:1745–48. There is some limited evidence in more recent years that current prescribing trends are beginning to match better the evidence-based recommendations to use cheaper, older drugs first; see, for instance, R. S. Stafford, C. D. Furberg, S. N. Finkelstein, et al., "Impact of Clinical Trial Results on National Trends in Alpha-Blocker Prescribing, 1996–2002," *JAMA* 2004; 291:54–62.

13. M. D. Rawlins, "The Role of the Pharmaceutical Industry in Postgraduate Medical Education," *Br J Clin Pharmacol* 1977; 4:257–58; N. M. Kaplan, "Sounding Board: The Support of Continuing Medical Education by Pharmaceutical Companies," *N Engl J Med* 1979; 300:194–96; M. D. Rawlins, "Doctors and the Drug Makers," *Lancet* 1984; 2:814; R. Smith, "Doctors and the Drug Industry: Too Close for Comfort," *Br Med J* (Clin Res Ed) 1986; 293:905–6; D. Kessler, "Drug Promotion and Scientific Exchange: The Role of the Clinical Investigator," *N Engl J Med* 1991; 325:201–3; F. Rosner, "Ethical Relationships between Drug Companies and the Medical Profession," *Chest* 1992; 102:266–69; C. K. Kasper, "Publication of Sponsored Symposiums in Medical Journals" [letter], *N Engl J Med* 1993; 328:1197; R. C. Noble, "Physicians and the Pharmaceutical Industry: An Alliance with Unhealthy Aspects," *Perspect Biol Med* 1993; 36:376–94; N. A. Bickell, "Drug Companies and Continuing Medical Education," *J Gen Intern Med* 1995; 10:392–94. For fairly typical rebuttals, see K. J. Boyce, J. N. Parochka, and K. M. Overstreet, "Industry Sponsorship of Continuing Medical Education" [letter], *JAMA* 2003; 290:1149; A. F. Holmer, "Industry Strongly Supports Continuing Medical Education," *JAMA* 2001; 285:2012–14.

14. Accreditation Council for Continuing Medical Education, annual financial report, 2003, www.accme.org/dir_docs/doc_upload97dd7a39-9746-4a5d-8c01-e56a9ffc0c8b_uploaddocument.pdf (accessed January 7, 2005).

15. S. Hensley, "Remedial Lessons: When Doctors Go to Class, Industry Often Foots the Bill," *Wall Street Journal*, December 4, 2002:A1.

16. M. A. Bowman, "The Impact of Drug Company Funding on the Content of Continuing Medical Education," *Mobius* 1986; 6:66–69; M. A. Bowman and D. L. Pearle, "Changes in Drug Prescribing Patterns Related to Commercial Company Funding of Continuing Medical Education," *J Contin Educ Health Prof* 1988; 8:13–20; J. Lexchin, "Interactions between Physicians and the Pharmaceutical Industry: What Does the Literature Say?" *Can Med Assoc J* 1993; 149:1401–7; M. E. Dieperink and L. Drogemuller, "Industry-Sponsored Grand Rounds and Prescribing Behavior," *JAMA* 2001; 285:1443–44; R. W. Spingarn, J. A. Berlin, and B. L. Strom, "When Pharmaceutical Manufacturers' Employees Present Grand Rounds, What Do Residents Remember?" *Acad Med* 1996; 71:86–88.

17. Hensley, "Remedial Lessons." At least one physician, apparently, has found giving these lectures more than a break-even venture. Dr. James R. Little, a family physician from Portland, Oregon, reported encountering a family physician who gave 160 presentations annually at $1000 each; he had reorganized his practice so as to leave extra time free during the middle of the day to allow him to give noon-time talks within a one-hour driving radius; J. R. Little, "When a Doctor Is the Rep" [response to *Ann Fam Med* on-line discussion], April 12, 2005, http://annalsfm.highwire.org/cgi/eletters/3/1/82#1690 (accessed May 5, 2005); and personal communication.

18. T. Randall, "New Guidelines Expected in 1991 for Relationship of Continuing Education, Financial Support," *JAMA* 1990; 264:1080.

19. Hensley, "Remedial Lessons."

20. Associated Press, "Pfizer Pleads Guilty in Drug Case," *Philadelphia Inquirer*, June 8, 2004.

21. Hensley, "Remedial Lessons."

22. See for instance J. A. Blumenthal, M. A. Babyak, K. A. Moore, et al., "Effects of Exercise Training in Older Patients with Major Depression," *Arch Intern Med* 1999; 159:2349–56.

23. Bowman, "Impact of Drug Company Funding."

24. Bowman and Pearle, "Changes in Drug Prescribing Patterns."

25. Spingarn, Berlin, and Strom, "When Pharmaceutical Manufacturers' Employees Present."

26. E. Hemminki, T. Karttunen, S. L. Hovi, and H. Karro, "The Drug Industry and Medical Practice: The Case of Menopausal Hormone Therapy in Estonia," *Soc Sci Med* 2004; 58:89–97.

27. Dieperink and Drogemuller, "Industry-Sponsored Grand Rounds."

28. L. Walker, "ROI for Meetings Beats Detailing and DTC," *Medical Meetings*, July 1, 2001. http://mm.meetingsnet.com/ar/meetings_roi_meetings_beats/index.htm (accessed January 7, 2005).

29. S. Krimsky, *Science in the Private Interest: Has the Lure of Profits Corrupted Biomedical Research?* (Lanham, MD: Rowman and Littlefield, 2003), 137. This letter came to light as a result of a legal investigation into alleged conflict of interest, related to Tugwell's service on a court-appointed scientific panel on silicone breast implants.

30. A. S. Relman, "Separating Continuing Medical Education from Pharmaceutical Marketing," *JAMA* 2001; 285:2009–12; quote p. 2010.

31. Relman, "Separating Continuing Medical Education."

32. A. S. Relman, "Defending Professional Independence: ACCME's Proposed New Guidelines for Commercial Support of CME," *JAMA* 2003; 289:2418–20.

33. D. J. Popeo and R. A. Samp, *Comments of the Washington Legal Foundation to the Accreditation Council for Continuing Medical Education Concerning Request for Comments on the January 14, 2003, Draft "Standards . . ."* (Washington, DC: Washington Legal Foundation, 2003).

34. ACCME, *Standards for Commercial Support* (Chicago: Accreditation Council for Continuing Medical Education, April 1, 2004), 1–3; www.accme.org/incoming/174_Standards%20for%20Commercial%20Support_April%202004.pdf; J. H. Tanne, "US Accrediting Agency Tightens Rules for Continuing Medical Education," *BMJ* 2004; 329:819.

35. Social scientist Jennifer Fishman, examining the industry's efforts to "sell" female sexual dysfunction as a disease requiring drug treatment, argues that even these apparently stringent new "firewall" requirements will fail, because of the multiple levels at which the industry now exercises influence over medical research. In the case of female sexual dysfunction, industry sponsored the research of an elite group of ten to twenty academic investigators to "discover" the disease and the efficacy of drug therapy, and then sponsored the "consensus conferences" at which those investigators met and put forward scientific criteria for diagnosing the "disease." These same investigators, in their role in industry-funded speakers' bureaus, then fanned out across the country to give CME presentations about this new "disease" and its "treatment." A "firewall" put in place at the CME level to try to disentangle any commercial influence is, according to Fishman, bound to fail, because the industry influence occurred so far upstream; J. R. Fishman, "Manufacturing Desire: The Commodification of Female Sexual Dysfunction," *Soc Stud Sci* 2004; 34:187–218. For more on these concerns, see the discussion of astroturf and disease mongering in chapter 13.

36. On the general implications of this and related measures involving physicians' conflicts of interest, see D. M. Studdert, M. M. Mello, and T. A. Brennan, "Financial Conflicts of Interest in Physicians' Relationships with the Pharmaceutical Industry—Self-Regulation in the Shadow of Federal Prosecution," *N Engl J Med* 2004; 351:1891–1900.

37. Office of the Inspector General, *Compliance Program Guidelines for Pharmaceutical Manufacturers* (Washington, D.C.: Department of Health and Human Services, April, 2003).

38. Office of the Inspector General, *Compliance Program Guidelines*, 20–21.

39. M. Chernock, "The State of CME: Light at the End of the Tunnel," *Pharma Voice* 2004; 4:22–31.

40. As I was completing work on this book, a major article appeared by a group of prominent academic physicians, urging much more stringent guidelines to prevent conflicts of interest in academic medical centers. They offered the opinion that even the new ACCME guidelines needed to be further strengthened; T. A. Brennan, D. J. Rothman, L. Blank, et al., "Health Industry Practices That Create Conflicts of Interest: A Policy Proposal for Academic Medical Centers," *JAMA* 2006; 295:429–33.

41. An early suggestion that the tougher new guidelines is not dampening industry interest in funding CME is F. Vrazo, "When Doctors Learn, Drug Firms Often Pay the Tab," *Philadelphia Inquirer*, June 8, 2005.

42. D. Bok, *Universities in the Marketplace: The Commercialization of Higher Education* (Princeton, NJ: Princeton University Press, 2003).

43. Bok, *Universities in the Marketplace*, 206.

12

PROFESSIONAL ORGANIZATIONS AND JOURNAL ADVERTISING

Of course [industry support] is going to bias us—the question is whether the bias is benign. [Without the funding from industry, instead of the annual meeting being held at the Philadelphia Convention Center,] we'd be sitting in the basement of the YMCA.

—Dr. David McDowell, Columbia University psychiatrist, on the American Psychiatric Association's dependence on pharmaceutical money to support its 2002 annual convention[1]

Recall Dr. E. Fuller Torrey's concluding comment in his "postcard" from the Berlin Psychiatric Congress, in chapter 11.[2] He hoped to reform the excesses of industry sponsorship of CME, but he feared that professional organizations, such as the American Psychiatric Association, were too dependent on industry funding for too much of their operating funds to take up the cudgel. Officials of the American Psychiatric Association have admitted that the industry supplies about one-third of the organization's annual budget.[3]

Since professional organizations commonly sponsor CME conferences, there is a good deal of overlap between the topics of the last chapter and this one. Also, many professional organizations also publish their own journals, and one way that the industry can defray the expenses of the organization is to purchase advertising space in the journal. It will therefore be convenient to discuss journal advertising and support for professional organizations together in this chapter.[4]

Despite the overlap, there is one major difference between the topics. CME, as we saw, was a discrete, well-reported activity. It proved easy to find specific figures on pharmaceutical industry support. By contrast, professional organizations conduct their business with relatively little disclosure of how much their operating budgets depend on industry.[5] Nor does the industry report support for professional organizations as a separate line item in any of their financial disclosures. The industry reports the total amount spent on journal advertising. But the publishers of medical journals also tend to regard the detailed operations of their journals as proprietary information. This makes it difficult to relate the sum received for journal advertising to the total costs of publishing the journal.

SOME STORIES OF PROFESSIONAL ORGANIZATIONS

One advantage to being a senior, well-respected figure in internal medicine—the editor of the *New England Journal of Medicine*, let us say—is that one finds oneself on a first-name basis with the presidents and board members of many of the most important medical-professional societies in the United States. Thus, when Dr. Jerome Kassirer came to write his book about problems with the pharmaceutical industry, he could draw on an insider's knowledge of a field that necessarily remains obscure to those of us less well placed.

Kassirer first turned his attention to the Society of Critical Care Medicine:

> The Web site for the 32nd meeting of the [Society of Critical Care Medicine] in San Antonio held early in 2003 contained a 20-page insert entitled *Sponsorship Opportunities*. The more than 50 opportunities for sponsorship add up to approximately two million dollars. They included the opening reception (can be purchased by a company for $100,000), the President's reception ($30,000), the Rustlers Rodeo Roundup ($150,000), the Chili Cook-off ($5,000 each), the Internet Pavilion ($40,000), and various educational grants ($125,000 for the President's Circle, $75,000 for Platinum level, $50,000 for Diamond level, etc.). For various smaller sums, companies can buy tote bags, pens, highlighters, and notepads for all the participants.[6]

The society, however, wished to make it abundantly clear that they were very concerned with ethics:

> An entry on the [Society of Critical Care Medicine] Web site entitled "Advertising and Sponsorship Opportunities" reads: "Are you looking for a winning strategy to enhance patient care by making state of art medical information available to more critical care professionals? One that is consistent with ethical guidelines concerning gifts to healthcare practitioners? Look no further, the Society of Critical Care Medicine has a practical way to demonstrate that your company cares about the patients it serves." If one did not know that the Web site belonged to a professional society, it could easily be mistaken for a commercial education enterprise.[7]

It is worth noting that the society is essentially using "ethics" as a bargaining tool to compete with its own members for handouts from the industry. The message seems to be: If you give freebies directly to our member physicians, you might run afoul of the new PhRMA or AMA guidelines or even the HHS-OIG anti-kickback warnings. Much better to give the boodle to us directly. You can then be confident that you are not violating any ethical rules—while still ensuring that our members have their arms twisted to prescribe your drug.

Kassirer next turned his attention to the American Society of Nephrology, the kidney specialists.

In 1999, Dr. William Bennett, then president of the American Society of Nephrology . . . , established a committee to define the key ethical issues in education, research, and clinical practice raised by the interaction of the profession and industry. . . . The committee identified major conflicts of interest involving education, research, and patient care. Issues were raised about compensation of directors of dialysis units, the quality of care given to dialysis patients, the structure of research projects, financial incentives that tempt clinical investigators to pressure patients to participate in research, and influence by industry on educational efforts. The committee proposed that the council of the society obtain systematic data about the extent of the ethical problems. . . . Late in 2003, Dr. Bennett provided a follow-up. He said, "The [American Society of Nephrology] decided not to pursue this matter further. I was outvoted 5 to 2. The [society] and academic 'researchers' are far too tight with industry for me. I was frustrated and took a great deal of flack from industry and colleagues for even suggesting the issue."[8]

When I read Kassirer's accounts of what he had found on the websites of various national medical-professional societies, I realized that I had been remiss in not checking out the website of my own national organization, the American Academy of Family Physicians. The 2004 scientific assembly in Orlando had just been completed, but the "exhibit prospectus" was still posted on the web. The prospectus boasted to would-be advertisers and renters of exhibit booths how many family physicians would be attending, how the attendees were considered the local opinion leaders and trend-setters, and how many of them had purchased or picked up items at booths at last year's assembly. Among the places firms were invited to advertise: the AAFP assembly TV program that ran eighteen hours a day in each attendee's hotel room; the "Shuttlevision," a promotional tape playing constantly in the shuttle bus taking attendees back and forth from the convention center; and the "Doctor's Bag door hanger" delivered to attendees' hotel rooms ("This is the official . . . hotel door delivery program; absolutely no materials may be delivered to registrants' hotel rooms by any other means").[9]

THE ECONOMICS OF THE PROFESSIONAL ORGANIZATION

The organizations that Kassirer and I have described appear to be responding to economic realities. Historically, medical-professional organizations have been supported primarily by the dues paid by their members—though as we saw, as far back as the late 1940s, the AMA had to confront the challenge of whether to raise dues in the face of dwindling advertising revenues or cave in to industry pressures in order to sell more ads.

Many medical organizations today follow the old dues-paying model for a simple reason—they have no choice. Many organizations are very small. They are either local or regional in scope (a county medical society or the state chapter of a national specialty society) or else they appeal to a very narrow subspecialty interest, so that only a few hundred physicians across the country would be interested in joining. No drug company may have much to gain by supporting such an organization.[10] (Some smaller societies are more open to commercial entanglements with the medical device industry—if, for example, the subspecialists who are members of the society form the principal market for a certain expensive surgical instrument or imaging device.)

By contrast, the larger or better-positioned organizations may negotiate their name and reputation and easy access to their members in exchange for operating revenue. The advantage to the organization is that it can offer more services to its members—better CME meetings, better-quality journals or newsletters, a larger and more efficient office staff—while keeping membership dues low.

One cannot assume that physicians make sufficient income so as to be willing to pay relatively high dues to their medical societies without resistance. For one thing, medical society dues are large enough to attract the notice of even quite well-off individuals. The current dues for membership in the AMA and its constituent state and county medical societies, for instance, is over $1000 annually in many cases.[11] For another, there may be little natural limit to the number of organizations that might claim the loyalty of any individual physician. Imagine, for instance, an internist who is director of an intensive care unit and who also focuses a good deal on kidney disease. Arguably, she ought to be a member of the American College of Physicians, the Society of Critical Care Medicine, and the American Society of Nephrology—even before she decides whether or not to join the AMA and her state and county medical societies.

Even if physicians ideally should not mind paying higher dues to their professional societies, they commonly discontinue their membership when dues are increased. Therefore, any organizational leader contemplating an increase in dues will have to factor in likely lost membership as part of the equation. Moreover, many societies have their dues policies set democratically, through a mechanism such as a house of delegates, and the membership is unlikely to vote higher dues for itself, even if the leadership thinks it worthwhile.

Finally, past habits shape present policies. The willingness of the pharmaceutical industry to shoulder a good portion of the costs of running many medical organizations has shaped the average physician's sense of what level of dues he "ought to" be willing to pay. The culture of entitlement has extended to the dues deemed acceptable. It is in this context that we can best assess Dr. McDowell's complaint about what it would mean for the American Psychiatric Association to have to hold its annual meeting in the basement of the YMCA. Physicians have come to feel *entitled* to a certain level of luxury in the settings in which their meetings are held. When Dr. McDowell made his comment to *Washington Post* reporter Shankar Vedantam, he clearly never anticipated the reply, "And what, exactly, is wrong with meeting in the basement of the YMCA?" And these same physicians have come to feel entitled to paying a level of dues and registration fees to support the American Psychiatric Association that would not, by themselves, allow the organization to hold its meetings at venues of the desired quality. Paying Pontiac prices to drive a Lexus seems to be what physicians now demand.

CURRENT DEPENDENCE OF ORGANIZATIONS ON INDUSTRY[12]

I was able to obtain detailed estimates of pharmaceutical funding received by one organization, the American Academy of Family Physicians (AAFP). The leadership of AAFP is perhaps more willing to disclose its internal finances because it believes that it has successfully created firewalls and conflict-of-interest policies to prevent undue influence of pharmaceutical funding over Academy activities. The AAFP is somewhat privileged in this regard. As a large organization whose members prescribe a very wide variety of drugs, its goodwill is actively sought by the pharmaceutical industry, giving the AAFP more control even in the face of large pharmaceutical contributions.[13]

Estimates provided by AAFP leadership suggest the breakdown of pharmaceutical support shown in table 12.1.[14]

Table 12.1. Estimated Pharmaceutical Support, American Academy of Family Physicians, 2002

Category	Percentage of total revenue	Estimated annual amount (in millions)
CME (all commercial support)	5	$3.02
Advertising in AAFP journals	22.5	$13.6
Special project support	10	$6.04
Total pharmaceutical support	37.5	$22.6
Total AAFP revenue	100	$60.4

AAFP derived approximately 22.5 percent of total revenue from journal advertising in 2002. This compares to a mean percentage among the six medical organizations of 15.3 percent (range, 2.1 to 31.3 percent), according to one of the rare published studies on this question.[15] It appears that medical societies are very heterogeneous in their reliance on journal advertising. It was reported that the AMA, in 1999, received approximately fifty-four million dollars in journal advertising revenues.[16]

Because so few data on medical organization finance have been published, my colleagues and I conducted a brief mail survey in 2003. We identified 222 organizations offering CME programs and appearing to be national in scope. From this list we randomly chose fifty organizations to receive a mailed survey form. We received seventeen responses, of which sixteen provided revenue estimates, as shown in table 12.2.

Table 12.2. Pharmaceutical Support for Fifty Randomly Selected National Medical Organizations, 2003 (n = 16 responding)

Total membership	165,950
Total annual revenue	$95,156,000
Pharmaceutical support: CME	$5,816,900
Pharmaceutical support: Journal ads	$5,717,840
Pharmaceutical support: Grants, other	$1,278,000
Total pharmaceutical support	$12,812,740
Percent of total revenue	13.5

Beside the low response rate, our informal survey had several limitations. We may have surveyed a disproportionate number of organizations whose main source of commercial support is the medical device or equipment industry rather than the pharmaceutical industry.[17] The median membership of the organizations responding to our survey was 2,500, suggesting that we had a disproportionate number of responses from smaller organizations. On the other hand, as we noted previously, many professional societies may be relatively small, in which case we sampled a fairly typical group.[18]

If these rather sparse data are to be believed, professional medical societies in the United States may form a bimodal population. For the "average" society, if such a thing exists, only about 10 to 15 percent of total operating revenue may come from the pharmaceutical industry. For a select group of larger organizations, who therefore represent highly desirable marketing targets from the industry standpoint, industry support may range around one-third.

In terms of ethics and policy, it probably does not matter much which exact form the pharmaceutical contribution takes. These organizations have fairly flexible budgets and governance structures, making it relatively easy to shift excess funds from one area to make up for a deficit in another. More ads sold for one's journal might translate into lower registration fees changed for the group's CME conferences, or could be used to lower future dues. Special grants means that the group can offer new services to members, or engage in new activities that yield positive publicity, without having to raise dues to cover the activity. So, when concerned about conflict of interest and trustworthiness, we appear justified in looking at total pharmaceutical support as a percentage of the organization's revenue.

THE ETHICS OF THE PROFESSIONAL ORGANIZATION

Calling an entity a "professional medical organization" might mean two different things. One possible meaning is that the organization is made up of individual members, each of which is a medical professional. As individuals, each member is bound by whatever ethical responsibilities define the professional "code of ethics." But the organization, as such, has no special ethical responsibilities of its own. It is no different from a trade union, say. At the *organizational* level, the fact that its members are "professionals" carries no special ethical weight.

This is not the understanding of "professional" that informed the guidelines proposed by Drs. Edmund Pellegrino, a senior physician-ethicist, and Arnold Relman, former editor of the *New England Journal*. Quite clearly, a "professional" organization in their view was required to have its own set of ethical standards, independent of the individual ethical character of its members. The ideal of professionalism entails "a commitment to the effacement of self-interest. . . . When physicians form professional associations, they should make this promise collectively."[19] Pellegrino and Relman argued that the organization should adhere to rather strict rules:

- Focus relatively more attention on the general public good, and less upon the specific economic interests of the membership.
- Avoid any tendency to become a trade union.
- Fund activities solely from members' dues or grants received from nonprofit entities.
- If the organization publishes a journal, ensure reasonable editorial independence.

Pellegrino and Relman see a significant conflict between the ethical ideas of professionalism and the economics of the medical society that we previously reviewed. They view seeking funding from for-profit entities, as a means of keeping dues low, an unacceptable conflict of interest. They propose to resolve the conflict by siding with ethics over economics.

Drs. Pellegrino and Relman, in putting forth their proposed guidelines for organizations, named no names. The proverbial visitor from Mars might conclude that they just happened to become curious about organizational ethics when they did. American physicians, by contrast, immediately associated their paper with the AMA's Sunbeam case.[20] In 1997, a group of top AMA leaders had made a deal with Sunbeam, manufacturer of home appliances, to allow the company exclusive use of the AMA name and logo on a line of health-related products, such as scales, air cleaners, massagers, and thermometers. In exchange, the AMA would receive royalties on sales, an amount estimated to be several million dollars annually. The AMA had taken no steps to review the appliances that would bear its name, to determine either their quality or their true medical need. The leaders who concluded the initial deal also failed to consult with the AMA board of directors and other key groups. When the deal became known, the negative publicity caused the AMA to back out, resulting in a twenty-million-dollar lawsuit from Sunbeam for breach of contract. Three of the involved leaders were forced to resign.[21]

JOURNAL ADVERTISING

It is reported that the first printed advertisement in history, in a German news book published in 1591, was for a medicinal herbal preparation.[22] Thus pharmaceutical advertising has a venerable history. In more recent times, pharmaceutical advertising has become a significant factor in the financial support of medical journals. More than thirty years ago, an editorial in the *New England Journal of Medicine* decried the increasing dependence of organized medicine and medical journals upon pharmaceutical industry funding.[23] The sorts of concerns raised in this editorial are well illustrated by the case of the *Annals of Internal Medicine*.

The *Annals* Story

In the early 1990s, Dr. Michael Wilkes, an internist, was a Robert Wood Johnson Clinical Scholar at the University of California-Los Angeles medical center. The

Clinical Scholars Program is designed for young physicians who show promise of later distinguished careers in academic medicine, and who wish to gain some additional experience in research methods. Over the years, Clinical Scholars have shown themselves to be willing to take on challenges and to think outside the box, as the common phrase has it. Dr. Wilkes proved to be no exception.

Dr. Wilkes and a fellow Clinical Scholar, Dr. Bruce Doblin, were casting about for a suitable research project under the direction of their supervisor, Dr. Martin Shapiro. They decided to do a carefully structured study of the quality of pharmaceutical ads in medical journals. They approached the study as a journal editor would approach the review of a scientific paper submitted for publication—they identified first a panel of reputed experts in the relevant fields of medicine and pharmacy, and developed review forms to make sure that the same criteria were reliably assessed for each advertisement. They used multiple reviewers to correct for individual bias.

Their initial results were quite unflattering to the advertising. They found numerous instances of unbalanced and misleading ads, and ads with no discernible educational value. Dr. Shapiro worked with Wilkes and Doblin to reanalyze and review their data numerous times—they knew their findings would be challenged and wanted to be absolutely sure that they could defend their results.

When they were finally satisfied with the paper, they submitted it for publication. The two "top" journals, the *New England Journal of Medicine* and *JAMA*, turned down the paper. For internists, the next-highest prestige journal was the *Annals of Internal Medicine*, which is published by the American College of Physicians.

Since 1990 the editorship of *Annals* had been jointly occupied by Drs. Robert and Suzanne Fletcher. The editorial board looked carefully at the Wilkes paper, decided that it addressed an important issue using careful research methods, and recommended publication. They elected to give it a rather prominent visibility, with the Fletchers writing an accompanying editorial, and also soliciting a commentary from the commissioner of the FDA, David Kessler. (The FDA has the authority to police fraudulent or misleading pharmaceutical advertising.) As the Fletchers wrote in their own editorial comment, if misleading or inaccurate ads appear frequently in journals, all of these parties—the drug companies, the journal editors, and the FDA—bear some responsibility for this state of affairs. So they saw the study as an indictment of themselves and of the FDA as much as a slam against the drug industry.

The research study and the two editorial commentaries were published in the June 1, 1992 issue of *Annals*.[24] All parties were unprepared for the avalanche that followed. The media picked up the story and ran vigorously with it. Regents of the American College of Physicians started to receive phone calls from reporters, members, and pharmaceutical industry executives, and wondered why the editors of their own journal had not at least given them some warning. (This being the first time such a thing had happened during the Fletchers' editorial tenure, they had no existing policy in place.) The spokespeople for the industry (the Pharmaceutical Manufacturers Association, predecessor organization to PhRMA) were outraged that they had not been treated as an equal party to the transaction and invited in advance to provide a comment or guest editorial, as had the FDA. The organization issued a statement claiming that it was unfair to impugn the reputation of the entire industry based on a small sample of 109 ads.

As a condition of the government grant funding they had received, Wilkes and his colleagues agreed to keep confidential which specific ads and which drug companies they had surveyed. This, however, did not stop Dr. Sidney Wolfe of the Public Citizen's Health Research Group, an activist and longtime critic of the industry. Wolfe filed suit under the Freedom of Information Act and was able to obtain the identification of the 109 ads. Despite the objections of the Fletchers and Wilkes and colleagues that the study had not been designed to judge the behavior of any specific firm, Dr. Wolfe publicized the ads and the companies responsible in a letter to Senator Edward Kennedy of Massachusetts, who had held hearings on pharmaceutical industry promotional practices.

Dr. Wilkes, as chief author, found that instead of being able to finish his Clinical Scholars work and start off on his career in health services research, he was suddenly the target of a massive industry counterattack, and had his time fully occupied with angry letters, phone calls, and hostile panel discussions.[25] Our concern, however, is with the Fletchers. Several large pharmaceutical companies pulled their ads from *Annals*, and the drop in advertising revenue worsened after Public Citizen's publicity. Between 1992 and 1995, *Annals* lost an estimated $1 to $1.5 million in ad revenue. It was impossible to prove cause and effect; during these years, advertising on the whole in medical journals was declining. But the drop for *Annals* appeared to be steeper than elsewhere, even though the journal's circulation was increasing; and the word on the street, at any rate, was that *Annals* was being punished for publishing the Wilkes study.

While no one in the American College of Physicians directly questioned the Fletchers' editorial judgment, the Fletchers nevertheless felt that many viewed their continued editorship as a liability to *Annals*. They resigned the editorship in December 1993 and accepted appointments at Harvard Medical School.[26] It was generally reported that following the Fletchers' departure, pharmaceutical ads in the *Annals* increased to levels near those prior to the Wilkes publication.[27]

In one way, the *Annals* affair appears to have had a longstanding impact on medical journal publication in the United States. Anyone reading the medical journals with an eye toward the role of the pharmaceutical industry will be struck by how regularly any article or editorial that is in any way critical of the industry is accompanied by an invited commentary from a pro-industry source, usually PhRMA. It is never explained why the pharmaceutical industry gets this favored treatment. It does not appear to be standard practice, for example, to offer the tobacco or the beef and dairy industries immediate rebuttal opportunities every time a journal prints something critical of smoking or cholesterol. If representatives of those industries take exception to what is written, they have to submit a letter to the editor, just like any average reader—and they often do. Since the Fletchers' failure to give the industry advance notice of, and an immediate chance to reply to, the Wilkes study was apparently a huge source of umbrage in the *Annals* case, one wonders whether the fate of the Fletchers and the financial fate of *Annals* served as a warning to other editors.

JOURNAL ADVERTISING REVENUE

The industry funds medical journals in three ways: purchasing advertising space, funding special journal supplements, and purchasing reprints of individual articles or of entire journal issues. The figures in table 12.3, obtained from the commercial firm IMS Health, appear to reflect the costs of journal ads only.[28]

Table 12.3. Industry Expenditures on Journal Advertising

Year	Amount ($ millions)
1996	459
1997	510
1998	498
1999	470
2000	484
2001	425
2002	437
2003	448

Ads are, at least in theory, clearly labeled as ads, and so might be thought to present less of an ethical concern than most other promotional activities. Nonetheless, Americans generally appear prone to the myth that just because one sees something in print, some official body has decided that it must be true. The FDA has jurisdiction over journal advertising, and can order an ad rescinded and the company to circulate a corrective letter. In practice, the FDA authority is seldom invoked, in part because by the time the FDA can investigate an ad, the ad's natural life span in the journals has usually expired. In one unusual case, the FDA notified Aventis Pharmaceuticals in December 2002 that its injectable cancer drug, Taxotere, was described to doctors in promotional material that overstated effectiveness, understated safety concerns, and suggested a broader set of uses for the drug than the FDA had approved. The company responded that it had ceased its campaign and that all promotional material of that type had been destroyed. The FDA complained on two subsequent occasions that the promotion was still in use and that the company had launched an ad campaign with the same misleading information. The company finally paid attention in November 2003, when the FDA threatened to seize the firm's entire supply of the drug.[29]

When a strongly pro-industry administration came to power in Washington in 2001, the FDA policing of drug ads decreased. The FDA filed about one-fourth as many warning letters between 2001 and 2004 as it had in the four years before 2001, and the staff assigned to ad review was cut.[30] At the same time as the FDA was working hard to streamline the process of approving new drugs, it extended the time it took to issue a warning letter regarding a misleading drug ad, by requiring that high-level FDA officials sign off on each such letter.[31]

JOURNAL SUPPLEMENTS

Pharmaceutical companies frequently sponsor conferences or symposia at which papers friendly to their drugs are presented—like the one at which David Healy heard another expert reading the paper that had originally been ghostwritten for him. The papers are often collected and printed in a special journal supplement. The editorial standards of the supplement are ordinarily much less stringent than the regular journal; a temporary guest editor of the company's choosing may make all the decisions on which papers to include. However, a reprint or photocopy of an article from the supplement looks at first glance exactly like an article printed in that journal that has gone through the more rigorous scientific peer-review process. When reprints of papers published in these supplements appear on a physician's desk, or are summarized verbally by a sales rep, the company enjoys the prestige of a reputable journal name without necessarily having to meet the quality standards the journal usually demands.[32] According to Richard Smith, editor of the *BMJ*, companies are willing to pay an extra bounty—the lower the quality and more favorable to selling the drug that the editors are willing to allow papers to be in the special supplement, the more the company will pay the journal for the privilege of publishing it.[33]

We saw how the handing out of journal article reprints was an important part of the ceremonial pas-de-deux between drug rep and practitioner. Smith states that companies may pay as much as a million dollars for reprints of a single major study, most of which is pure profit for the journal. Smith concludes, "The major journals try to counterbalance the might of the pharmaceutical industry, but it is an unequal battle—not least because journals themselves profit from publishing studies funded by the industry."[34] A handful of the most widely circulated journals—including the four major weekly English-language journals, the *New England Journal of Medicine*, the *Lancet*, *BMJ*, and *JAMA*—can afford to spurn the publication of any supplements. But even those journals depend for part of their revenues on reprint sales and ads. The more financially vulnerable a journal is, the less of a struggle it can put up against encroachment by industry. When editors know they can receive lucrative payments by allowing a slightly less rigorous study to be published, or a study that is spun in favor of a particular drug, and that sticking to the highest scientific standards will, by contrast, result in impoverishment, it is not surprising if the average editor caves in. This trend may account for the fact that many journals still lack disclosure policies for authors' conflicts of interest, and that even journals that have a disclosure policy tend to police it very poorly.[35]

When we tried to make sense of the extent to which medical organizations' ethics were compromised by support from industry, we asked what percentage of the total annual budget came from drug companies. The answer to this question, for medical journals, turns out to be shrouded in equal secrecy. Lawrence Altman noted in the *New York Times* in 1999 that most of the twenty-five thousand scientific journals are secretive about their profits and their advertising budgets, and that even when figures are released, different accounting methods make it hard to compare across journals.[36] Therefore, the total level of dependence of medical journals on pharmaceutical advertising appears to be unknown. The three pieces of data that are hardest to track down, when assessing the overall influence of the drug industry on medicine, are:

- total amount spent by industry on gifts to and hospitality of physicians,
- portion of medical organization budgets that derive from industry, and
- portion of medical journal publication costs that derive from industry.

If lack of transparency is an ethical warning bell, these three areas ring most loudly.[37]

NOTES

1. S. Vedantam, "Industry Role in Medical Meeting Decried; Symposiums Sponsored by Pharmaceutical Companies Trouble Some Psychiatrists," *Washington Post*, May 26, 2002:A10.

2. E. F. Torrey, "The Going Rate on Shrinks: Big Pharma and the Buying of Psychiatry," *The American Prospect*, July 15, 2002, 15–16.

3. D. Borenstein, "Pharmaceutical Companies," *Psychiatric News* (American Psychiatric Association) 2000; 35 (November 17): 3, 27.

4. The conflicted relationship between the *American Journal of Hypertension* and the American Society of Hypertension highlight both the difficulties in these relationships and the present-day pressures to reform. The conflict appears at one level to be a dispute between two prominent academic experts in hypertension—Dr. John H. Laragh, professor at Cornell and editor of the *Journal*, and Dr. Thomas D. Giles of Louisiana State University, president of the society. According to Laragh, it was necessary for the *Journal* to sever its ties with its long-time parent organization because the society was becoming too dominated by industry ties and by individual physicians who accepted fees from the industry. This, Laragh claimed, was especially having an impact on society-sponsored CME. According to Giles, the problem is rather the refusal of Laragh to allow the society any appropriate role in oversight of the *Journal*'s editorial mission, and the fact that Laragh receives an annual stipend of $229,000 for his roles in connection with the *Journal*, much of this supported indirectly by pharmaceutical advertising revenues. As of July 2005, the *Journal* and the society seemed to be in a race to see which would get to sever its ties with the other first; R. Winslow and R. Zimmerman, "High Blood Pressure: A Medical Journal, Doctors Sever Ties," *Wall Street Journal*, July 29, 2005:B1.

5. Glassman et al. reported on the percentage of revenue that six professional medical organizations derive from pharmaceutical advertising in their journals; P. A. Glassman, J. Hunter-Hayes, and T. Nakamura, "Pharmaceutical Advertising Revenue and Physician Organizations: How Much Is Too Much?" *West J Med* 1999; 171:234–38. They found in the process that medical organizations are generally unwilling to reveal the extent to which they receive funding from industry; P. A. Glassman, personal communication, January 7, 2003.

6. J. P. Kassirer, *On the Take: How Medicine's Complicity with Big Business Can Endanger Your Health* (New York: Oxford University Press, 2005), 120.

7. Kassirer, *On the Take*, 121.

8. Kassirer, *On the Take*, 124–25.

9. AAFP, exhibit prospectus: Scientific assembly 04 Orlando. American Academy of Family Physicians, 2004; www.aafp.org/PreBuilt/MarketingPages2004.pdf (accessed October 18, 2004).

10. On the other hand, these smaller societies have one major advantage—their total budgets are very small, hence a small contribution can make all the difference for their continued viability. This makes them a good target for local drug reps and their district managers, from whom a contribution of a few thousand dollars can go far in buying the good will of a few key local physicians who are officers of the society. This aspect of industry support for professional societies is therefore best addressed under the heading of gifts given by reps to individual physicians, although of course that distinction is somewhat arbitrary.

11. As of January 2005, the dues structure I was offered as a physician practicing in Ingham County, Michigan, would have me paying a total of $1,265 annually if I chose to join the AMA and the state and county medical societies, as a package deal.

12. The data in this section were developed as part of a research project that I undertook along with Andrew Hogan, John Goddeeris, and Anders Kelto of Michigan State University.

13. For this and later points I am indebted to electronic mail communications from the AAFP vice president for science and education, Dr. Norman Kahn, January 6 and April 28, 2003.

14. Support shown for CME programs is all commercial support, not specifically support from the pharmaceutical industry. According to the ACCME annual report for 2003, 96 percent of all commercial support for CME is from the pharmaceutical industry. I use that conversion factor to estimate the pharmaceutical share of commercial support for CME here.

15. Glassman, Hunter-Hayes, and Nakamura, "Pharmaceutical Advertising Revenue."

16. L. Altman, "Inside Medical Journals, A Rising Quest for Profits," *New York Times*, August 24, 1999:F1.

17. In most ways, the ethical and policy issues raised by financial relationships between physicians and medical device companies mirror the pharmaceutical issues addressed in this book. For purely practical reasons I have elected not to extend my analysis to the device industry, but would hope that most of the solutions I shall propose in future chapters could also be applied to problems that exist there.

18. At least one measure suggests that we may have obtained somewhat representative data. According to the ACCME, physician specialty and nonspecialty organizations collectively received about $119 million in CME support from the pharmaceutical industry in 2002; so it would appear that our survey revealed about 5 percent of that activity. Sixteen organizations responded out of a possible universe of 222 (7.2 percent), so it would not be unexpected to account for approximately 5 percent of total revenues.

19. E. D. Pellegrino and A. S. Relman, "Professional Medical Associations: Ethical and Practical Guidelines," *JAMA* 1999; 282:984–86; quote p. 984. See also T. K. Hazlet and S. D. Sullivan, "Professional Organizations and Healthcare Industry Support: Ethical Conflict?" *Camb Q Healthc Ethics* 1994; 3:236–44.

20. A further reason to publish a paper of this sort at the time was the firing of *JAMA* editor George Lundberg early in 1999, presumably because the AMA board wished to assert more control over the editorial contents of the *Journal*—a move that apparently backfired, since, again due to negative publicity, the board was able to secure the services of a new editor only by reaffirming the principles of editorial independence in a highly public manner. A firing that was more directly due to a clash over commercial funding of medical organizations was Jerome Kassirer's departure from the *New England Journal* later in 1999; J. P. Kassirer, "Goodbye, for Now," *N Engl J Med* 1999; 341:686–87. He had apparently disagreed with the Massachusetts Medical Society's plans to promote the *New England*

Journal "brand" in a series of spinoff products. It would seem, however, that Kassirer's departure came after the paper by Pellegrino and Relman would have been completed.

21. J. Kaiser, "Furor over Company Deal Roils AMA," *Science* 1997; 278:26; J. P. Kassirer and M. Angell, "The High Price of Product Endorsement," *N Engl J Med* 1997; 337:700. Many observers thought that the AMA proved it had learned little from the Sunbeam debacle when, in 2001, it accepted grants from large drug companies to help educate physicians about its new code of ethics on gifts from drug companies; S. Okie, "AMA Blasted for Letting Drug Firms Pay for Ethics Campaign," *Washington Post*, August 30, 2001:A3.

22. K. B. Leffler, "Persuasion or Information? The Economics of Prescription Drug Advertising," *Journal of Law and Economics* 1981; 24:45–74, citation p. 48 (in turn citing F. Presbrey, *The History and Development of Advertising* [New York: Doubleday, 1929], 289).

23. R. Seidenberg, "Advertising and Abuse of Drugs," *N Engl J Med* 1971; 284:789–90.

24. M. S. Wilkes, B. H. Doblin, and M. F. Shapiro, "Pharmaceutical Advertisements in Leading Medical Journals: Experts' Assessments," *Ann Intern Med* 1992; 116:912–19; D. A. Kessler, "Addressing the Problem of Misleading Advertising," *Ann Intern Med* 1992; 116:950–51; R. H. Fletcher and S. W. Fletcher, "Pharmaceutical Advertisements in Medical Journals," *Ann Intern Med* 1992; 116:951–52.

25. Critiques of the methods used by Wilkes and colleagues can be found in J. Jacoby, "Misleading Research on the Subject of Misleading Advertising: The Wilkes et al. Investigation of Pharmaceutical Advertising in Leading Medical Journals," *Food and Drug Law* 1994; 49:21–36; P. H. Rubin, "Are Pharmaceutical Ads Deceptive?" *Food and Drug Law* 1994; 49:7–20. Perhaps the most pertinent critique was that it was inappropriate to apply to drug ads the same standards of scientific peer review that one would apply to journal articles. Against this critique could be lodged the counterpoint, that the industry itself frequently emphasizes the "educational" and "scientific" nature of the "information" it provides to physicians.

26. A. C. Tsai, "Conflicts between Commercial and Scientific Interests in Pharmaceutical Advertising for Medical Journals," *Int J Health Serv* 2003; 33:751–68. Tsai's detailed account of this episode is based on interviews with the principals as well as on published sources.

27. The bounce-back of *Annals* ads to previous levels after the Fletchers left was confirmed by a count of advertising pages; e-mail communication from Dr. Seth Landefeld, January 19, 2005.

28. M. B. Rosenthal, E. R. Berndt, J. M. Donohue, R. G. Frank, and A. M. Epstein, "Promotion of Prescription Drugs to Consumers," *N Engl J Med* 2002; 346:498–505.

29. T. Pugh, "FDA's Review System Has Its Problems," *Lexington Herald-Leader*, January 29, 2004.

30. T. Pugh, "FDA Policing of Drug Ads Fades as Numbers Grow," *Lexington Herald-Leader*, January 29, 2004; M. Kaufman and B. A. Masters, "FDA Is Flexing Less Muscle: Some Question Its Relationship with Drugmakers," *Washington Post*, November 18, 2004: A1.

31. R. Pear, "Investigators Find Repeated Deception in Ads for Drugs," *New York Times*, December 4, 2002; Kaufman and Masters, "FDA Is Flexing Less Muscle"; Associated Press, "Waxman: FDA Lax on Drug Ads," *Richmond Times-Dispatch*, January 30, 2004; M. T. Gahart, L. M. Duhamel, A. Dievler, and R. Price, "Examining the FDA's Oversight of Direct-to-Consumer Advertising," *Health Aff (Millwood)* 2003; Suppl:W3-120-3; T. Frank, "Erasing the Rules, Part II. Friends on the Inside: Bush-Appointed Administrators at the FDA Have Consistently Sided with the Interests of Business," *Long Island Newsday*, October 11, 2004:A4.

32. L. A. Bero, A. Galbraith, and D. Rennie, "The Publication of Sponsored Symposiums in Medical Journals," *N Engl J Med* 1992; 327:1135–40; P. Lurie, T. B. Newman, and S. B. Hulley, "Caution over Journal Supplements," *BMJ* 1993; 307:1140–41; P. A. Rochon, J. H. Gurwitz, C. M. Cheung, J. A. Hayes, and T. C. Chalmers, "Evaluating the Quality of Articles Published in Journal Supplements Compared with the Quality of Those Published in the Parent Journal," *JAMA* 1994; 272:108–13.

33. R. Smith, "Medical Journals and Pharmaceutical Companies: Uneasy Bedfellows," *BMJ* 2003; 326:1202–5.

34. Smith, "Medical Journals and Pharmaceutical Companies," 1204.

35. S. Krimsky and L. S. Rothenberg, "Conflict of Interest Policies in Scientific and Medical Journals: Editorial Practices and Author Disclosures," *Science and Engineering Ethics* 2001; 7:205–18. Another and probably bigger reason for poor policing, however, is the fact that many journals are run by skeleton staffs and rely heavily on time volunteered by busy professionals.

36. Altman, "Inside Medical Journals."

37. As this book was going to press, one of the most thorough and thoughtful analyses of medical journal advertising appeared: A. Fugh-Berman, K. Alladin, and J. Chow, "Advertising in Medical Journals: Should Current Practices Change?" *PLoS Med* 2006; 3:e130. This paper reveals the lengths to which medical journals go to "sell" themselves, and by implication their readers, to pharmaceutical advertisers—for instance, by the ads that the journals themselves place in magazines such as *Medical Marketing and Media*. Fugh-Berman and colleagues argue that journals would better serve the profession if they either funded themselves from a source other than advertising or at least diversified their ads so that other items physicians buy—automobiles, for instance—were advertised alongside of drugs. The reason most medical journals do not accept the latter sort of "lifestyle" ad is that they have policies restricting advertising to items that directly affect or form a part of medical practice. "Lifestyle" ads make the journal seem less "professional." Ironically, by preserving this veneer of professionalism, the journals may actually be allowing professionalism to be seriously challenged at a deeper level.

13

THE INDUSTRY AND THE CONSUMER

Advertising serves not so much to advertise products as to promote consumption as a way of life.

—Christopher Lasch, 1978[1]

Some activities that the pharmaceutical industry views as its public service and educational function are aimed at the general public and not directly at the medical profession. These functions might seem irrelevant to this volume, which is about the interaction between medicine and the industry. Critics of the industry, however, charge that it is one large marketing machine. That machine is especially adept at interweaving seemingly disparate activities into a seamless marketing campaign. More important, marketing to consumers effectively alters the culture of America life, and those cultural changes in turn alter the way that patients and physicians relate to each other. The cultural changes and the consequent alteration of the physician-patient interaction appear to be precisely what the industry intends. The industry's ability to achieve cultural change on such a large scale is yet another measure of its power.

DIRECT-TO-CONSUMER ADVERTISING

We have seen how the label "ethical drug company" shaped the relationship between medicine and the pharmaceutical industry during the twentieth century. One aspect of "ethical" drug company behavior was advertising only to physicians and never to the general public. Physicians might have imagined that the industry would never threaten the goodwill it had built up with them over all those years by shifting its ground and marketing directly to consumers. Industry, however, clearly had no commitment to this historical artifact, and was eager to jettison the tradition as soon as it seemed fiscally worthwhile.

Direct-to-consumer (DTC) ads, especially on television, were not feasible under the FDA rules that held sway before 1997.[2] The rules required an exhaustive listing of drug side effects and warnings, making most mass media ads unwieldy and prohibitively expensive. In 1997 the FDA altered its rules, in keeping with the agency's increasingly pro-industry stance. So long as the requisite laundry list of side effects was available elsewhere (such as in a print ad or on a website), DTC ads were now allowed—a practice that only one other developed country, New Zealand, has seen fit to emulate. DTC ads in the United States increased fortyfold between 1994 and 2000; by 1999 the average television viewer was exposed to nine ads for prescription pharmaceuticals each day.[3] In the early years of the twenty-first century, DTC ads were the fastest growing segment of pharmaceutical marketing costs, during a time when the industry was spending less on print advertising aimed at physicians. In 2004, the industry was reported to have spent $4.45 billion on advertising to consumers.[4] Nevertheless, the total costs of DTC ads represent only a fraction of the amount companies continue to spend on all marketing to physicians.[5]

In the fall of 2003, the FDA held open hearings on DTC policy. The hearings were heavily dominated by industry-funded social scientists, effectively drowning out any voices of doubt.[6] The industry was perhaps motivated by fears that the FDA would crack down on the underdisclosure of drug risks in DTC ads.[7] One speaker after another presented data to show that consumers accrued major benefits from DTC advertising, which led them to become aware of serious, treatable diseases they did not realize that they might have, and to seek timely medical advice from their physicians. Reportedly, DTC ads had succeeded in destigmatizing some conditions, for which patients had previously been too embarrassed to seek medical advice; so some needy patients were for the first time receiving effective treatment.

The general quality of this research is suggested by a critique of one paper that was published in the journal *Health Affairs*. Joel S. Weissman of Harvard University and several colleagues performed a telephone survey. Thirty-five percent of those surveyed reported going to their physicians after seeing a product advertised. Fully a quarter of those received a new diagnosis at their visit with the physician, and nearly half of those new diagnoses were viewed by the authors as being of high priority. Only about half of the time did the physician prescribe the advertised drug—evidence, according to the authors, that DTC ads were not exerting an undue influence on physician prescribing and that physicians still retained freedom of judgment.[8]

Thomas Bodenheimer, a critic of the industry, noted some rather basic design flaws in Weissman's study. Most notably, there was no control group. Perhaps patients who have never seen a DTC ad also have new diagnoses made 25 percent of the time when going to see their physicians. Without a comparison group, none of the beneficial consequences attributed to DTC ads can be confirmed. Indeed, when all the research design inadequacies of Weissman's paper (plus a companion paper in the same journal) are added up, these "studies" appear to be less research and instead themselves advertisements for DTC ads. Bodenheimer saw the same strategy at work here as we saw earlier with the CLASS study—place the paper in a distinguished journal, despite major flaws in the study design, and trust that readers will be sufficiently impressed with the journal that the paper is printed in and do not bother to read the fine print later on when the flaws are exposed.[9]

The fact is that we do not know very much about the impact of DTC ads, for good or for ill. The question of whether DTC ads lead to increased costs of drugs as more consumers demand a higher-priced product, or as consumers seek drug therapy for a condition they previously were willing to live with, is very difficult to determine, again due largely to the problem of identifying a control for experimental purposes. There is clearly an association between how much a given drug adds to total expenditures and the likelihood that the drug will be heavily advertised.[10] Toshiaki Iizuka of Vanderbilt University and Ginger Z. Jin of the University of Maryland tried to assess the impact of DTC ads by comparing advertising practices to a large database of national health expenditures. They found that more DTC advertising led to more patient visits and more drug prescribing, and that physicians spent somewhat more time with patients. Physicians, however, did not appear to alter their choices of drugs within any given therapeutic class in response to advertising levels. Iizuka and Jin concluded that the industry is essentially correct in its claims—that more patients seek help after seeing DTC ads but that physicians retain discretion over which drug to prescribe. As they summarized, DTC ads are market-expanding rather than business-stealing.[11] An ad for a particular drug such as Nexium, a proton-pump inhibitor for acid reflux, might increase sales of all proton-pump inhibitors, but does not prompt physicians who used to prescribe a different proton-pump inhibitor to prescribe Nexium instead. Iizuka and Jin admit, however, that their data cannot exclude the possibility that any class of drugs might be overprescribed (compared to whatever might be judged to be the ideal practice), or that physicians treat conditions with drugs when a nondrug approach might be better. In any event, one group concluded in 2003 that the industry recoups $4.20 in sales for each $1.00 spent on direct-to-consumer ads.[12]

A somewhat different picture emerged when Barbara Mintzes and colleagues at the University of British Columbia administered a brief questionnaire to patients both before and after a physician visit, and also queried physicians about their medication choices. They compared data for Sacramento, California, and Vancouver, British Columbia, to include samples that presumably were and were not exposed to DTC ads, respectively. (Since Vancouver residents routinely watch U.S. television, 87 percent of their Canadian sample had seen at least one DTC ad, however.) Mintzes and colleagues found that about 3 percent of the Vancouver patients, and 7 percent of the Sacramento patients, requested an advertised drug during that day's visit—a statistically significant difference. Overall, patients who requested advertised drugs ended up leaving the office with more prescriptions for that visit than other patients. Physicians acceded to the patients' request about three-fourths of the time in both cities, though in as many as half the cases the physicians indicated that they would not personally have recommended that drug.[13] Mintzes and colleagues concluded that DTC ads tended to shift medical practice away from drugs that physicians preferred and toward more use of drugs generally.

Physicians, for their part, have been generally negative about DTC ads.[14] A typical complaint is that patients now arrive belligerently demanding drugs that they have seen advertised. It takes valuable time that the physician does not have to talk them out of their supposed need for this drug; and even after spending the time, the patient often leaves dissatisfied.

One might dismiss the physicians' complaints as revealing the profession's unwillingness to address the real needs of patients. After all, if patients now have questions about drugs that they did not have previously, what is a better use of the physicians' time than to educate the patient and to answer these questions? On this view, it is significant that most surveys of patients reveal a generally positive attitude toward DTC ads.[15] If patients find such ads valuable, how can physicians oppose them and still view themselves as patient advocates?

John Abramson, a family physician at Harvard, has been perhaps the most eloquent in making the physicians' argument against DTC ads. First he highlights the disingenuousness of the industry's claim that these ads are a form of public-service education.[16] The industry has not retained health educators to manage its DTC portfolio; it has instead, not surprisingly, engaged the services of advertising agencies. Abramson quotes Ernestine McCarren, the general manager of one of these ad agencies, Ehrenthal & Associates: "We want to identify the emotions we can tap into to get that customer to take the desired course of action. If you can't find that basic insight, you might as well forget everything else."[17]

What does the DTC ads' appeal to the patient's emotions, and the more subtle "selling" of a culture of consumption, do to the relationship between physician and patient? Abramson explains his worry:

> At its best, the trust between doctor and patient creates the opportunity for open discussion of symptoms, fears, models of disease, life circumstances, and expectations. Once all of these are on the table, an optimal approach can be developed to meet individual patients' needs. Often approaches and solutions had not been previously apparent to either the doctor or the patient. Rarely can the best solutions be achieved simply by prescribing a drug and being done with the issue.
>
> From my perspective as a family doctor, I found the requests for specific drugs deleterious to both the process and content of good doctoring. Once a patient made a request for a specific drug, the success of the visit from the patient's point of view became defined by whether or not the drug was prescribed. At that point, it became hard to recoup the full potential of the encounter. I was less able to broaden discussion beyond the use (or not) of the latest drugs to more effective ways to control symptoms and preserve health—like avoiding allergens or adopting a more active lifestyle.[18]

Anyone reading Abramson's book is likely to conclude that this family physician is eager to serve as a patient educator and informant. He sees spending extra time with his patients to answer their questions as his main agenda, not as an extra hurdle in the middle of a hectic day. His complaint is not that DTC ads force him to spend time talking with patients. He claims rather that the quality and nature of that time have been subverted by the message of consumption. The patient no longer leaves feeling cared for because the physician has involved the patient in the optimal management of his own problems.[19] Rather the patient now leaves frustrated because he is sure that the physician's job is to hand him a commercial product that he can passively consume, thereby solving all his problems for him. The same advertising culture works hard to persuade all of us that we become smart, successful, and sexy not by dint of our own hard work—far less by dint of character—but rather by spending our money on the right consumer goods. It would be very odd indeed if that advertising culture gave the patient a message that reinforced Abramson's style of doctoring.[20] Yet the available evidence (as Abramson's own book demonstrates comprehensively) proves that Abramson's type of doctoring produces better results than does taking a lot of pills.[21]

THE CELEBRITY SALESPERSON

The pharmaceutical industry did not invent the consumerist advertising culture.[22] Now that the culture exists, the industry merely wishes to use it to its full advantage. But when an industry has as much money to spend as this one, that alone distorts the market and adds immensely to the power of the pharmaceutical firms. As Abramson further notes, television and magazines now receive hefty profits from DTC ads and have every incentive to ensure that the flow of these ads continues. Is it therefore a coincidence that the coverage of "news" about new drugs in these media sources tends to be so uncritical?[23] As magazine editor Gloria Steinem once said, "You don't get product ads unless you praise the product."[24] By purchasing DTC ads, the industry has also bought for itself another route to disseminate its message to the public (including physicians)—a route that has the added advantage of purporting to be "news coverage" or informed, expert commentary rather than paid advertising.

In March 2002, actress Lauren Bacall appeared on the NBC *Today* program in a rare interview. She spoke about a good friend who had gone blind recently from macular degeneration, and mentioned Visudyne, a new treatment for the condition. Neither Bacall nor NBC revealed that she had been paid for her time by Novartis, the maker of Visudyne.[25] On the same day that reporter Melody Petersen revealed the Bacall incident in the *New York Times*, actress Kathleen Turner talked about her battle with rheumatoid arthritis in a CNN interview. The next day, after finding out that Turner had been paid by Amgen and Wyeth, makers of the rheumatoid arthritis drug Enbrel, CNN issued a new policy promising to reveal any such financial links in future news broadcasts.[26]

The year following, Petersen revealed another ploy to peddle ads as news. A Boca Raton, Florida company called WJMK Incorporated was producing video "news breaks" that local public television stations could broadcast in between regular programs. The firm originally hired Morley Safer of CBS News, then tried to secure the services of Aaron Brown of CNN and Walter Cronkite. Standing on a typical TV-news-style set, the host introduced health-related segments that last two to five minutes. No mention was made in the broadcast of the fact that companies were paying WJMK $15,000 per segment and were allowed to edit and approve the contents.[27]

Another excellent way to sell drugs is to turn a scientific investigator into a celebrity. Dr. Jennifer Berman, a urologist, and her sister Dr. Laura Berman, a clinical psychologist, are codirectors of the Female Sexual Medicine Center at the University of California at Los Angeles. After they appeared twice on the Oprah Winfrey television show in February 2001, their book, *For Women Only: A Revolutionary Guide to Overcoming Sexual Dysfunction and Reclaiming Your Sex Life*, shot to the top of the bestseller charts. The photograph of the two sisters, young, smiling, and attractive, graces the cover of their book, as well as their commercial website.

The Bermans' materials freely recommend Viagra and testosterone replacement as treatments for female sexual dysfunction. Neither drug is approved for this use by the FDA. Consequently, no drug company can legally market these drugs for that purpose. But the companies can give research grants to the Bermans' center at UCLA and advertise freely on their website. In turn the Bermans make more money from their book sales and from other related entrepreneurial activities. The companies buy marketing for their drugs' off-label use without paying directly and so avoid any possible legal penalty.[28]

ASTROTURF

In a society with deeply rooted democratic and egalitarian values, we tend to pay special attention to the words of average people who have experienced a disease or its treatment. Grassroots organizations made up of such "real people" therefore have a special status, and are often deferred to by reporters and by legislators.

The pharmaceutical industry has mastered a basic rule of social change. People seldom change their behavior because they hear a single message from a single source. By contrast, people quickly change when they hear the same message a number of times from many different sources. Grassroots organizations are a highly effective means of getting the message out, provided that they can be persuaded to do the industry's bidding. When a group already exists, compliance can be ensured by a generous grant to support "educational" work. But sometimes no group exists and the industry needs to invent one. The term "astroturf" refers to a phony grassroots organization that is a mouthpiece fully funded by the industry.[29]

One early example of astroturf dates to the 1980s. During the previous decade, emergency rooms in the northern United States, during the winter flu and virus season, would routinely treat a few dozen cases of Reye syndrome. Children recovering uneventfully from a cold or other virus would suddenly worsen and would be found to have serious liver damage. When evidence began to mount that giving aspirin during the viral illness might be the cause of Reye syndrome, the makers of aspirin decided to launch a counterattack to head off the feared FDA demand for a warning label. Thus appeared a new organization, the American Reye's Syndrome Association. The association created and distributed an elaborate brochure to instruct parents on how to recognize the symptoms of

Reye syndrome, and how to tip off the physician that the disease might be the correct diagnosis. The brochure failed to mention, however, that aspirin might be a risk factor, and parents were given no warning to avoid the use of aspirin-containing products for wintertime viruses. Hidden at the bottom of the brochure was the information that the entire campaign had been funded by Glenbrook Labs, the manufacturer of Bayer Aspirin for children.[30]

Later, the biotechnology firm Genentech, which had licensed to Eli Lilly the distribution of its human growth hormone, discovered that sales would remain very limited as long as prescriptions were written only for children with diagnosed growth hormone deficiency. A huge market, by contrast, existed among hormonally normal children who were short, and whose parents wished them to be taller. Two existing charities, the Human Growth Foundation and the Magic Foundation, began to sponsor height screenings for children at schools, malls, and fairs. Parents of children shown to be shorter than average received follow-up letters suggesting that they see their physicians for evaluation. Neither school officials nor parents were told that drug company money was supporting the effort.[31]

In 2003, the state of Kentucky, trying to cut costs in its Medicaid program, tried to eliminate the psychiatric drug Zyprexa from its preferred drug formulary, based on arguments that considerably cheaper drugs would work quite satisfactorily for the vast majority of patients. Consumer groups, especially advocacy groups for the mentally ill, bombarded the state agencies with mails and faxes. Demonstrations were held and witnesses testified at hearings that removing Zyprexa from the formulary would drastically affect patients' quality of life. Only some time later was it revealed that Eli Lilly, the manufacturer of Zyprexa, had bankrolled the entire campaign. Gardiner Harris noted in the *New York Times* that other states had already shied away from addressing psychiatric drugs in their Medicaid formularies, fearful of exactly this sort of pressure tactic.[32] One article by pharmaceutical industry insiders referred to patient organizations as the "ground troops" in the industry's lobbying war to get governmental agencies to include various drugs on their approved formulary lists.[33]

The year 2003 also saw the extended debate over passage of a Medicare drug benefit. The American Association of Retired Persons (AARP), a large and influential organization representing older Americans, opposed some features that were voted into the bill, notably an industry-friendly provision that prohibited the Medicare administration from bargaining for volume discounts in drug prices. AARP found itself up against several well-funded groups with names such as the United Seniors Association, 60 Plus Association, and Seniors Coalition. Investigation revealed that all of these organizations were created *de novo* to lobby for the industry version of the Medicare drug benefit, and were funded almost entirely by public relations firms that in turn received their funding from industry. The groups had no office addresses of their own and no membership lists.[34]

Dr. David Healy, the psychiatrist, took time off from telling us about ghostwriting to review a brochure he received for a conference held in London in 1996. For a fee of about $1,000 per day, attendees could be instructed by representatives of the major pharmaceutical companies on how to set up patients' groups and patient education campaigns.[35]

THE LOTRONEX STORY

Alosetron (Lotronex), manufactured by Glaxo Wellcome (later GlaxoSmithKline), was approved for sale by the FDA in February 2000. The drug was designed to control symptoms in the more severe cases of a common condition, irritable bowel syndrome (IBS). Patients who had severe abdominal cramps and diarrhea got significant benefit from this drug.

During the remaining months of 2000, cases were reported of a potentially fatal condition called ischemic colitis. Some patients had such severe constipation after taking Lotronex that stool impacted in their large bowels, shutting off blood flow. In November 1999, when the drug was under review by an FDA advisory committee, Glaxo Wellcome claimed that there was no causal link between their drug and ischemic colitis. By June 2000, the company admitted that ischemic colitis might be linked to Lotronex but that the condition was "transient and self-limiting," and no deaths had been reported. Starting in September, reports of fatalities began to appear. (By April 2002, at least seven deaths had been attributed to the drug.) In November 2000, Dr. Paul Stolley, a senior consultant at the FDA, wrote a twenty-page internal memo giving reasons why the problem would not be solved simply by better educating doctors about the risks, the course of action favored by Glaxo Wellcome. On November 28, 2000, Glaxo Wellcome voluntarily stopped selling Lotronex.

Usually a drug that is withdrawn remains unavailable. By June 2002, however, Lotronex was back on pharmacy shelves. As journalist Ray Moynihan reported in the *BMJ*, there are two versions of how the drug made it back on the market.[36] According to FDA leaders, the agency was doing its job—balancing its duty to keep unsafe drugs off the market with the needs of patients for effective treatment. IBS patients themselves lobbied hard with the FDA to keep Lotronex available. The agency worked closely with the manufacturer and came up with the best possible compromise. They allowed the drug to be sold, but required that only physicians who were certified experts in its use could prescribe it.

Dr. Stolley told Moynihan a rather different story. Before coming to the FDA, Stolley had a distinguished academic career at Johns Hopkins, the University of Pennsylvania, and the University of Maryland, and was a former president of the American Epidemiological Society. He noted that the FDA's own statistics showed that perhaps 5 percent of the public had IBS, and of that group, only 5 percent had symptoms severe enough to consider Lotronex. Glaxo Wellcome claimed that as many as 20 percent of the U.S. population are affected. The company, partly by funding organizations such as the International Foundation for Functional Gastrointestinal Disorders, sought to shape opinion about the severity of the disease, and also hired *Frasier* star Kelsey Grammar as a celebrity spokesperson.

Despite the hype, Lotronex seemed at best to be only about 10 to 20 percent more effective than placebo treatment. FDA evidence suggested that of two hundred patients taking Lotronex for three months, one would probably develop ischemic colitis.

Two major lobbies for IBS patients, the Lotronex Action Group and the International Foundation for Functional Gastrointestinal Disorders, began a protest campaign as soon as the drug was withdrawn in November 2000. Moynihan's investigations showed that the Lotronex Action Group appeared to be independent of the drug company. The International Foundation for Functional Gastrointestinal Disorders, by contrast, openly proclaimed its funding from the company on its website.

The combined grassroots activity and astroturf had the desired effect. Dr. Stolley and another senior expert in adverse drug reactions were taken off the Lotronex case, and Stolley resigned from the FDA. In April 2002, an FDA advisory committee recommended that the drug should be specifically labeled for use only by IBS patients who had failed other therapies, and could be dispensed only by gastroenterologists who had been specially certified as experts in IBS treatment. Three members of the advisory committee were "furious" when the FDA leaders overruled them, and allowed any physician to proclaim herself an IBS expert for purposes of prescribing Lotronex.[37]

LOBBYING BY THE PHARMACEUTICAL INDUSTRY

On December 15, 2004, PhRMA announced that it had named its new president and CEO, former Louisiana congressman Billy Tauzin (R). The news release highlighted Tauzin's record in Congress as a leader of bipartisan cooperation and Tauzin's own successful fight with intestinal cancer, which he attributed to newly developed pharmaceuticals.[38]

The PhRMA news release did not mention that this was the second time that Tauzin's name was linked to the pharmaceutical industry's major lobbying organization. It had first been announced the previous January that Tauzin intended to resign from his congressional post and take up the million-dollar-a-year CEO position at PhRMA after the current president, Alan Holmer, had announced his decision to retire.[39] Tauzin and PhRMA were immediately deluged with negative press coverage. Tauzin had been a key architect in the House of Representatives of the Medicare prescription drug benefit passed at the end of 2003. In January 2004, reporters were still pointing out the various hidden features of the new law that all seemed to favor the industry, most notably the provision that prohibited Medicare from using its volume purchasing power to negotiate drug price discounts. To critics, this sweetheart deal looked like classic political payola—congressman writes the sort of bill the industry wants; industry rewards congressman with well-paid sinecure from which he can proceed to lobby his former colleagues on behalf of the industry.

The pressure proved too much at the time, and Tauzin and PhRMA both backpedaled.[40] Presumably, by December of the same year, people had had time to forget the negative publicity of January, and the Republicans had also won big in the November elections and appeared to have unassailable positions in both the House and Senate in the new Congress. The Billy Tauzin case illustrates how well placed the industry is in a government that is still awash in special-interest funds and where campaign finance reform has made relatively little headway.

In June 2003, as planning began in earnest for the 2004 elections, Public Citizen reported that the pharmaceutical industry had deployed 675 lobbyists, more than one for each senator and congressperson, specifically to influence legislation.[41]

Billy Tauzin will be in good company; 26 of these lobbyists were former congress-men, and nearly half of the 675 lobbyists had previously worked for the federal government. The industry spent more than $91 million on lobbying in 2002, an 11 percent increase from the previous year. With the Medicare drug benefit before Congress in 2003, the industry pulled out all the stops and spent a reported $139 million.[42]

A survey of federal lobbying using figures from 2000 showed that health care was the single biggest lobbying sector, with the $237 million spent in health lobbying amounting to 15 percent of the total lobbying budget. Within the health sector itself, pharmaceutical and health products companies accounted for the largest proportion, with a total of $96 million.[43]

With more than one lobbyist per member of Congress, it might seem that the industry could be totally bipartisan in its approach. Pharmaceutical lobbying actually tends heavily to favor the Republican side of the aisle.[44] The cordial working relationship is hinted in a letter written by Jim Nicholson, chair of the Republican National Committee, to Charles Heimbold, chair and CEO of Bristol-Myers Squibb, in April 1999. Nicholson suggested forming a "pharmaceutical coalition" to provide "the perfect vehicle for the Republican Party to reach out to the health care community and discuss their legislative needs. . . . We must keep the lines of communication open if we want to keep passing legislation that will benefit your industry." Nicholson then requested a $250,000 donation to the Republican National Committee.[45]

At least through the end of 2004, the lobbying clout of the industry has largely guaranteed that no major governmental unit in the United States would take any action that seriously compromised the industry's interests. State governments trying to cut Medicaid costs through the extended use of drug formularies or by forming multistate coalitions to bargain for lower prices, regularly were descended upon by herds of lobbyists, and their legislators were bullied into backing off.[46] While a bill to allow the reimportation of cheaper drugs from Canada and other countries surprisingly passed the House of Representatives and gained the vocal support of key senators of both parties, this legislation somewhat mysteriously disappeared into the committee system and never reemerged.[47] And as we have already seen, the Medicare prescription drug benefit that had passed at the end of 2003 turned out to have several provisions that appeared to have been written by industry lobbyists. At this writing it is too soon to tell if the events of 2004 that stirred public opinion against the industry—the antidepressant-suicide and the Vioxx scandals—will begin to counteract the industry's lobbying clout in the corridors of government and lead to a window of opportunity for tighter regulation.

DISEASE MONGERING

Drug companies obviously make drugs, but less obviously they make views of illnesses. . . . It may often be far more effective to sell the indication than to focus on selling the treatment.

—David Healy[48]

Dr. John Abramson's critique of DTC advertising is that it alters the way patients view medical care, so that it becomes harder for a conscientious physician to work with the patient. Instead of a participatory posture that accepts responsibility for teamwork in maintaining health, and that relates a good deal of ill health to lifestyle choices, DTC ads encourage a consumerist view that the mere ingestion of the correct medication (ideally, an expensive one) will ensure good health and a symptom-free existence.

This shift by itself is sufficient evidence of the industry's power to alter our society. But from the industry's point of view, it is not enough. Why wait until the patient has a disease that the physician recognizes and then try to convince both patient and physician that the company's blockbuster drug is the answer? Instead it is better to convince regular people that they are patients. People must be persuaded that problems in their lives that they had previously regarded as nonmedical are actually diseases—so long as a drug the company sells can then be hawked as the therapy.[49]

In a refreshingly frank how-to guide for marketers, Vince Parry refers to "the art of branding a condition." This practice is not new, he claims. Warner-Lambert, back in the 1920s, tried to market Listerine for everything from dandruff to wound irrigation, with no luck. Then they hit upon the brilliant stroke of renaming bad breath "halitosis." This new condition, Parry recounts, "was demonized for a range of social casualties from lack of career advancement to divorce. As the antidote, Listerine saw sales increase from $100,000 to $4 million over the next six years, and helped to make halitosis a household word."[50] The fact that "halitosis" does not exist in any meaningful medical sense does not mar Parry's glowing account.

Today, the conditions calling for this same approach are anxiety and depression, "where illness is rarely based on measurable symptoms and, therefore, open to conceptual definition." Parry assigns much of the credit for the fact that psychiatry's *DSM*, the *Diagnostic and Statistical Manual of Mental Disorders*, has grown to its "current phonebook dimensions" to the fact that "newly coined conditions were brought to light through direct funding by pharmaceutical companies, in research, in publicity or both." As a "legendary example" of condition branding, Parry offers the example of panic disorder. Upjohn, through its strategic funding, managed to disentangle panic disorder from the broader category of anxiety neuroses and at the same time install its drug alprazolam (Xanax) as the first-choice drug to treat the new disease.[51]

We now have drugs proven, to varying degrees of efficacy, to treat baldness, shyness, childhood hyperactivity, adolescent adjustment problems, lackluster sex, premenstrual moodiness, incontinence, and ugly toenails. All these conditions, once the normal burdens of living inside an aging or imperfect human body, have been transformed into pathologies, because they can now be treated with medications. The drug companies did not create these clinical realities; they uncovered them in their desperate search for the next drug they could make, test, and sell. In the process, they have done a brilliant job of medicalizing human unhappiness. An insured American suffering from one of these problems is grateful to have a medical remedy—purchased with the tax-advantaged status of a health care transaction—that did not exist ten years ago.[52]

As we saw in the case of Lotronex, we must exercise care in discussing "medicalizing human unhappiness," or more specifically, "disease mongering" by the pharmaceutical industry, as Australian journalist Ray Moynihan has dubbed it.[53] All human misery exists along a spectrum, or better, along two spectra. One ranges from mild to severe; the other ranges from resistant to management with medications to very accessible to management with medications. If we look only at cases that are at the severe end of the first spectrum, and also toward the treatable end of the second spectrum, it will seem cruel and callous to talk about the industry "selling disease." Instead, we will be struck by the extreme misery that the individual suffered from before drug therapy was available, and the significant improvement in the individual's life that occurred after drug therapy was administered. On what basis could a physician claim that the drug ought not be used? Or that the industry should not have taken steps to inform the sufferer of the medication?

This benign portrayal, however, becomes harder to sustain if we accept that the industry is primarily interested in the relief of human suffering insofar as that entails selling drugs. Companies choose never to sell only a few drugs; whenever possible their goal is to sell a lot of drugs. No company can succeed by sending the message that only the most severe cases merit medical attention and drug therapy. The industry hopes that use of the medication will be extended as far as possible toward the other end of each spectrum—the milder-suffering end and the less-responsive-to-medication end. Due to the shape of the typical disease bell curve, lowering the severity threshold at which people think they have a "real" disease and need drug treatment typically expands the potential market by a factor of ten or more. It is only with a low severity threshold that a PR firm can whip up a proper scare campaign about a hidden epidemic of disease that afflicts ten, twenty, or fifty million people.

Physicians know that as one starts to offer drug treatment to people with progressively less severe conditions, bad things usually happen. The chance of suffering a serious drug side effect starts to become greater than the chance of substantial benefit. This, in a nutshell, was the tragedy of chloramphenicol. At the same time that patients are exposed to greater risks of drug toxicity, the society as a whole is paying a much higher prescription drug bill, again with little benefit to show for it. J. D. Kleinke, a health economist, questions the fairness of this situation: "While forty-three million Americans go without health insurance, at least as many are swallowing pills for smaller waistlines, quieter children, better erections, and stronger presentation skills."[54] Ray Moynihan and Alan Cassels, in their book, *Selling Sickness*, raise the fairness question to the international level, questioning the aggressive "selling" of attention deficit/hyperactivity disorder in both children and adults: "In this age of globalization, is it conceivable that we in the wealthy developed world will continue to spend billions every year diagnosing and medicating children whose symptoms include 'often fidgets with hands or feet' and prescribing lifelong speed to adults who 'drum their fingers,' when each year millions of children and adults just across our borders die early from preventable and treatable life-threatening diseases? Surely this is one obscenity too many."[55]

The committee of the British House of Commons that reported on the influence of the drug industry in 2005 found documents describing one company's "strategic planning process." The company targeted the nearly two million people in Britain who do not currently go to see a physician or take prescription medication, noting that these "missing millions" represented a "significant opportunity." They engaged a PR firm to study these people, find out what was keeping them away from the physician's office, and "identify hooks and drivers to encourage them to seek advice both emotional and rational."[56] The possibility that these people were not seeing a physician because they were well, and that they were not taking prescription medicines because they needed none, was apparently dismissed.

As a rule, astroturf and disease mongering go hand in hand today, and are often linked with other industry activities as well. Consider the campaign to promote "social phobia" (what previous generations would have referred to as "shyness") as an indication for the use of SSRI antidepressants. The campaign featured all of the following:[57]

- Industry-sponsored research by so-called academic experts, purporting to prove that social phobia is a real mental illness and responds to the recommended drugs
- Industry-sponsored seminars at professional meetings, to promote the above "research" findings
- Industry-sponsored supplements to major psychiatric journals, again to publicize the "research"
- Newly formed organizations of sufferers from social phobia (funded solely by the industry), complaining of the discrimination they suffer at the hands of uninformed psychiatrists who fail to recognize and treat their "disease"
- Direct-to-consumer advertisements listing possible symptoms of social phobia and encouraging viewers to "ask your doctor" about the advertised medicine

We have seen in this chapter how the pharmaceutical industry, through its unmatched financial resources, is able to have a significant influence not only on the messages that Americans hear about drugs, but on the very ideas Americans entertain about the nature of disease and its treatment. This is a sizable concentration of power in the hands of an industry that has proven very adept at using that power to maximize profits. It has then used its huge profits to flood the public sector with lobbyists and campaign contributions, further increasing its economic and political power.

Who can rein in that power? As we saw in the Lotronex case, the FDA is generally responsible for controlling the excesses of the large drug companies. As the Lotronex case also showed, industry critics have questioned the FDA's current effectiveness. We next need to address how the FDA got to where it is today and what role it plays in managing the interface between medical practice and the pharmaceutical industry.

NOTES

1. C. Lasch, *The Culture of Narcissism: American Life in an Age of Diminishing Expectations* (New York: Norton, 1978), 137.

2. On the history of DTC ads, see W. L. Pines, "A History and Perspective on Direct-to-Consumer Promotion," *Food Drug Law J* 1999; 54:489–518; A. Lyles, "Direct Marketing of Pharmaceuticals to Consumers," *Annu Rev Public Health* 2002; 23:73–91. I am grateful to Anders Kelto for these references. Pines argues that in principle the FDA accepted DTC ads back in the late 1970s when it moved to require patient package inserts in all drugs sold. Once the wall of medical paternalism had been breached and patients were seen as having the right to information about drugs without having to apply to physicians for it, there was no logical reason not to allow advertising to consumers by industry as well. Pines also notes how the AMA neutralized itself as a voice against DTC ads. In 1993, the AMA launched a weekend cable TV network on health issues, aimed primarily at physicians but accessible by consumers. To finance the network, the AMA turned to industry advertising and developed guidelines for ads aimed directly at consumers. The network eventually folded; but the AMA was now on record as supporting DTC ads and could not easily change its tune, even later when many physicians viewed the ads with ire.

3. J. Abramson, *Overdosed America: The Broken Promise of American Medicine* (New York: HarperCollins, 2004), 151.

4. S. Hensley, "Some Drug Makers Are Starting to Curtail TV Ad Spending," *Wall Street Journal*, May 16, 2005:B1. This may represent a high point as indications were that spending was set to decline in 2005; see the following note.

5. M. B. Rosenthal, E. R. Berndt, J. M. Donohue, R. G. Frank, and A. M. Epstein, "Promotion of Prescription Drugs to Consumers," *N Engl J Med* 2002; 346:498–505. By early 2005 there was some evidence that these ads were having less impact on consumers and that the industry might soon begin to cut back on them due to multiple factors—pressure from the FDA in the wake of the Vioxx withdrawal, and preference to advertise more via the Internet where more extensive information could be provided; J. Schmit, "Drugmakers Likely to Lob Softer Pitches," *USA Today*, March 16, 2005:3B; S. Hensley, "Some Drug Makers Are Starting to Curtail TV Ad Spending," *Wall Street Journal*, May 16, 2005:B1. The industry also started to backtrack on its "right" to advertise as it wished following the Vioxx debacle, and spoke of developing a stronger voluntary code of advertising conduct; R. Pear, "Drug Industry Is Said to Work on an Ad Code," *New York Times*, May 17, 2005:A17. Comparisons between 1999 and 2002 surveys of American consumers indicated a relative dropping off of favorable opinions toward DTC drug ads; K. J. Aikin, *The Impact of Direct-to-Consumer Prescription Drug Advertising on the Physician-Patient Relationship* (Washington, D.C.: FDA Division of Drug Marketing, Advertising, and Communications, September 22, 2003) www.fda.gov/cder/ddmac/aikin/aikin.PPT.

6. M. Kaufman, "Drug Ads Do More Good Than Harm, FDA Told," *Washington Post*, September 23, 2003:E4; N. Ives, "F.D.A. Reviews Ads for Drugs," *New York Times*, September 29, 2003:C11.

7. C. Rowland, "A Dose of Reality: FDA to Push Firms to Make Ads Clearer about Drug Risks," *Boston Globe*, September 23, 2003:D1.

8. J. S. Weissman, D. Blumenthal, A. J. Silk, K. Zapert, M. Newman, and R. Leitman, "Consumers' Reports on the Health Effects of Direct-to-Consumer Drug Advertising," *Health Aff (Millwood)* 2003; Suppl:W3-82-95.

9. T. Bodenheimer, "Two Advertisements for TV Drug Ads," *Health Aff (Millwood)* 2003; Suppl:W3-112-5.

10. Barents Group LLC, *Factors Affecting the Growth of Prescription Drug Expenditures* (Washington, D.C.: National Institute for Health Care Management Research and Educational Foundation, 1999).

11. T. Iizuka and G. Z. Jin, "The Effects of Direct-to-Consumer Advertising in the Prescription Drug Markets," Social Science Research Network Electronic Library, 2003. http://papers.ssrn.com/sol3/papers.cfm?abstract_id=365140 (accessed July 23, 2004).

12. M. B. Rosenthal, E. R. Berndt, J. M. Donohue, A. M. Epstein, and R. G. Frank, "Demand Effects of Recent Changes in Prescription Drug Promotion," Kaiser Family Foundation, June 2003; www.kff.org/rxdrugs/6085-index.cfm.

13. B. Mintzes, M. L. Barer, R. L. Kravitz, et al., "How Does Direct-to-Consumer Advertising (DTCA) Affect Prescribing? A Survey in Primary Care Environments with and without Legal DTCA," *CMAJ* 2003; 169:405–12.

14. J. Frey, "Selling Drugs to the Public—Should the UK Follow the Example of the US?" *Br J Gen Pract* 2002; 52:170–71; R. J. Cooper and J. R. Hoffman, "Selling Drugs to Doctors: It's Marketing, Not Education," *Br J Gen Pract* 2002; 52:168–69; "Europe on the Brink of Direct-to-Consumer Drug Advertising" [editorial], *Lancet* 2002; 359:1709. In an interesting twist on physician condemnation of DTC ads, Larson and colleagues studied ads broadcast by U.S. academic medical centers and found many of the same features that critics decry in drug-company advertising; R. J. Larson, L. M. Schwartz, S. Woloshin, and H. G. Welch, "Advertising by Academic Medical Centers," *Arch Intern Med* 2005; 165:645–51.

15. M. Perri and W. M. Dickson, "Direct to Consumer Prescription Drug Advertising: Consumer Attitudes and Physician Reaction," *Journal of Pharmaceutical Marketing and Management* 1987; 2:3–23; J. H. Powell, "Survey Positive on Ads Pushing Drugs," BusinessToday.com, January 14, 2003, www.businesstoday.com/business/business/drug01092003.htm (accessed January 14, 2003).

16. A. F. Holmer, "Direct-to-Consumer Advertising—Strengthening Our Health Care System," *N Engl J Med* 2002; 346:526–28.

17. Abramson, *Overdosed America*, 155; the quotation is from W. Ross, "Why Rubin-Ehrenthal Sticks Exclusively to DTC Accounts," *Medical Marketing & Media* September 1999; 34:136ff.; www.cpsnet.com/reprints/1999/09/McCarren.pdf (accessed November 14, 2004). The fact that DTC ads focus so much on emotional appeals to patients, rather than objectively imparting information about health, was the primary reason the House of Commons Health Committee in Britain strongly opposed having the United Kingdom follow the U.S. lead in allowing such ads; House of Commons Health Committee, *The Influence of the Pharmaceutical Industry* (London: The Stationery Office Limited, April 5, 2005), 77; www.parliament.the-stationery-office.co.uk/pa/cm200405/cmselect/cmhealth/42/42.pdf (accessed April 20, 2005).

18. Abramson, *Overdosed America*, 156–57.

19. Evidence leading to a different conclusion might be provided by a survey of patients conducted by FDA staff in 2002. Of those going to the physician to request a specific brand-name drug, 69 percent stated that they received a prescription for it, but 45 percent said that the physician also recommended changes in behavior or lifestyle; Aikin, "The Impact of Direct-to-Consumer Prescription Drug Advertising."

20. Michael Oldani, the anthropologist and former drug rep, described a friend who has become very frustrated with her primary care physician. The friend has several times com-

plained of feeling "stressed out." Instead of asking for a detailed history about the sources of the stress, the physician keeps offering the woman a drug to "ease her stress," which the woman refused to take on discovering that it was an antidepressant. The friend, who is slightly overweight, also becomes angry when the physician continues to push the antidepressant with the argument that one if its common side effects is weight loss, but never offers her any advice on either stress reduction or weight control otherwise. Oldani adds that reps are commonly trained to "spin" a drug's side effects into positive selling points; in this case the physician appears to be parroting the rep's script to the patient. M. J. Oldani, "Thick Prescriptions: Toward an Interpretation of Pharmaceutical Sales Practices," *Med Anthropol Q* 2004; 18:325–56, quote p. 352.

21. Evidence that this problem predates the rise of DTC ads in the late 1990s comes from a much earlier mass-marketing campaign, for estrogen as a replacement hormone therapy in menopausal women. Robert A. Wilson, a gynecologist heavily funded by the pharmaceutical industry, wrote a bestseller, *Feminine Forever* (1966), extolling the virtues of estrogens and glossing over the lack of scientific evidence supporting their use. Another physician reported sometime later—after Wilson's book had been reinforced by a spate of stories in women's magazines—that "the situation has gotten ridiculous. Women come in asking for 'the youth pill,' and they say, 'check my estrogen level.' From what they've read they think it's as simple as driving into a gasoline station and having their oil checked"; S. M. Rothman and D. J. Rothman, *The Pursuit of Perfection: The Promise and Perils of Medical Enhancement* (New York: Vintage, 2004), 79.

22. Tomes argues that the intersection between American medicine and the consumer culture goes at least as far back as the first half of the twentieth century. She cites ads from the 1920s and 1930s focusing on the rise of heart disease and other diseases of overindulgence, as contrasted with the infectious diseases that posed the main threat to life only a few decades earlier; these ads suggest that by consuming the right over-the-counter medications, Americans can indulge as much as they wish and still remain healthy. Also, suspicions of the medical profession as being too closely allied with the pharmaceutical industry date back to early consumer-activist campaigns of the 1930s; N. Tomes, "Merchants of Health: Medicine and Consumer Culture in the United States, 1900–1940," *J Am Hist* 2001; 88:519–47.

23. R. Moynihan, L. Bero, D. Ross-Degnan, et al., "Coverage by the News Media of the Benefits and Risks of Medications," *N Engl J Med* 2000; 342:1645–50.

24. Abramson, *Overdosed America*, 166.

25. M. Petersen, "Heartfelt Advice, Hefty Fees," *New York Times*, August 11, 2002.

26. M. Petersen, "CNN to Reveal When Guests Promote Drugs for Companies," *New York Times*, August 23, 2002.

27. M. Petersen, "A Respected Face, but Is It News or an Ad?" *New York Times*, May 7, 2003: B1.

28. J. R. Fishman, "Manufacturing Desire: The Commodification of Female Sexual Dysfunction," *Soc Stud Sci* 2004; 34:187–218. The Bermans' website (currently dominated by Dr. Laura Berman's photo) is www.newshe.com (accessed April 10, 2005).

29. R. O'Harrow Jr, "Grass Roots Seeded by Drugmaker: Schering-Plough Uses 'Coalitions' to Sell Costly Treatment," *Washington Post*, September 12, 2000:A1, A8–9.

30. P. J. Hilts, *Protecting America's Health: The FDA, Business, and One Hundred Years of Regulation* (New York: Knopf, 2003), 221.

31. L. Marsa, *Prescription for Profits: How the Pharmaceutical Industry Bankrolled the Unholy Marriage between Science and Business* (New York: Scribner, 1997), 208.

32. G. Harris, "States Try to Limit Drugs in Medicaid, but Makers Resist," *New York Times*, December 18, 2003:A1.

33. House of Commons Health Committee, *The Influence of the Pharmaceutical Industry*. The report in turn referred to an article published in *Pharmaceutical Marketing* in May, 2000.

34. R. Moynihan, "U.S. Seniors Group Attacks Pharmaceutical Industry 'Fronts,'" *BMJ* 2003; 326:351.

35. D. Healy, "Shaping the Intimate: Influences on the Experience of Everyday Nerves," *Soc Stud Sci* 2004; 34:219–45. The conference, "Creating Targeted Patient Education Campaigns," was sponsored by the Institute for International Research.

36. R. Moynihan, "Alosetron: A Case Study in Regulatory Capture, or a Victory for Patients' Rights?" *BMJ* 2002; 325:592–95.

37. Dr. Jerry Avorn, of Harvard, generally a critic of the pharmaceutical industry, adopts a view of the Lotronex case that tends to side with the FDA "version." He notes that this case broke new ground, in that the FDA responded to a side-effect problem in a way that was not a simple dichotomy of either allowing unfettered sales of the drug or taking it completely off the market. Avorn believes that drug problems are too complicated for simplistic solutions and that most of the time we need a graded response that splits the difference between the drug's advocates and its detractors. J. Avorn, *Powerful Medicines: The Benefits, Risks, and Costs of Prescription Drugs* (New York: Alfred A. Knopf, 2004), 179–80. It is hard to see, however, how the eventual resolution of the Lotronex case represents the "graded response" that Avorn advocates, instead of the return to largely unfettered prescribing.

38. www.phrma.org/mediaroom/press/releases/15.12.2004.1104.cfm (accessed December 21, 2004).

39. F. Ahrens, "Tauzin Expected to Leave House for Trade Group," *Washington Post*, January 24, 2004:E1.

40. W. M. Welch, "Tauzin Pulls Out of Talks to Become Lobbyist," *USA Today*, February 26, 2004:4A; B. Walsh, "Tauzin Halts Job Talks with Drug Group," *New Orleans Times-Picayune*, February 27, 2004:5.

41. "The Other Drug War 2003: Drug Companies Deploy an Army of 675 Lobbyists to Protect Profits," Public Citizen Congress Watch, June 2003, www.citizen.org/congress/reform/drug_industry/contribution/articles.cfm?ID=9922 (accessed December 21, 2004).

42. M. Forsythe, "$139 Million Lobby Blitz Thrown at Medicare Bill," *Bergen County* [NJ] *Record*, November 21, 2003:B1. A later report put the 2003 figure at $116 million; Center for Public Integrity, "Drug Lobby Second to None: How the Pharmaceutical Industry Gets Its Way in Washington," Center for Public Integrity, 2005, www.publicintegrity.org/rx/report.aspx?aid=723&sid=200 (accessed July 7, 2005).

43. S. H. Landers and A. R. Sehgal, "Health Care Lobbying in the United States," *Am J Med* 2004; 116:474–77. These authors note that an additional $12 million was spent in lobbying by patients' organizations. As we have noted above, some of this spending may be "astroturf" and thus a form of disguised industry lobbying as well.

44. R. Toner, "Democrats See a Stealthy Drive by Drug Industry to Help Republicans," *New York Times*, October 20, 2002; S. Theimer, "Drug Companies Wooing GOP Pols at RNC," *Las Vegas Sun*, September 1, 2004.

45. Quoted in Abramson, *Overdosed America*, 91. The letter was made public as part of the legal challenges to the McCain-Feingold campaign finance reform amendment. The full letter is available at www.publici.org/dtaweb/downloads/story_01_062403_BCRA7.pdf (accessed November 10, 2004).

46. R. Gold, "Regional Report: Drug Makers Win State Medicaid Fight," *Wall Street Journal*, March 20, 2002:B14; Harris, "States Try to Limit Drugs"; P. Stith, "Drug Makers Lobby, State Does U-Turn," *Raleigh News & Observer*, April 6, 2004.

47. F. J. Frommer, "Drug Group Spent $8.5 Million Lobbying against Importation," *Philadelphia Inquirer*, October 13, 2003; R. Pear, "Group of Senators Agrees on Drug Imports," *New York Times*, April 22, 2004:A23; C. T. Zaneski, "Support Grows on Hill for Drug Imports: A Third Senate Chairman Comes Out for Opening U.S. Borders to FDA-Approved Medicines from Canada and Other Countries," *Baltimore Sun*, June 3, 2004:1D. While this legislative push seemed to die out in the waning days of the 2004 legislative season, it gained new life early in 2005; Bloomberg News, "More Republicans are Backing Drug Imports," *Boston Globe*, January 27, 2005. However, as proofs for this book were being corrected (July 2006), the legislation had not moved forward and remained apparently bottled up in committee.

48. D. Healy, *The Anti-Depressant Era* (Cambridge, MA: Harvard University Press, 1997), 181, 198.

49. A particularly bald statement of this business strategy is: "The medicalization of many natural processes is creating markets for lifestyle drugs for those who want to 'optimize quality of life' . . . pharmaceutical companies are searching for new disorders, based on extensive analysis of unexploited market opportunities. . . . The coming years will bear greater witness to the corporate sponsored creation of disease"; J. Coe, "The Lifestyle Drugs Outlook to 2008, Unlocking New Value in Well-being," Datamonitor, *Reuters Business Insight, Healthcare*, PLC, 2003; 12:148; quoted in R. Moynihan and A. Cassels, *Selling Sickness: How the World's Biggest Pharmaceutical Companies Are Turning Us All into Patients* (New York: Nation Books, 2005), 179.

50. V. Parry, "The Art of Branding a Condition," *Medical Marketing and Media* 2003; 38:43–49, quote p. 44.

51. Parry, "The Art of Branding a Condition," 46.

52. J. D. Kleinke, "Access versus Excess: Value-Based Cost Sharing for Prescription Drugs," *Health Aff (Millwood)* 2004; 23:34–47, quote p. 41.

53. E.g., R. Moynihan, I. Heath, and D. Henry, "Selling Sickness: The Pharmaceutical Industry and Disease Mongering," *BMJ* 2002; 324:886–91; Moynihan and Cassels, *Selling Sickness*. If the industry hopes to sell so-called "lifestyle drugs" that explicitly aim to reduce human unhappiness rather than treat disease, "medicalization" is indeed a necessary step, as the FDA will typically demand proof that a new drug addresses a "medical" condition before it will grant approval; Fishman, "Manufacturing Desire."

54. Kleinke, "Access versus Excess," 42.

55. Moynihan and Cassels, *Selling Sickness*, 81 (reference in original omitted).

56. House of Commons Health Committee, *The Influence of the Pharmaceutical Industry*. In selecting this particular campaign for comment, I do not mean to appear to discount the great public health benefits of identifying, for example, undiagnosed cases of hypertension or diabetes that might at present be causing no symptoms; but I would assume that sending out a PR firm to sell more medicines is hardly the ideal way to conduct public health screening.

57. S. V. Argyropoulos, S. D. Hood, and D. J. Nutt, "Social Phobia: Illness or Illusion?" *Acta Psychiatr Scand* 2001; 103:241–43; V. Starcevic, "Opportunistic 'Rediscovery' of Mental Disorders by the Pharmaceutical Industry," *Psychother Psychosom* 2002; 71:305–10; Moynihan, Heath, and Henry, "Selling Sickness"; P. Conrad, and V. Leiter, "Medicalization, Markets and Consumers," *J Health Soc Behav* 2004; 45 Suppl:158–76.

14

THE FDA: FROM PATENT MEDICINES TO AIDS DRUGS

Apparently they just throw drugs together and if they don't explode they are placed on sale.

—FDA agent investigating the Massengill company
following the Elixir Sulfanilamide disaster, 1937[1]

I do not think we need to be particularly proud that it took an international ca-tastrophe to make us realize that the first thing with drugs is safety.

—Rep. Peter Rodino (D-NJ), on how the thalidomide disaster
resulted in passage of the Kefauver-Harris amendments in 1962[2]

MAD COWS AND SAFE DRUGS

In December 2003, the first U.S. case of bovine spongiform encephalopathy, or mad cow disease, was identified in a slaughtered dairy cow. The U.S. Department of Agriculture (USDA) rushed to reassure Americans and the world that the U.S. beef supply was safe, while other countries quickly banned imports of American beef. Skeptics accused the USDA and the beef industry of inadequate safeguards. *Consumer Reports*, for example, posted on its website a list of measures that food safety advocates had been pushing for a number of years, and that would have provided better protection.[3]

The beef industry found itself confronting the irony of "regulatory capture." Policy analysts have long argued that any government regulatory agency tends in the long run to be captured by the industry it is supposed to regulate.[4] But, like the proverbial dog that likes to chase trucks, the industry must decide what to do with what it has captured. In the short run, it no doubt seemed a great success for the beef industry that it had fought off onerous and expensive regulations. Then a crisis arrives, and the industry realizes—too late—that it may lose millions of dollars that it might have saved had it been willing to embrace somewhat stricter safeguards.

The mad-cow crisis, during one month in 2003, comprises in a nutshell much of the history of the FDA from its inception in 1906. The pharmaceutical industry has spent most of those years lobbying energetically to get FDA regulators off its back as much as possible, and a few of those years realizing belatedly, usually in the face of a catastrophe, that its own financial interests are ill served by overly weak regulation. A brief review of the FDA's history shows that the competing forces at work today have existed all along, with periodic pendulum swings as one set of forces temporarily dominates.

THE FDA'S DILEMMA

In the ideal world, the FDA would walk a fine line—standing aside quickly to allow valuable, lifesaving new drugs to reach the market, while cautiously blocking unsafe and ineffective drugs. The great difficulty in assessing the FDA's success is that we, the public, require that it do contradictory things. What Silverman and Lee wrote in 1974 could easily be said today:

> The government . . . has been denounced for harassing the drug industry, and for being too soft on industry; for letting unsafe drugs reach the market, and for banning useful drugs; for moving too slowly, and for moving too fast; for tampering with the freedom of the press by interfering with drug advertising, and for letting advertisers pollute the environment with misleading drug claims; for allowing drug profits to soar, and for trying to keep drug prices low; for interfering with the seemingly divine right of the physician to prescribe as he alone sees fit, and for failing to control disastrously irrational prescribing; and, in general, for being bureaucratic, vacillating, dictatorial, inconsistent, addicted to nit-picking, and basically incompetent.[5]

What exactly counts as "regulatory capture"? Braithwaite's discussion of corporate crime in the pharmaceutical industry suggests some of the nuances. Braithwaite asks what government regulation is supposed to do—seek the punishment of wrongdoers, or protect public safety? He then argues that these goals are often in conflict. The best way to punish wrongdoers is to keep taking the industry to court and trying to single out individuals for criminal prosecution whenever misdeeds become known. But this strategy may easily drive industry wrongdoing farther underground and create an adversarial environment between the regulators and those within industry who have the most power to clean things up. On Braithwaite's analysis, industry is always divided within itself, and there are powerful forces within the drug companies that want the same things that the hardest-headed FDA bureaucrat wants. The safety of the public can often better be protected when the FDA adopts a more conciliatory stance and works with those positive forces inside industry. That in turn lays the agency open to charges that it is coddling the drug companies. (Braithwaite suggests backing up this conciliatory posture with the proverbial big stick. Occasional, carefully chosen criminal prosecutions work wonderfully in ensuring that industry pays careful attention to the FDA.)[6]

The history of the FDA through the course of the twentieth century suggests that the ship has often tacked on its course, frequently getting too cozy with industry and occasionally adopting an adversarial posture.[7] Today, the big stick seems notable for its absence.

ORIGINS

The movement toward FDA-type government regulation began first in England, and focused on impure foods long before people became concerned with impure drugs.[8] In the United States, the Department of Agriculture took up the adulterated foods issue in the late nineteenth century. The head of that department's Chemical Division, Harvey W. Wiley, extended the department's reach to drug safety in 1903. Wiley was a member of the AMA's Council on Pharmacy and Chemistry and tried to coordinate his efforts at Agriculture with the AMA's work fighting patent medicines.

Thanks to the work of Wiley and the AMA, and muckraking books like Upton Sinclair's *The Jungle* and articles in *Collier's* and the *Ladies' Home Journal*, the 1906 Pure Food and Drug Act was passed.[9] The Food and Drug Administration was born, as a division of the Department of Agriculture, with Wiley as its first chief.[10]

In the next few years, the difficulty of balancing the obligations of a regulatory agency became evident. Wiley was exactly the sort of crusader and zealot who could effectively move the nation to create the FDA; those same traits made him a poor choice to manage it. He tried to solve every problem by dragging manufacturers into court. After many pitched battles with his superiors he resigned in 1912. In that same year, the young FDA was reminded of the limits of its powers. One "Dr. Johnson" was selling a "Mild Combination Treatment for Cancer." The FDA showed that its claims to cure cancer were based on no scientific evidence whatsoever. The court, however, ruled that the 1906 act gave the FDA no power to assess the *effectiveness* of any drug; all it could do was prevent the sale of unsafe drugs. The FDA asked for, and got from President Taft and Congress, a 1912 amendment to the Pure Food and Drug Act to fill in this gap. But the new amendment set a very high bar, because the FDA had to prove not only ineffectiveness but also intent to defraud.[11] Further, the FDA had no authority to regulate advertising, or to require that a product's ingredients were listed on the label. Most important, a company could sell an unsafe drug and the FDA could take no action until it was already in public use.

In a pattern that would repeat itself over the years, a disaster was needed for the FDA to get the expanded regulatory powers it sought.[12] In 1937, 106 people died as a result of taking a new antibiotic liquid, Elixir Sulfanilamide, manufactured by a Tennessee firm, Massengill and Company. Their chemist had trouble dissolving the sulfa drug in water or alcohol, and so used as a vehicle diethylene glycol—better known today as automobile antifreeze—with some raspberry flavoring.[13] The public and Congress galvanized for action when they realized that under current law, the worst crime Massengill could be charged with was mislabeling the drug; they violated no laws by bringing a blatantly poisonous substance to market without prior testing.

THE NEW FDA, 1938–1960

In the wake of Elixir Sulfanilamide, Congress passed the 1938 Food, Drug, and Cosmetic Act. It broadened the definition of "drug" to include additional medical substances and devices and the FDA was also given control over cosmetics. Proof of safety was required before a new drug could be marketed, and complete and accurate labeling was required.

The FDA was shifted in 1953 from its original home in the Department of Agriculture to the new Department of Health, Education, and Welfare (DHEW), the predecessor of today's Department of Health and Human Services (DHHS). In 1954, George P. Larrick, who had begun work at the FDA thirty-one years earlier as a food inspector, became commissioner. As Larrick had risen through the FDA ranks, he became convinced of the need for harmony with the drug industry. He was a genial man who wanted to be liked. The White House and DHEW were deluged with phone calls and mail originating from Larrick's industry friends, supporting him for commissioner. As he saw it, his constituency was the industry, and he believed that the industry was basically honest and decent.[14]

Silverman and Lee's characterization of Larrick's tenure was that the "FDA had worked without fanfare because it had not been doing much work at all—certainly in the case of drugs—and that the regulators had become entirely too friendly with the industry to be regulated."[15] At Larrick's FDA, "drug company officials were able to simply walk into the building, find the desk of the medical officer reviewing the company's drug application, and wade in with questions and arguments about the evidence. At the same time, if a consumer came to the agency asking for data on the safety of a drug, even one already approved and on the market, he was denied access completely."[16]

One FDA medical officer recalled many years later that Tuesday nights at Georgetown's Rive Gauche restaurant were well known to FDA staffers—one could go there assured that pharmaceutical company representatives would be on hand to pick up the tab.[17] Dr. Barbara Moulton, an FDA medical officer known as one of the agency's "young Turks" for her willingness to stand up to industry pressure, recalled later that she had once tried to hold up a new drug application until the manufacturer agreed to a label warning that the drug was potentially addictive. She was overruled by the head of the FDA Bureau of Medicine, who told her, "I will not have my policy of friendliness with industry interfered with."[18]

In 1958, Tennessee Senator Estes Kefauver (D) began hearings into the practices of the pharmaceutical industry. The hearings initially were prompted by suspicions of price fixing and the realization that the prices of popular drugs commonly represented a 400 to 500 percent markup over manufacturing costs.[19] Kefauver initially had no interest in showing up or blindsiding the FDA; in fact, his eventual goal was to increase its regulatory authority over the industry. He went to FDA headquarters and personally briefed them on the strategy he hoped to follow in the hearings. The response from the FDA leadership was chilly. The former deputy commissioner, Winton B. Rankin, recalled years later, "Larrick didn't want to have a damn thing to do with Kefauver's bill. He saw it as just a lot of trouble . . . that was not going to help the agency."[20]

As the Kefauver hearings started to expose secrets that the drug companies would have preferred to keep hidden, said historian Philip Hilts, "If the agency were an official arm of the drug industry, it could not have been more quiet, puzzled, and embarrassed."[21] It was not merely that there was a dispute between the drug industry and its critics and the FDA took the side of industry. Rather, as Hilts describes it, the FDA simply did not understand what the dispute was about in the first place. There was no awareness, it seemed, that drug firms that had originally been storefront operations now had become huge industrial conglomerates and could afford to spend millions of dollars in marketing their products and manipulating medical opinion. The FDA had no clue how big the problems were.

THE HENRY WELCH SCANDAL

If Larrick was embarrassed by the mere fact that Kefauver was holding hearings, he soon had reasons to be even more embarrassed over specific revelations. The Senate committee revealed in 1960 that the head of the FDA's Division of Antibiotics, Henry Welch, had, unknown to his superiors, earned during the previous seven years a total of $287,142 for outside work.[22] Welch had publishing interests and edited a journal. He had shared articles in press with the drug companies, letting them know that he would make changes that they suggested so long as the companies purchased reprints or monographs and steered advertising revenue his way. Since his division had to approve all new antibiotics, it is fair to assume that the companies believed that by contributing to Welch's publishing empire, they were also buying favor with the agency that would approve or deny them the right to market their new products.

At the 1956 Antibiotics Symposium, cosponsored by the FDA, while Welch and his partners retained the rights to publish and sell the conference proceedings, Welch declared that combination antibiotics ushered in "a third era of antibiotic therapy." This position outraged academicians like Charles May, who knew that there was virtually no scientific evidence to support the use of these heavily marketed drugs. It was later revealed that Pfizer was planning to use that "third era" phrase in an advertising campaign for its new combination antibiotic, Sigmamycin. Welch allowed Pfizer staff to insert that phrase into his speech, and Pfizer obligingly purchased 260,000 copies of reprints of that speech for international distribution.[23]

Welch became adept at exploiting the financial potential of the evolving relationship between the drug rep ("detail man" in that era) and the practicing physician. Both parties to the transaction had a strong interest in maintaining a charade, and the handing out of reprints of scientific papers was a key element in the charade. By giving the physician a reprint, the detail man made two statements: "You can trust what I say because I am backing it up by giving you the original scientific literature that supports my claims"; and, "I respect you as a critical, independent-thinking, thoughtful practitioner, who would never take anything I say at face value without checking out the facts for yourself." The physicians themselves would be among the first to admit that they seldom, if ever, had time actually to read the reprints; or if they did, in those days, that they had any inkling of how to separate real science from pseudoscience. So the giving of reprints functioned as theater even as it provided the veneer of an exchange of information and of physician education. And selling the drug companies those reprints was becoming big business.

The FDA "young Turk," Dr. Barbara Moulton, who had excellent academic credentials in antibiotics and infectious diseases, attended the 1956 symposium. She later testified before the Kefauver committee, "Dr. Welch's opening remarks . . . produced a most unfavorable reaction on the part of the more reputable clinical investigators. I heard most derogatory comments on the part particularly of the foreign participants in the symposium, who were shocked by the obvious commercialism of the whole program, and who stated unequivocally that the United States Government seemed to be dominated by the pharmaceutical industry in a way that would not be tolerated abroad."[24]

Dr. Welch may have enriched himself at the expense of the FDA's reputation, but there is no evidence that he *directly* did anything to threaten the safety of drugs. Indeed, when faced with the problem of an unsafe antibiotic (chloramphenicol) that was being inappropriately marketed by its manufacturer, Welch listened sympathetically to the physician who first tried to focus attention on the issue and turned over FDA records that documented the extent of the injuries produced by the drug.[25] But at the same time that the Welch case was unfolding, another case showed that some parts of the U.S. pharmaceutical industry had not advanced very much since the 1937 Massengill debacle.

The drug firm Richardson-Merrell was a subsidiary of the Vick Chemical Company, best known today as the manufacturer of the perennial favorite, Vick's Vapo-Rub.[26] Richardson-Merrell saw its big chance with a new drug called triparanol—or, as the company's internal coding system labeled it, MER-29, one of the first cholesterol-lowering drugs. The company marketers prepared to tell people that they could eat all the high-cholesterol foods they craved, so long as they took one triparanol pill a day for the rest of their lives. They calculated huge potential profits.

The FDA approved MER-29 in 1960, over the objection of the medical officer who reviewed the company's submission data. By the time the company voluntarily withdrew the drug in 1962, its users had been suffering from cataracts at about three times the normal rate. A later investigation by the FDA field staff (who had been tipped off as a result of a chance encounter between one of their agents and the husband of a disgruntled Richardson-Merrell lab technician) revealed that most of the "safety" data, derived from animal studies, had been faked.[27] Eventually the investigation led to criminal charges against the company and three top officials, resulting in the rather paltry fine of $80,000. The company fared less well in the civil courts, and faced about fifteen hundred lawsuits from those claiming to have been damaged by taking MER-29; it paid out an estimated $45–55 million in awards.[28]

MER-29, coming after a decade of news about the rapid proliferation of new "miracle" pharmaceuticals, might easily have turned into a scandal equal to the 1937 Elixir Sulfanilamide affair, leading to demands to give the FDA increased powers to protect the public. As it turned out, MER-29 was eclipsed by a greater scandal. Triparanol was dubbed MER-29 presumably because it was the twenty-ninth chemical in the Richardson-Merrell company pipeline to reach a certain stage of pharmaceutical development. Waiting in the wings at the same firm was another compound called MER-32, which the world was soon to know much better under its generic name, thalidomide.[29] The stage was now set for the event that shaped the FDA for the next twenty years.

THALIDOMIDE AND FRANCES KELSEY

The German pharmaceutical industry, once the envy of the world, lay in shambles after World War II. One surviving company, Chemie Grünenthal, elected to rebuild in a particularly ruthless manner. Between 1953 and 1954 it had introduced two new antibiotics that turned out to have severe side effects, which the company either failed to discover or else tried to cover up.[30]

In 1954, the company discovered a new compound, thalidomide. The drug appeared to have potential as a sleeping pill and tranquilizer. Scientists found that they could feed massive doses to rats and other animals without killing them, or indeed without their showing any signs whatsoever.[31] Grünenthal never conducted controlled trials in humans. Physicians on retainer to the company simply tried it out on patients and supplied testimonials of glowing success in curing insomnia and anxiety. On the other hand, even before the drug was marketed, Grünenthal received reports of a variety of side effects, including nausea, giddiness, constipation, excessive wakefulness, and allergic reactions.

Despite these reports, Grünenthal decided to promote its new medication as the first "completely safe" sedative, since the most popular sedatives then on the market, barbiturates, were habit-forming and deadly in overdose. The company pushed the safety record partly because they wished to make thalidomide available without a doctor's prescription. Since the drug was purported to be so safe, a particularly appealing market was pregnant women. Grünenthal also combined thalidomide with aspirin, cough medicine, and other substances, selling these mixtures under a variety of brand names—later making it extremely difficult to find out exactly who had taken the drug.

Between 1958 and 1960, physicians began to contact Grünenthal with reports of a new side effect, peripheral neuritis—numbness or tingling in the arms or legs that often failed to get better even after the person quit taking the drug. The company responded with lies. Even after they had received one hundred such reports (which were stored in a secret "bunker" hidden beneath an old factory chimney), the company responded to new reports by denying any knowledge of the problem.[32]

As reports of side effects mounted, Grünenthal stepped up the intensity of its defenses. Its sales department adopted the slogan, "We must succeed, whatever the cost."[33] It promoted research trials by physicians likely to publish favorable results. Some physicians who tried to publish reports of side effects found themselves being harassed by private detectives hired by the company. When one medical journal received a manuscript reporting side effects, the company exerted pressure on the editor and managed to stop publication.[34]

Grünenthal also tried to promote overseas sales. Distillers, better known as a manufacturer of liquor than as a drug firm, bought the license to distribute thalidomide in Britain and Australia. But Grünenthal had trouble entering the U.S. market. The first firm they contacted, Smith, Kline, and French, had a competent research staff and quickly determined that the Grünenthal data on efficacy and safety were full of holes. Lederle also turned them down. Finally the Germans began to do business with Richardson-Merrell, which, as the MER-29 episode proved, lagged behind the industry leaders in the quality of its research apparatus. Richardson-Merrell was granted the license for U.S. and Canadian sales of thalidomide.

Richardson-Merrell planned to market the drug especially for nausea and vomiting in pregnancy. They discovered they had no knowledge of how women and fetuses would be affected by the drug. Instead of doing the necessary research, they sought a public relations solution. The company approached an obstetrician, Dr. Ray Nulsen, to submit a ghostwritten article to the *Journal of Obstetrics and Gynecology* to promote the drug for use in pregnancy. The editor of the journal balked, and asked for information on whether the drug crossed the placenta to enter the fetal circulation. The company had to admit that it had no idea.[35]

In countries where thalidomide was being used, infants were being born with a condition known as phocomelia—absent or severely shortened arms or legs that sometimes looked like the flippers of seals. By early 1961, Dr. William McBride, a Sydney obstetrician, had become convinced that there was a direct connection between the drug and the defect. McBride published a paper describing his findings in the prominent British medical journal, the *Lancet*, in December 1961.[36]

The larger public became aware of thalidomide when a second physician, a Hamburg professor of pediatrics, Dr. Widukind Lenz, made the same association that Dr. McBride had observed earlier (but had not yet published). Lenz undertook a systematic canvassing of his area of Germany and located fourteen recent cases of phocomelia—a number much greater than would be predicted by chance—all apparently linked to thalidomide.[37] On November 15, 1961, Lenz notified Grünenthal of his suspicions, and five days later reported his findings at a meeting of German pediatricians.[38] Grünenthal sent three company executives along with the firm's legal adviser to harass Lenz, whom they later attacked publicly as a "half-wit."[39] But the Hamburg health authorities were alarmed by Lenz's data and asked Grünenthal voluntarily to withdraw the drug from the market. The company instead sent out seventy thousand promotional letters to German physicians declaring that their drug was safe.[40] But within the week, after negative newspaper stories, the company decided to withdraw thalidomide from the market in Germany. It was later estimated that forty thousand Germans had suffered from peripheral neuritis as a result of taking thalidomide and that between eight and twelve thousand deformed babies had been born.[41]

Grünenthal had thrown in the towel in Germany, but was not prepared to lose its international profits. The drug remained on the market for a number of months in many other countries. A reporter in Sao Paulo, Brazil, became aware of the recent births of limbless babies and was informed by authorities that no thalidomide was being sold in that city. He eventually discovered that the drug was indeed being sold in local pharmacies, under five different brand names, none of them labeled "thalidomide." After the reporter published his findings, authorities finally confiscated 2.5 million tablets of thalidomide in Sao Paulo alone.[42]

THALIDOMIDE AND THE FDA

The FDA's role in the thalidomide affair began on September 12, 1960, fourteen months before Lenz's revelations in Hamburg. The FDA had received the request from Richardson-Merrell to market thalidomide in the United States under the trade name Kevadon. The application landed on the desk of Dr. Frances O. Kelsey, a recently hired medical officer. At first glance she looked like a new Washington hand who was unlikely to know the ropes very well, and her supervisors perhaps planned to hand her an "easy" file like thalidomide. After all, the drug had been widely sold over the counter in many other countries, so its U.S. approval seemed a foregone conclusion.

"Frankie" Kelsey, then forty-seven years old, had been born in Canada and became a U.S. citizen on her marriage to Dr. F. Ellis Kelsey. She met him at the University of Chicago where she had earned both an M.D. and a Ph.D. in pharmacology. During World War II the Drs. Kelsey worked on a government malaria project and conducted research on quinine (an antimalarial drug) using rabbits. They found that quinine had toxic effects on rabbit fetuses while the mothers remained free of any damage; the mothers' livers broke the compound down rapidly but the fetal liver could not do the same. Frances Kelsey therefore had early experience with a drug responsible for birth defects that might not show any obvious signs in the adult animal.[43] Some of these earlier experiments also indicated a possible linkage between a drug that caused peripheral neuropathy in adults and the same drug's potential to damage the fetus.[44]

After the war, Dr. Ellis Kelsey became head of physiology and pharmacology at the University of South Dakota. Frances helped him write a basic textbook of pharmacology, then settled down as a family physician in a rural area of the state. Finally Ellis Kelsey was appointed a special assistant to the Surgeon General, and the family moved to Washington, D.C. Frances first found work as an editor for the *Journal of the American Medical Association*, and then became a medical officer at the FDA.

When Dr. Frances Kelsey opened the four-volume thalidomide file, she immediately noticed two things. First, it appeared that the company had not anticipated that the file would receive any serious scrutiny; they seemed to have slapped it together on the assumption that it would get a simple rubber stamp. In her stint at the AMA *Journal*, Kelsey had become familiar with a group of physicians whom the editors regarded as little more than paid shills for the drug companies. They constantly submitted letters and articles that were nothing more than glowing testimonials for various drugs, and Kelsey became used to weeding out their submissions. Kelsey's suspicions rose when she saw many of these same names on the company list of physicians who had done "research" on thalidomide.

Second, she decided that there were serious gaps in the scientific basis for the application. Whereas the Grünenthal scientists had been pleased when no rats showed any signs whatever after taking thalidomide, interpreting this as evidence of the drug's safety, Kelsey wondered if the rats were even absorbing the drug at all—no one at Grünenthal had ever thought of testing the rats' blood to see if any thalidomide was present.[45] The FDA pharmacologist who had reviewed the data before the files were handed to Kelsey had noted that the data on long-term use of the drug were totally inadequate to prove safety.

The law then in effect gave Kelsey two options. She could reject the application within the next sixty days if she found solid evidence that the drug was unsafe. Otherwise the drug would automatically be approved. Kelsey's next move showed that she knew the Washington game better than anyone would have imagined. She waited fifty-eight days and then declared that the application was incomplete. Legally, it was as if Richardson-Merrell had submitted nothing at all and had to start over.

The drug company should have had no way of knowing who the medical officer was who had blocked their application. But Kelsey's boss, Dr. Ralph Smith, obligingly sent Richardson-Merrell Kelsey's name and phone number. The company then started to contact her directly (Kelsey eventually documented fifty-one such contacts), to persuade her to approve the application—the company had ten million thalidomide tablets sitting in warehouses waiting to be shipped.

Dr. E. Joseph Murray, Richardson-Merrell's director of scientific relations, undertook to deal with the Kelsey problem. He first tried a cooperative approach, phoning her to ask what data she was lacking. But Kelsey smelled a rat when Murray kept trying to make revisions in the application over the phone but not on paper, and also when the documents the company sent contained different information than what she had previously been told. She began to believe that the company's posture was more than arrogance and sloppiness; they must actively be withholding key information.

When Kelsey repeated her fifty-eight-day "incomplete" gambit a second time, Murray switched to intimidation. New faces began to appear at the FDA demanding approval for Kevadon, among them Dr. Louis Lasagna, a nationally prominent pharmacologist. Once a sharp critic of industry practices, Lasagna had since become a paid consultant for various companies.[46] But now Kelsey had a new weapon. A letter had appeared in the *British Medical Journal* documenting reports of peripheral neuritis caused by thalidomide.[47] The overseas publications were often weeks late getting to the United States, but this issue fortunately showed up on time. When Murray called to badger her some more, Kelsey casually mentioned the *BMJ* letter. Murray's reaction suggested strongly that the company had known about the peripheral neuritis problem and had omitted this information from its FDA application.

For over a year Dr. Kelsey managed to play her delaying game, aware that her superiors had the authority to sign off on the thalidomide approval despite her objections (as had happened with MER-29). Both her colleagues and at least some of her key superiors at the agency backed her up and resisted company pressure on her behalf.[48] Finally came the public announcement of Dr. Lenz's discovery in November 1961. Even though Grünenthal withdrew thalidomide from the German market that month, Richardson-Merrell did not stop Canadian sales of the drug until March 2, 1962, and only withdrew its FDA application on March 8.

Dr. Kelsey, who until now had been careful to stay out of the limelight, became useful for Senator Estes Kefauver's campaign to give the FDA major new authority to regulate drugs. Kefauver had been getting nowhere with the bill, the Kefauver-Harris amendments, that had resulted from his Senate hearings. The White House staff under John Kennedy viewed their fellow Democrat from Tennessee as a loose cannon. At one point, the White House went behind Kefauver's back and promoted a watered-down bill. So the chances for passage of a bill with real teeth looked grim, unless something triggered an outpouring of public sentiment. Thalidomide arrived at the psychologically ideal moment for Kefauver and his allies. Kefauver's office tipped off the *Washington Post*, and the newspaper carried a story on July 15, 1962: "Heroine of FDA Keeps Bad Drug off Market." Kefauver followed up with a speech to the Senate three days later in which he urged that Dr. Kelsey be given a gold medal for Distinguished Federal Civilian Service.[49] President Kennedy now had little choice but to jump on the bandwagon, award the medal to Kelsey, and support the stronger version of the Kefauver-Harris amendments.

Richardson-Merrell distributed 2.5 million tablets of thalidomide to 1,267 U.S. physicians, who in turn gave them to perhaps 20,000 patients. Supposedly this was all part of a clinical testing program, though in actuality it was pure marketing, what would in later parlance be called a "seeding trial." Under existing regulations, no one had any idea who these patients were, or how to track down either the patients or the remaining tablets. It is still unknown how many afflicted infants may have been born in the United States as a result of this distribution of the drug.[50]

The public prosecutor in Aachen, Germany, conducted a four-year investigation and eventually filed criminal charges against nine Grünenthal executives. The trial did not begin until 1968. The company called expert witnesses who testified that there was no conclusive proof that thalidomide caused birth defects, and claimed further that unborn fetuses had no legal protection under German law anyway. The company also continued its intimidation tactics, and five journalists who had written unfavorably about the company received threats. Grünenthal managed to keep the trial going into 1970, then invoked a form of blackmail against the prosecutor—if you keep this trial going any longer, we will go bankrupt, and then there will be no money left to pay any compensation to victims.[51] Eventually a settlement was reached in which the company agreed to pay thirty-one million dollars in compensation to German thalidomide children and the criminal prosecution was dropped. Richardson-Merrell settled most U.S. and Canadian civil suits out of court.[52] Braithwaite, writing in 1984, considered the inability of the existing legal apparatus to punish those responsible for the thalidomide disaster a "staggering" admission of the law's ineffectiveness in dealing with pharmaceutical company wrongdoing.[53]

The thalidomide affair marked a milestone not only for the FDA, but also in the relationship between medicine and the pharmaceutical industry. It was now clear how much damage could be caused by an unsafe drug coming onto the market. It was also clear how the drive for profits might tempt a company to cut corners and also to cover up evidence that was unfavorable to continued sales.

Finally, it was clear that the great advances of pharmaceutical science from the 1930s to the 1960s were not by themselves a guarantee that serious problems would not arise. Medical science could not promise the public that its advances would necessarily result in the betterment of health. As Paul Starr famously observed in another context some two decades later, "The dream of reason did not take power into account."[54]

Almost all of the practices in the research, development, and marketing of drugs that we find problematic today had appeared before the MER-29 and thalidomide cases became widely known.[55] What is surprising is not how much, but rather how little has changed since 1962.

THE FDA AFTER THALIDOMIDE

The 1962 Kefauver-Harris Amendments mostly completed the process begun in 1906 of giving the FDA the power that it possesses today. The major change was that the FDA could demand scientific data from the manufacturer to prove that any new drug was effective as well as safe. Even more important, this provision was made retroactive to 1938. The FDA also gained new authority to inspect drug manufacturing and testing facilities.

Much of this actually had very little to do with the thalidomide disaster, which was, after all, more about safety than effectiveness. One provision in the new law that spoke directly to the recent tragedy, however, was a requirement that all company promotional material include the generic name of the drug as well as the trade name. The FDA was given more authority to make generic names easier to remember and understand. (Before this, companies often deliberately made generic names gobbledygook, so that physicians could remember only the simpler trade name and could not request a generic drug instead.)[56]

The FDA did little to exercise its new powers until Larrick retired at the end of 1965.[57] The next FDA commissioner, Dr. James Goddard, was a young career administrator in the Public Health Service. He instituted the massive Drug Efficacy Study of 1966–1969, supplementing the thin staff ranks at the FDA with expert committees appointed by the National Academy of Sciences. About four thousand drugs on the market in 1962 (actually about twenty-eight hundred *different* drugs) were reviewed for efficacy. Seven percent of the drugs were found to be totally ineffective, and about three hundred drugs were removed from market. Companies challenged these rulings in the courts, which upheld the FDA's authority in almost all aspects. The fact that this huge task of review was completed at all, let alone relatively close to schedule, says a good deal for the energy of the FDA staff and its commissioner in those years.[58]

THE PENDULUM SWINGS BACK

After Goddard left in 1968, the FDA had begun a gradual swing away from the Frances Kelsey legacy and back toward a more permissive posture regarding the industry. John Abraham performed case studies of the approval process for some nonsteroidal anti-inflammatory drugs (NSAIDs) during the 1970s and 1980s: "The case studies . . . do not support the complacent industry viewpoint that commercial interests can be relied upon to deliver the best marketing decisions for patients."[59] He found numerous examples of company scientists going to extremes to deny findings that cast their drug in a bad light. For example, in a 1985 review, company scientists insisted that the drug suprofen posed no risks of cancer in humans despite animal testing in which benign tumors were found:

> Here again we see senior industrial scientists seeking to undermine the significance and fundamental purpose of their own carcinogenicity testing in animals when the results are positive. For a crucial principle of chemical toxicological testing (especially carcinogenicity testing) is that the tests are conducted in animals in order to inform an assessment of the cancer risk in humans. If a positive result in such animal tests can be considered as "no evidence" that a drug could cause cancer in humans, then there seems to be little point in undertaking the tests in the first place.[60]

Most important, Abraham found that the permissive posture toward industry increased as the FDA moved from the 1970s into the 1980s.[61]

Scandal again plagued the FDA in the late 1980s, this time involving the generic drug approval process. It had for many years been an article of faith—one that eventually even the large drug companies ceased to challenge—that FDA-approved generic drugs were functionally equivalent to the brand-name drug in almost all instances. This faith was temporarily shaken when two FDA officers in the generics division, Charles Y. Chang and David Brancato, were discovered to be receiving gifts from generics companies in exchange for speedy approvals of bioequivalence data. The take included tens of thousands of dollars, free travel, a fur coat, and a VCR. Mylan, an honest generics firm that felt discriminated against by the chicanery, hired a private detective, who eventually discovered pieces of an incriminating photo in Chang's garbage. The scandal was revealed in congressional hearings held by Representative John Dingell in May 1989. As a result, two hundred generic drugs were temporarily or permanently withdrawn from market, and fifty-five company officials and five FDA staff were convicted of felonies. The scandal forced Frank Young, the apparently honest FDA commissioner, out of office.[62]

During the George H. W. Bush administration, Congress gave the FDA new responsibilities, but budgets lagged behind. Staff and enforcement reductions added to the demoralization caused by the generics scandal. "The situation was so bad that even leaders of the pharmaceutical industry created a support fund for the beleaguered agency. The companies acknowledged privately that they depend for their credibility on the FDA's reputed toughness. If the FDA falters, the reputation of their own products falters with it."[63]

AIDS, ACT UP, AND CHANGES IN THE FDA'S MANDATE

In the early days of the AIDS epidemic, there seemed little reason to imagine that the activists demanding more research into the new disease would find any common ground with the drug industry. The industry's recalcitrance was a major barrier to effective treatment. Industry analysts believed that the epidemic would soon wane. In 1984, with ten thousand HIV cases in the United States, the drug companies predicted that unless two hundred thousand were affected, profits would be too small to justify investment in research.

Leadership in AIDS treatment came from the government sector, dragging industry along reluctantly. Dr. Samuel Broder at the National Cancer Institute was convinced that viruses, including HIV, could be successfully attacked with the right molecule. The most promising molecules, however, were owned by the industry. Broder went to a number of companies for assistance and was turned down by most. Finally, Burroughs Wellcome, who manufactured acyclovir (a drug effective in treating the herpes virus infections), reluctantly agreed to make some of its compounds available to government researchers for testing for anti-HIV activity.

Because of the dangers to laboratory workers posed by HIV, this work required a specially designed lab dedicated to virus research. Burroughs Wellcome had no such lab, nor did any government or university scientist then working on AIDS. In a notable act of courage, scientists at the NIH and at Duke University announced they would accept the risk, and work in their own, less well protected labs.

One of the compounds sent by Burroughs Wellcome for testing ("compound S") turned out to be the first effective anti-HIV drug, AZT. At first Burroughs Wellcome agreed to do laboratory analyses on samples shipped from government and university labs, but the company then reneged on that agreement. Broder was able to reassign scientists from other NIH labs to do the necessary work. Despite the general impression that the FDA during that era was incredibly slow and cautious in approving new drugs, it took the agency all of one week to approve human tests of AZT after the initial, promising laboratory results. When AZT produced dramatic responses in early human trials, the FDA quickly approved the drug for marketing.[64]

Though most of the heavy lifting (as well as the serious personal risks) had been assumed by government and university scientists, Burroughs Wellcome retained the rights to sell AZT, and immediately triggered a backlash by pricing the new drug at about $10,000 for a year's treatment. The company calculated that it had spent about eighty-six million dollars of its own money on the drug and feared either that the epidemic would wane or that competing drugs would soon eat into their market share. They made one hundred million dollars on the drug in its first year of sales, and since the epidemic cooperated fully with the private marketplace, Burroughs Wellcome recouped their investment many times over within a few years.[65]

The AIDS community became angry first at the high cost of treatment and the fact that many sufferers could not afford the new life-extending drug. Later anger focused on the scientific studies that the FDA had decided to forgo in order to bring AZT to market quickly (although that was not how the activists saw it). It turned out that the initial recommended dose of AZT was too high, and patients suffered serious side effects until a better dose was determined. Some activists declared that AZT was killing more people than it was saving.

The radical group ACT UP, "AIDS Coalition to Unleash Power," became the point group for the protests. When ACT UP decided on a major Washington rally to be held in October 1988, there was initial disagreement as to the ideal target. Since President Ronald Reagan had been so slow to recognize the AIDS crisis, the White House was at the top of some protestors' list. But eventually the group chose the FDA. For one thing, the agency had the power to approve or delay new drugs, and that seemed critical, even though at the time there were no new drugs to approve. (Some AIDS activists realized the danger to HIV sufferers if the approval process were sped up too much, but their voices were largely drowned out.) For another, the FDA had shown itself to be flexible, and its top officials had been willing to meet with AIDS activists, causing some split within FDA ranks and within the scientific community. Ironically, by showing that it might respond more quickly than other agencies to continued pressure, the FDA earned the privilege of being in ACT UP's bullseye. The ACT UP protests, all artfully designed for maximum media exposure, carried a simple message: HIV sufferers were dying because the FDA was too slow in approving new drugs.

In the wake of the protests, activists and scientists worked hand in hand to design new methods to complete drug testing adequately while at the same time allowing the maximum number of patients to have access to drugs of real promise. The activists in the end had to agree that their charges against the FDA had been in large part baseless—they saw firsthand how much damage could be done when unsafe, partially tested drugs were rushed into use.[66] But whether they wanted to or not, ACT UP had succeeded in singing in harmony with the pharmaceutical industry. It no longer seemed that the American public wanted the FDA to protect them above all else from the next thalidomide. Rather, the public increasingly seemed to be saying that the FDA should get out of the way and allow new drugs to be used quickly. It was no longer acceptable (as the popular lore portrayed the situation) that European patients should be able to use the latest drugs years in advance of Americans. Congress, it turned out, was listening.

THE DRUG LAG

Back in 1972, the term "drug lag" had entered into the national vocabulary. It resonated with John Kennedy's proclamation of the "missile gap" between the United States and the Soviet Union. The "drug lag" is the claim that Europeans typically have access to new prescription drugs many years before Americans do. Like the missile gap, the drug lag turned out to be mostly a myth. The initial scholarly paper that addressed the issue found that forty-three drugs had been introduced in Britain before the United States, but thirty-nine had first come onto the market in America. But the mythical drug lag took on a life of its own when the concept was picked up by conservative, antiregulation economists. Later the drug industry was happy to fund more studies that purported to show the "drug lag" steadily widening. Coming from the opposite end of the political spectrum, ACT UP reenergized this claim just as a more pro-business, antiregulatory group was increasingly exercising power in Congress.[67]

David Kessler, a Harvard-trained pediatrician with a law degree and considerable Washington policy-making experience, became FDA commissioner in 1990. Although he had previously worked for such conservatives as Senator Orrin Hatch of Utah, he began his tenure with strong signals that he intended to be an activist FDA commissioner and that the old mission of protecting the public from unsafe drugs or mislabeled food was alive and well.[68] But Kessler was also a pragmatist and was committed to doing what he could to eliminate the "drug lag," to the extent that the problem was real.

If anything, the problem seemed to be shrinking. The median approval time for a new drug went from thirty-three months in 1987 to twenty-two months in 1991. Back in 1980, a report from the nonpartisan Government Accounting Office had clearly identified three major contributors to the "drug lag"—understaffing at the FDA, incompetent and uninterested industry research teams that often submitted incomplete or inadequate data, and a lack of communication between the two. To Kessler it seemed that these problems could all be addressed in a nonideological and pragmatic fashion. The FDA began quiet negotiations with industry representatives and with staffers from key congressional committees.[69]

What eventually passed Congress in 1992 (though some conservative ideologues tried to scuttle it, claiming that an excessively bureaucratic FDA was the sole problem), was the Prescription Drug User Fee Act (PDUFA). The drug industry would pay a fee for each new drug submitted for approval. The FDA would hire more reviewers to speed up the process. Various safeguards were built into the law to ensure that the FDA used the new money to speed review and did not divert the funds for other purposes.[70] The law requires renewal every five years. Including provisions of the 2002 renewal, a total of some fifteen hundred new employees have been added to (or are planned for) the FDA staff, virtually all for dealing with new drug approvals, and very few for reviewing the safety of drugs already approved.[71] Under the provisions of PDUFA, the pharmaceutical industry now supplies about 50 percent of the FDA funding for reviewing new drug applications.[72]

In 1992, a new Democratic administration was voted into office. But general FDA policy did not change. (Indeed, when conservative Republicans seized control of the House in the 1994 elections, an attempt was made to eliminate the FDA totally and let the drug industry regulate itself.) During the 1990s it seemed that both political parties agreed that job one at the FDA was to speed up new drug approvals and that a more cooperative posture between the FDA and industry was the desirable route to take. Looking at Kessler's entire career as FDA commissioner, it is hard to see him being as "activist" in the regulation of the drug industry as he was in his battle to gain regulatory authority over the tobacco industry.[73]

To mention just one example of industry-friendly tilt, the FDA initially used a classification system for new drugs. Drugs were categorized as 1A (significant therapeutic advance), 1B (marginal therapeutic advance), or 1C (no therapeutic advance). In 1992, the agency, under pressure from industry, abandoned this classification. New approvals are now classified as "significant new drugs" or "other," to avoid the 1C category that companies view as a marketing disadvantage.[74]

With the FDA taking what appeared to be a decided pro-industry slant, and with new drug approvals being speeded up due to an infusion of funds obtained from the industry, critics began to charge that more and more unsafe drugs were being approved, and that the number of drugs later withdrawn for safety concerns was increasing. The FDA leadership disputed those charges.[75] Unfortunately, their reply was of little value because they took literally the question of whether the FDA was approving new drugs "too quickly" and discussed only the actual length of time spent on review as a variable associated with whether or not a drug later was shown to have a safety concern. The more pertinent questions are whether the reviews were *sufficiently* thorough and whether *enough* time was spent, given the specific issues raised by that drug.[76] In the next chapter we will investigate the details of these criticisms and bring our account of the FDA up-to-date.

NOTES

1. H. F. Dowling, *Medicines for Man: The Development, Regulation, and Use of Prescription Drugs* (New York: Alfred A. Knopf, 1970), 193.

2. R. Brynner and T. Stephens, *Dark Remedy: The Impact of Thalidomide and Its Revival as a Vital Medicine* (Cambridge, MA: Perseus, 2001), 108.

3. "Mad Cow Update: How to Limit Your Risk," *Consumer Reports*, December 2003, www.consumerreports.org/static/0312mad0.html (accessed 1/2/04).

4. J. Abraham, *Science, Politics and the Pharmaceutical Industry: Controversy and Bias in Drug Regulation* (London: UCL Press, 1995), 22–23; J. Abraham, "The Pharmaceutical Industry as a Political Player," *Lancet* 2002; 360:1498–1502.

5. M. Silverman and P. R. Lee, *Pills, Profits and Politics* (Berkeley: University of California Press, 1974), 234–35.

6. J. Braithwaite, *Corporate Crime in the Pharmaceutical Industry* (Boston: Routledge & Kegan Paul, 1984), 291–347.

7. My major source for this chapter is Philip J. Hilts's *Protecting America's Health: The FDA, Business, and One Hundred Years of Regulation* (New York: Knopf, 2003).

8. Dowling, *Medicines for Man*, 188.

9. For example, Samuel Hopkins Adams's investigative series for *Collier's* on patent medicines were collected as: S. H. Adams, *The Great American Fraud* (New York: P. F. Collier, 1907).

10. In the larger scheme of things, the political forces responsible for passage of the Act of 1906 focused almost exclusively on impure food and were concerned very little with drugs. Initially Roosevelt distrusted Upton Sinclair's account of the horrors of the meatpacking industry, given the author's pronounced socialist leanings; he challenged Sinclair to give specifics and then sent his own spy into the plants. When the spy reported outrages even more severe, and less printable, than had appeared in *The Jungle*, Roosevelt put further pressure on Congress to pass the bill; E. Morris, *Theodore Rex* (New York: Modern Library, 2001), 435–48.

11. Dowling, *Medicines for Man*, 188–91.

12. Dowling, *Medicines for Man*, 192–93.

13. Details of the Elixir Sulfanilamide story can be found in Hilts, *Protecting America's Health*, 89–92; Dowling, *Medicines for Man*, 193; Silverman and Lee, *Pills, Profits and Politics*, 86–87; and Brynner and Stephens, *Dark Remedy*, 40.

14. Hilts, *Protecting America's Health*, 119–20 (based on an interview with former deputy commissioner Winton B. Rankin).

15. Silverman and Lee, *Pills, Profits and Politics*, 237.

16. Hilts, *Protecting America's Health*, 120.

17. Brynner and Stephens, *Dark Remedy*, 40.

18. J. Lear, "Drugmakers and the Govt.—Who Makes the Decisions?" *Saturday Review*, July 2, 1960, 37–43; quote p. 42.

19. R. Harris. *The Real Voice* (New York: Macmillan, 1964), 3–6.

20. Hilts, *Protecting America's Health*, 137.

21. Hilts, *Protecting America's Health*, 136–37.

22. The best source on the Welch case is R. E. McFayden, "The FDA's Regulation and Control of Antibiotics in the 1950s: The Henry Welch Scandal, Felix Marti-Ibanez, and Charles Pfizer & Co.," *Bull Hist Med* 1979; 53:159–69. McFayden in turn derived almost all of his information from the documents of Kefauver's Senate committee. See also a series of exposés written by John Lear, the science editor of the *Saturday Review*: J. Lear, "The Certification of Antibiotics," *Saturday Review*, February 7, 1959, 43–48; J. Lear, "Public Health at 7-1/2 Percent," *Saturday Review*, June 4, 1960, 37–41; Lear, "Drugmakers and the Govt." See also Harris, *The Real Voice*, 108–12.

23. Harris, *The Real Voice*, 111. One week before the Kefauver committee revealed the true extent of his business dealings, Welch filed for early retirement from the FDA for health reasons. This allowed him to collect his federal pension, even though his superiors fired him after they learned the truth; McFayden, "The FDA's Regulation and Control of Antibiotics in the 1950s."

24. Lear, "Drugmakers and the Govt.," 38.

25. Hilts, *Protecting America's Health*, 110–11.

26. As explained by the Insight Team of the *Sunday Times* of London in their later book on thalidomide, Vick Chemical Company was originally the parent company of the drug firm William S. Merrell; in 1960 Vick changed its name to Richardson-Merrell, Inc. Most published sources refer to the company as Richardson-Merrell during the period we are considering; Insight Team of *The Sunday Times* of London, *Suffer the Children: The Story of Thalidomide* (New York: Viking, 1979), 64.

27. Hilts, *Protecting America's Health*, 144–46; Braithwaite, *Corporate Crime*, 61–65; Silverman and Lee, *Pills, Profits and Politics*, 89–90; Insight Team, *Suffer the Children*, 64–68.

28. Silverman and Lee, *Pills, Profits and Politics*, 91–92; Insight Team, *Suffer the Children*, 64–69.

29. Insight Team, *Suffer the Children*, 68.

30. Brynner and Stephens, *Dark Remedy*, 7.

31. Brynner and Stephens, *Dark Remedy*, 9.

32. Brynner and Stephens, *Dark Remedy*, 23–24.

33. Insight Team, *Suffer the Children*, 37.

34. Braithwaite, *Corporate Crime*, 67–69.

35. Hilts, *Protecting America's Health*, 150.

36. In one of the strange twists to this story, McBride claimed later that he had sent his letter to the *Lancet* much earlier in the year, and that the journal had initially rejected it, but that he received notification of this only by surface mail, thereby causing a huge delay in publicizing the problem. But the *Lancet* denied any record of an earlier submission and McBride could never produce any documentary evidence to back up this claim; Brynner and Stephens, *Dark Remedy*, 29. Nonetheless McBride's account was apparently accepted by the *Sunday Times* Insight Team, *Suffer the Children*, 87–91.

37. Brynner and Stephens, *Dark Remedy*, 30–31.

38. Harris, *The Real Voice*, 186.

39. Hilts, *Protecting America's Health*, 155.

40. Brynner and Stephens, *Dark Remedy*, 32.

41. Hilts, *Protecting America's Health*, 154–58.

42. Braithwaite, *Corporate Crime*, 67–71; Silverman and Lee, *Pills, Profits and Politics*, 94–96.

43. Brynner and Stephens, *Dark Remedy*: 44–5.

44. Silverman and Lee, *Pills, Profits and Politics*, 95.

45. Dr. Kelsey's hunch on this point was accurate. Richardson-Merrell performed some studies using a syrup form of the medicine on seventy-eight rats and one dog; nearly all the animals promptly died. It appeared that the liquid drug was much more easily absorbed than in its initial powder or tablet form. But the company never revealed these new, alarming data to the FDA. Insight Team, *Suffer the Children*, 70.

46. Hilts, *Protecting America's Health*, 153.

47. A. L. Florence, "Is Thalidomide to Blame?" *BMJ* 1960; 2:1954.

48. Harry Dowling, who tended to treat the FDA gently in his book, wrote that Dr. Kelsey "and her colleagues" had been worried about the drug's safety from the outset; Dowling, *Medicines for Man*, 201. Others classed Kelsey as one of the small band of FDA medical officers called the "young Turks" who, like Barbara Moulton, were zealous in carrying out their business and were therefore somewhat shunned by their colleagues; Brynner and Stephens, *Dark Remedy*, 47. Philip Hilts, in his history of the FDA, credits Ralph Smith and others for supporting Kelsey and resisting the company pressure; Hilts, *Protecting America's Health*: 152–54.

49. Harris, *The Real Voice*: 184–89.

50. Braithwaite, *Corporate Crime*, 72; Harris, *The Real Voice*, 188–89. Richardson-Merrell's own documents later revealed that the company had no illusions that it was doing legitimate research in distributing these tablets broadcast. A brochure to the company sales force said: "Bear in mind that these are not *basic* clinical research studies. We have firmly established the safety, dosage and usefulness of Kevadon. . . . This program is designed to gain widespread confirmation of its usefulness. . . . You assure your doctors that they need not report results if they don't want to. . . . Be sure to tell them that we may send them report forms or reminder letters but these are strictly reminders and they need not reply." (Insight Team, *Suffer the Children*: 73) At that date, while ethical review of research studies in humans was much less developed than it is today, the AMA had published a consent form that it suggested that physicians ask patients to sign before giving them a drug that was part of an experimental clinical trial. Richardson-Merrell did not give these forms to doctors to use as part of its "research"; Insight Team, *Suffer the Children*: 71.

51. Brynner and Stephens, *Dark Remedy*, 76.

52. Brynner and Stephens, *Dark Remedy*, 68–71; Insight Team, *Suffer the Children*.

53. Braithwaite, *Corporate Crime*, 310.

54. P. Starr, *The Social Transformation of American Medicine* (New York: Basic Books, 1982), 3.

55. For example, as we have already seen, a long article critical of the pharmaceutical industry, published in 1961, complained of nearly all the same practices highlighted by today's critics; C. D. May, "Selling Drugs by 'Educating' Physicians," *J Med Educ* 1961; 36:1–23. Silverman and Lee, *Pills, Profits and Politics* (1974) eerily presages such recent works as Marcia Angell's *The Truth about the Drug Companies: How They Deceive Us and What to Do about It.* (New York: Random House, 2004). The main exception is the current concerns about direct-to-consumer advertising, and secret drug company support of supposed patients' grassroots organizations ("astroturf"); in the 1960s and 1970s, the large companies still

adhered to the traditional "ethical" label which meant that marketing directly to consumers was not allowed.

56. Dowling, *Medicines for Man*, 202–3.

57. According to friendly and critical accounts, Larrick either laid the groundwork for the administrative structure at the FDA that would enforce the new law (Dowling, *Medicines for Man*: 204–5) or mostly sat on his hands and did nothing (Silverman and Lee, *Pills, Profits and Politics*, 238).

58. Silverman and Lee, *Pills, Profits and Politics*, 238; Dowling, *Medicines for Man*, 205–6; Hilts, *Protecting America's Health*, 170–77.

59. Abraham, *Science, Politics and the Pharmaceutical Industry*, 242.

60. Abraham, *Science, Politics and the Pharmaceutical Industry*, 235; the manufacturer in this case was Ortho-Silag.

61. Abraham, *Science, Politics and the Pharmaceutical Industry*, 249.

62. Hilts, *Protecting America's Health*, 252–4.

63. Hilts, *Protecting America's Health*, 256.

64. Hilts, *Protecting America's Health*, 242–45.

65. Hilts, *Protecting America's Health*, 245–46.

66. Hilts, *Protecting America's Health*, 246–52.

67. Hilts, *Protecting America's Health*, 190–95, 276. The original scholarly publication was W. M. Wardell, "Introduction of New Therapeutic Drugs in the United States and Great Britain: An International Comparison," *Clin Pharmacol Ther* 1973; 14:773–90. An early attempt to portray the problem from a conservative economist's point of view was S. Peltzman, "An Evaluation of Consumer Protection Legislation: The 1962 Drug Amendments," *J Political Economy* 1973; 81:1049–91.

68. Hilts, *Protecting America's Health*, 257–75.

69. Hilts, *Protecting America's Health*, 276–78.

70. Hilts, *Protecting America's Health*, 278–79.

71. Angell, *The Truth about the Drug Companies*: 208–9.

72. D. Willman, "The New FDA: How a New Policy Led to Seven Deadly Drugs," *Los Angeles Times*, December 20, 2000:A1.

73. On tobacco, see D. Kessler, *A Question of Intent: A Great American Battle with a Deadly Industry* (New York: Public Affairs, 2001). For examples of publications suggesting a tough stand against the drug industry, see D. A. Kessler, "Addressing the Problem of Misleading Advertising," *Ann Intern Med* 1992; 116:950–51; D. A. Kessler, J. L. Rose, R. J. Temple, R. Schapiro, and J. P. Griffin, "Therapeutic-Class Wars—Drug Promotion in a Competitive Marketplace," *N Engl J Med* 1994; 331:1350–53.

74. D. Drake and M. Uhlman, *Making Medicine, Making Money* (Kansas City: Andrews and McMeel, 1993), 78.

75. M. A. Friedman, J. Woodcock, M. M. Lumpkin, J. E. Shuren, A. E. Hass, and L. J. Thompson, "The Safety of Newly Approved Medicines: Do Recent Market Removals Mean There Is a Problem?" *JAMA* 1999; 281:1728–34.

76. A. J. Wood, "The Safety of New Medicines: The Importance of Asking the Right Questions," *JAMA* 1999; 281:1753–54.

⑮

THE FDA AND THE INDUSTRY, 1990–2004

The FDA is as obstructionist as the drug companies, if not more so. That may be the biggest scandal behind these drug stories.

—CBS News correspondent Sharyl Attkisson, on the difficulties she faced in 2002 trying to clarify the label warning about gastrointestinal bleeding for Celebrex[1]

In the previous chapter we saw how the FDA, stung by charges that it was standing in the way of the American public getting access to the very latest life-saving drugs, abandoned the "Frances Kelsey ethic" (if one could call it that) of the immediate post-thalidomide era, and put itself in a position as more of a partner to industry and less of a consumer watchdog. Given the conflicting pressures that the agency has faced since it was created, this immediately set up the criticism from the opposing direction, that public health and safety had now taken a back seat to company profits.

The best way to highlight the problems that have arisen in this recent period of the FDA's history is to look in detail at some of the more controversial drug reviews. In hindsight, it is hard to see why earlier incidents did not trigger the negative publicity and the calls for action that occurred during 2004, in the wake of (first) the revelation of the suppression of data on antidepressants and suicides in children, and (next) the withdrawal of Vioxx. For whatever reason, the "tipping point," that we discussed in the introduction, had not yet been reached.

THE FEN-PHEN STORY

The Fen-phen Controversy

"Fen-phen" is two drugs, fenfluramine and phentermine, taken in combination. For many years, each had been used separately for weight loss, but they were widely regarded as unsatisfactory. "Fen" caused drowsiness, whereas "phen," which was related to amphetamines or "speed," made the patient feel wired. Around 1979, Dr. Michael Weintraub of the University of Rochester decided that perhaps these problems could be solved if the two drugs were used in combination. Thus was born the idea of fen-phen. A 1992 study by Weintraub's team prompted the interest in fen-phen among the larger medical community.[2]

Later, another scientist, Richard Wurtman at the Massachusetts Institute of Technology, invented a new chemical version of "fen," dexfenfluramine. He claimed that this medication had the same obesity-fighting potential as "fen" but without the problematic side effects.

In 1996, Wyeth-Ayerst, a division of American Home Products, manufactured two drugs—Pondimin ("fen" or fenfluramine), prescribed as part of the fen-phen combination, and Redux, Wurtman's new drug, dexfenfluramine. The FDA had approved Pondimin as a single drug some years ago, although the fen-phen combination had never received FDA approval. This meant that physicians using fen-phen were using Pondimin in what is referred to as an "off-label" manner. Physicians can legally prescribe medications however they wish, and the FDA has no jurisdiction over physicians' use of combinations like fen-phen. But the FDA does have the regulatory authority to prevent drug companies from *marketing* their products for off-label uses. Redux, as a newly developed drug, was only just now going through the FDA approval process.

The marketing of a prescription diet pill is a ticklish business. Physicians have, on the whole, been leery of using medication for weight loss, fearing both side effects if the drug is continued long term and regaining of the weight once the medication is stopped. (Physicians are of course members of the larger society, and that society has traditionally regarded obesity as a problem of individual willpower, not a "disease" that ought to be treated with medication.) Getting a drug onto the market and into widespread use meant that the company would have to break down this physician resistance.

Physicians are most prone to prescribe a diet pill for the "morbidly obese" patient. This patient is hugely overweight, fifty to one hundred pounds or more, and suffers from medical diseases that are directly worsened by the obesity. But there are not enough morbidly obese patients to make this market alone lucrative for the drug manufacturer. The real profits come from the much larger group of patients who are only ten or twenty pounds overweight, who are not now medically ill as a result, but who just want to look and feel thinner. From a medical point of view, this latter group of mildly obese patients should not be going anywhere near a prescription diet pill. But the drug manufacturer could reasonably foresee that once a diet pill got onto the market and into common use, these mildly obese patients would make up the most lucrative market. To start off, physicians motivated more by greed than ethics would set up diet clinics and prescribe the new drugs for all paying customers. The bandwagon effect of these pills being widely available would then pressure the average family doctor to prescribe them for his or her patients who came in begging for help in losing a few pounds.

If the company wished to look scientific and prudent, while tapping into the most lucrative market, it might adopt a two-faced marketing strategy. To get the drug approved by the FDA and into general use in the community, the marketing strategy would stress the medical complications and dangers of morbid obesity and suggest that the drugs should be prescribed only for these medically needy patients. The company could then hope for the bandwagon effect to cause the use of the pills to spill over to women who wanted to fit into a smaller dress size. Whether by design or by good luck, this is the course Wyeth-Ayerst followed with its drugs, Pondimin and Redux. The strategy worked so well that while only 3.7 million prescriptions were written for Pondimin in the United States in 1992, by 1995, when the popularity of fen-phen was gathering steam, physicians wrote 18 million prescriptions.[3]

Wyeth-Ayerst could not directly urge physicians to prescribe the off-label fen-phen combo, but physicians' professional societies, through scientific continuing education, could recommend this approach for the medical therapy of obesity. Wyeth-Ayerst became a staunch supporter of several organizations that the investigative reporter Alicia Mundy dubbed "Obesity, Inc."—the American Association for the Study of Obesity, the American Obesity Association, and Shape Up America!, a new advocacy group led by former Surgeon General C. Everett Koop.[4] Before 1997, Wyeth-Ayerst gave $725,000 to Shape Up America! After its diet drugs had been taken off the market, however, Wyeth-Ayerst suddenly lost interest in Dr. Koop's work and made no further grants to his organization.

"Obesity, Inc." created a drum roll of concern within the medical profession and among the general public. One statistic that was widely repeated by its spokespersons (despite the fact that Wyeth executives admitted in an internal memo that no one knew where it came from or if it was true) was that obesity causes the deaths of three hundred thousand Americans every year. "Obesity, Inc." was well poised to do (with Wyeth financial backing) what Wyeth could not do itself—publicize fully the literature reports on the usefulness of fen-phen, and create a groundswell of support for the idea that obesity is a deadly chronic illness and so requires the long-term use of powerful drugs to combat it. Moreover, even if safety issues arose and fen-phen caused a few deaths, who could quibble, if the nation were entrenching to battle a huge epidemic of three hundred thousand deaths per year?

Two safety issues, in fact, did emerge in relation to fen-phen—primary pulmonary hypertension and heart valve damage. Primary pulmonary hypertension, or PPH, is a condition of the vessels that carry blood through the lungs. They become thickened and clamp down, blocking the blood flow. The heart has to work harder to push to blood through the lungs, and the blood cannot carry away as much oxygen as the body needs to function. The patient becomes short of breath, dizzy, and faint, fatigues easily, and begins to retain fluids. PPH, unless it is recognized and treated promptly, has no cure and is usually fatal within a few years. In Europe in the mid-1960s, there had been a substantial number of cases of PPH associated with the use of an earlier appetite-suppressant drug, Aminorex, which had a mode of action similar to fen-phen's.

The heart valve damage seen in some users of fen-phen involves fibrosis, the thickening of the heart valves with fibrous tissue so that they do not open and close properly and become leaky. This process is also irreversible once advanced. Unlike PPH, there is a potential treatment for the valve problem, but it involves open heart surgery to replace the defective valves with mechanical ones. According to one later study, valve problems were found among 1.3 percent of obese subjects who had not taken the drugs, but in 13 to 25 percent of those who had taken Redux or fen-phen for several months.[5]

To assess the importance of the risks, one would also wish to know just how effective fen-phen was in taking off and keeping off the pounds. Here Wyeth and "Obesity, Inc." were somewhat less vocal in spreading the statistics. The documentation Wyeth-Ayerst sent to the FDA for the approval of Redux included a study suggesting that Redux was 3 percent more effective than placebo as a weight-loss pill, and that the average patient taking it lost six pounds.

Despite these unimpressive data on effectiveness, Wyeth-Ayerst made profits of nearly $180 million on Pondimin and Redux in 1996. Wall Street analysts confidently predicted that in a year or so, Redux sales alone would reach $1 billion annually.

Fen-phen: What the Company Did

Wyeth-Ayerst was marketing two drugs that were only minimally effective for weight loss, and that had potentially serious risks, at huge profits. According to documents later made public after a wave of lawsuits, Wyeth-Ayerst tried its best to prevent news of the side effects from reaching the FDA and practicing physicians. It also funded its own studies to claim that the risks had been massively overblown.

The previous experience with Aminorex showed that PPH was a foreseeable risk factor. Beginning in 1990, Wyeth-Ayerst began receiving reports of PPH as a result of taking fen-phen and (later) Redux. The official label warning approved by the FDA stated that a few cases of PPH had occurred. As more cases arose, some at the FDA started to urge a stronger warning label—a so-called "black box," which would call specific attention to the warning by means of a bold black outline. Wyeth-Ayerst's marketing projections showed that many physicians would stop prescribing the drugs if they carried such a warning. The company's response was an internal "SWAT team" specifically to fight against the black box.

Later, when the fen-phen controversy hit the media, Wyeth-Ayerst maintained that there had been too few cases of PPH to prove conclusively that the disease was actually caused by fen-phen or Redux. Some European patients who had taken fen-phen also took a Chinese herbal "cocktail" said to assist weight loss. How was one to be sure that the herbs, rather than Wyeth's drugs, didn't cause PPH? As to the other risk, heart valve damage, Wyeth-Ayerst insisted that reports of that side effect emerged from out of the blue in 1997. No one could have anticipated beforehand that heart valve damage was a potential risk factor. Therefore, scientists and physicians had no reason to be looking for it.

The company documents released by the lawsuits painted a different picture. A European subsidiary of Wyeth-Ayerst performed a study on rats in 1990 to look for cancer risk. The company submitted data from this study as part of the FDA approval process for Redux. When independent scientists later reviewed the rat tissue slides, they found, indeed, no evidence for cancer. What they did find was a massive amount of fibrosis involving the entire heart, including the valves. Most likely this fibrosis was at the root of *both* PPH and heart valve damage. One scientist who looked at the slides said later that if the rats had not been sacrificed as part of the experiment, they would soon have died of their heart disease.

When Wyeth-Ayerst reported the data to the FDA, they highlighted the fact that there had been no cancer seen in any of the rats. In the small print, they noted that "focal fibrosis" had been observed. They did not say *where* the fibrosis was focused, and the word "heart" was never mentioned in the report.

As reports of adverse drug reactions started to roll in from real people, and not rats, the company pursued the same general policy—say just enough so that you can later claim that you made all the disclosure legally required, but say it in such a way that no one will notice its true significance. Wyeth-Ayerst dutifully sent reports of PPH and heart valve damage along to the FDA. But the heading on the report often concealed the key diagnosis. If a patient had PPH or heart valve damage and also experienced some minor side effects like constipation, the report might be headed "constipation." The company guessed, correctly, that overworked FDA staffers would read the heading and might not search the fine print carefully to find the more ominous diagnosis.

The company faced a more serious problem early in 1997, when reports of valve disease arrived from the unlikely location of Fargo, North Dakota. Pam Ruff, an echocardiogram technician, had become suspicious a couple of years earlier when she found herself diagnosing a lot of serious valve disease among young women taking diet pills, and she finally convinced her physician supervisors to take the issue seriously and to begin a formal study. The responsible person at Wyeth-Ayerst began dutifully to enter these reports, with their official code numbers, into the list of adverse reactions for the FDA. Then someone changed his mind, and the staffer was directed to overwrite the reports—use the same code numbers but for different, more minor side effects for different drugs. Apparently the company thought that receiving a batch of reports, all of one serious adverse reaction, would set off alarm bells at the FDA, while trickling the same reports to the FDA slowly over an extended period of time might not have the same effect. Eventually all the reports were in fact sent to the FDA, so that Wyeth-Ayerst could claim that the whole matter was a clerical slip, not evidence of concealment.

Meanwhile, Pam Ruff had interested one of the Fargo cardiologists, Dr. Jack Crary, in her cause, and he in turn found that Dr. Heidi Connolly at the Mayo Clinic had independently made note of the same problem. Eventually it was decided that the prestigious Mayo Clinic should take the lead in preparing an article for the *New England Journal of Medicine*.[6] When the article appeared, the FDA finally took action. Wyeth-Ayerst was allowed to withdraw Pondimin and Redux from the market voluntarily.

The company began a damage-control program to the tune of ninety million dollars in grants to investigators it knew to be sympathetic. Virtually all studies paid for by the company concluded that the risk of PPH or heart valve damage with the drugs was extremely low, and that (by implication) the FDA had overreacted by ordering the drugs off the market. Several of these studies were placed in major cardiology and medical journals, in a few cases without a clear statement as to where the funding had come from. This in turn led sympathetic commentators in the popular press (particularly in one *Wall Street Journal* piece) to portray the company and its drugs as unduly persecuted.[7] Virtually every study published in major journals, and *not* funded by Wyeth-Ayerst, concluded that there was a causal relationship between the diet pills and the side effects, while all company-funded studies downplayed or denied the relationship.[8]

As a result of this heavily funded Wyeth-Ayerst campaign, ensuring that favorable studies were placed in respectable journals and then trumpeted loudly in the popular media, many physicians remained puzzled as to whether the diet drugs were really as big a risk as they were said to be.

Fen-phen: The FDA's Role

The FDA had a number of opportunities to strengthen the warnings on the already-approved Pondimin and to hold up or reject the application for approval for Redux. Because the lawsuits that gained access to the Wyeth-Ayerst documents failed for the most part to release any internal FDA papers, Alicia Mundy, the investigative reporter who wrote a book about the fen-phen controversy, relied primarily on interviews with Dr. Leo Lutwak. Lutwak, an expert on endocrine and metabolic disorders, had been a professor at Cornell and joined the FDA in 1992 upon his retirement from his academic post. Eventually Lutwak was forced out of his FDA position by a boss who complained that he was insufficiently deferential to the needs of the FDA's "clients"—the pharmaceutical companies. Through the mid-1990s, Lutwak often found himself apparently alone within the FDA structure in insisting that the diet drugs were unsafe and ought to be off the market.

Dr. Lutwak attributed the FDA's pro-industry tilt partly to the revolving door. Virtually all pharmaceutical firms count among their executive ranks a number of former staffers from the FDA. These insiders know how all the FDA procedures work, whom to call to get anything done, and how all the players in the FDA hierarchy are likely to react. Thus each drug firm has its own mock FDA within its walls and can plan strategy accordingly. Moreover, the current FDA staff know that these well-paying industry jobs are waiting for them after their tour of duty at the federal agency ends. In terms of later career advancement, it's a good idea to curry favor with the industry while one is at the agency.

In addition to the revolving door, the companies know the value of congressional pressure. Several prominent congresspersons weighed in with phone calls to key FDA officials during the fen-phen saga. As a major contributor to these politicians' reelection campaigns, Wyeth-Ayerst could almost always find a willing senator or representative to make a phone call to urge faster action in approving Redux, or in keeping sensitive information away from the public gaze.[9] A phone call from the Hill carries with it an implied threat of a cut in next year's budget if the FDA official at the other end of the call fails to respond appropriately.

The major challenge for the FDA over Pondimin and Redux arose from the PPH problem. Pondimin, as we have seen, carried a very weak warning that only a handful of PPH cases had been reported—which was, in retrospect, false, since Wyeth-Ayerst already had on file a list of 101 PPH victims when the label still claimed only four cases. Redux was being pushed for approval with virtually no acknowledgment that PPH might be a serious risk. From the drug firm's point of view, the biggest problem was a European study called IPPHS, the International PPH Study. This study was undertaken when a marked rise in PPH cases occurred in Europe, where fen-phen had become popular a few years before. The IPPHS investigators were among the most prestigious epidemiologists and PPH experts in both Europe and America. In August 1996, the results were published in the *New England Journal of Medicine*.[10]

Before IPPHS was published, Dr. Lutwak attended hearings on Redux and Pondimin in which IPPHS representatives discussed their preliminary data. He listened to them describe the markedly increased risks of PPH among users of the diet pills, and imagined that these data would shake up the FDA panel charged with reviewing the Wyeth drugs. Instead, the attitude of the FDA staff and its outside experts seemed to be that these were only preliminary data, and Americans can't trust European studies anyway. In actuality, the final publication of the IPPHS showed even more striking risks than did the preliminary data presented to the FDA earlier.

Dr. Stuart Rich, a coauthor of IPPHS, was outraged when known consultants to Wyeth were allowed to write an accompanying editorial, downplaying the risks and recommending continued use of the drugs.[11] He agreed to be on the *Today* show to discuss his concerns. After his television interview, Rich received a phone call from a senior Wyeth executive who warned him not to speak to popular media any more or "bad things would happen." This scared Rich sufficiently so that he did not speak to any more media sources, until he talked with PBS *Frontline* in 2003.[12]

The FDA eventually approved Redux for the market with only one concession to the safety issue—a demand that Wyeth-Ayerst follow up release of the drug with a Phase IV study, or postmarketing survey, designed to get accurate numbers on risks after the drug was in widespread use in the community. Even then, Wyeth-Ayerst managed to postpone coming up with detailed plans for the design of the Phase IV study, and called on its congressional allies to pressure the FDA to keep all hearings on that matter closed to the public (using the excuse that trade secrets might be revealed at those meetings). After one FDA official called for Pondimin's label warnings to be reviewed, the agency took no action for two years.

Ironically, once the unexpected news about the heart valve damage from Fargo and the Mayo Clinic hit the press, some FDA officials were pleased and relieved. (At that time they had no way to know that the "focal fibrosis" revealed in the 1990 European rat study in fact had pointed years ago to the heart problem.) Some of Dr. Lutwak's colleagues had, all along, been worried about the safety of the drugs, but felt that there was no way that the FDA could buck the Wyeth-Ayerst juggernaut.

Now that the heart valve horse was out of the barn, maybe the agency could finally get the upper hand and force the drugs off the market—as indeed soon occurred.

The FDA's role in the controversy continued even after the drugs were pulled from the market. Wyeth-Ayerst pestered the FDA to alter the wordings of several of its public statements, in order to create a stronger legal defense for a wave of lawsuits from hundreds of PPH and heart valve victims. In several cases, the FDA obligingly altered those statements to insert language favorable to the company.[13] The company's attempt to shore up its legal defense nevertheless failed; as of mid-2000, Wyeth-Ayerst had not won a single lawsuit and had been forced to settle many for huge damages. The internal documents showing how the firm had suppressed and manipulated risk data to protect sales were simply too damning to juries. But the company nonetheless managed to hitch the FDA to its cause.

THE REZULIN STORY

We have seen that in 1999, criticisms of a too-speedy drug approval process caused the FDA commissioner and his top staff to author a paper denying the charges.[14] The year after this paper was published, the FDA was forced to take yet another recently approved drug off the market—Rezulin.

In 1982, scientists in Japan were investigating a new drug called ciglitazone, the first of a new class of chemicals called thiazolidinediones.[15] Beside bordering on the unpronounceable, the main claim to fame for this group of chemical agents was a resemblance to the anticholesterol drug, clofibrate. They were known to have effects on certain fat cells. Ciglitazone was tested as a possible anticholesterol drug but had to be abandoned because it was found to be too toxic to the liver. Along the way, the scientists noticed something interesting. Even though it appeared to be active in fat cells and to have nothing to do with the cells that controlled sugar and insulin in diabetes, ciglitazone demonstrated a strong glucose-lowering effect.

In Type II diabetes, the type that occurs most commonly in adults (and that accounts for about nine-tenths of all cases of diabetes in the United States), fat cells, insulin, and glucose participate in a delicate balance. We once thought that the main problem in adult-onset diabetes was the failure of the islet cells in the pancreas to make enough insulin. We now realize that a big part of the problem is that other tissues become increasingly resistant to the action of insulin.

One way that insulin resistance shows itself is whether muscle cells use glucose or small fatty molecules as their main source of energy. Diabetes commonly leads to high levels of these free fatty acid molecules, which muscle cells use instead of glucose, so that the level of glucose in the bloodstream rises. With the thiazolidinedione drugs present, the levels of free fatty acids drop and the muscle cells use up more glucose, so the level of glucose in the blood drops also.[16]

In 1994, the Parke-Davis division of Warner-Lambert found that its new thiazolidinedione drug, troglitazone (brand name: Rezulin), appeared to be much less toxic to the liver than ciglitazone. The NIH was about to begin a national diabetes study, involving four thousand subjects at twenty-seven sites. Companies lobbied hard to try to get their pet drugs included in the study. Warner-Lambert tried to sweeten the pot by promising the NIH twenty million dollars in additional funding for the trial if Rezulin was included. They were successful, and in 1996, Dr. Richard C. Eastman, director of the NIH diabetes division, made favorable comments about the drug in a news release from Warner-Lambert announcing the inclusion of Rezulin in the NIH diabetes study. What was not revealed was that Dr. Eastman had become a paid consultant to Warner-Lambert in November 1995. The *Los Angeles Times* later reported that Dr. Eastman had received at least $78,000 in consulting fees from that company, and that his total additional income, from a total of six drug firms, was more than $260,000. Dr. Eastman's superiors at NIH ruled that these consulting arrangements did not constitute a conflict of interest. The *Los Angeles Times* reported that twelve of the twenty-two experts who played a central role in designing the NIH National Diabetes Study had received consulting fees or research grants from Warner-Lambert.[17]

By 1997, the Warner-Lambert scientists had enough data to seek FDA approval for Rezulin. Because the drug was the first of an entirely new class, and diabetes experts were nearly unanimous in calling for improved drugs to treat this chronic disease, the FDA put Rezulin on a fast track and approved it in about six months. Apparently uncommented upon at the time was the fact that forty-eight of the twenty-five hundred subjects included in the company's data had shown considerable elevations in one liver enzyme, a common sign of impending liver damage.[18] When the drug was first marketed, the FDA required no special warnings about liver testing.

On December 1, 1997, the British agency charged with ensuring drug safety surveyed six reported deaths from Rezulin-induced liver failure, and ordered the drug removed from the market in that country. The American FDA did not order Rezulin withdrawn until March 21, 2000 (at which time the known U.S. death toll was sixty-three). Why these different reactions? *Los Angeles Times* reporter David Willman conducted numerous interviews and surveyed internal documents, and reported that there had been an internal struggle within the FDA between the higher-ups and a group that came to be known as "the Termites."[19]

The higher-ups were led by Dr. Janet Woodcock, director of the FDA's drug evaluation center, and her deputy, Dr. Murray M. "Mac" Lumpkin. Dr. Lumpkin had initially been in charge of the fast-track review that led to Rezulin being approved in only six months. Dr. Lumpkin came to typify a conflict that critics of today's FDA claim should never arise. He was later in charge of monitoring the safety of Rezulin and considering each respective challenge to its being allowed to remain on the market. That is, Dr. Lumpkin was supposed to be the one to decide whether he had initially been right or wrong in pushing for Rezulin's quick approval.

Arrayed against the higher-ups was a group of FDA scientists, the "Termites." The first of the Termites was Dr. John K. Gueriguian, a veteran medical officer who read the scientific studies as showing that Rezulin had relatively little advantage over other diabetes drugs to offset the threat of liver problems.[20] Warner-Lambert applied pressure and the higher-ups ordered Gueriguian off the Rezulin case.[21]

The next "Termite" was Dr. Robert I. Misbin, a diabetes specialist who had initially welcomed this promising new class of drugs. He started to doubt his initial enthusiasm when he discovered that the company had delayed eight months in notifying the FDA of some liver function abnormalities in Rezulin patients.[22] Eventually he shared his concerns with a congressional committee and was then subjected to an FDA disciplinary review.

The next major Termite recruit was Dr. David J. Graham, who would later receive greater notoriety as the Vioxx whistle blower in 2004. After some initial reporting of liver-failure deaths in the *Los Angeles Times*, FDA commissioner Jane E. Henney ordered a reevaluation of Rezulin in January 1999. The case was assigned to Dr. Graham, who was the first FDA person in the story so far to have nothing at all to do with new drug approvals. Graham's sole portfolio is the safety of drugs already on the market.

By the time Dr. Graham became involved, the main issue regarding Rezulin was the label warning calling for careful monitoring for liver toxicity. Wyeth-Ayerst had initially formed its "SWAT Team" to fight against the "black box" for fen-phen. Warner-Lambert realized that it had a serious enough problem with Rezulin that a label warning might be its best alternative to having the drug removed from the market. Working very closely with Dr. Lumpkin, the company ended up revising the label four times. The last warning said that all patients taking Rezulin should have monthly liver tests for the first year of treatment, and also added that Rezulin should not be used as the first drug to treat diabetes, but should be prescribed only after it had been shown that other drugs don't work.

Even then—as the British regulators had realized back in 1997—there was no reason to believe that monitoring would prevent deaths. The liver failure caused by Rezulin could occur so quickly that a patient who tested normal last month might be terminally ill by the next. For that reason, the NIH withdrew Rezulin from the National Diabetes Trial in June 1998 after a number of deaths among trial participants.[23]

On March 26, 1999, Dr. Graham presented his conclusions to the FDA advisory committee that had initially approved Rezulin. He showed that Rezulin raised a person's risk of developing liver failure by a factor of twelve hundred. One of every eighteen hundred patients taking Rezulin could be predicted to suffer liver failure—a much greater number than Warner-Lambert's claim that the incidence was only one in one hundred thousand. The monitoring program offered no guarantee of safety; and even if it did, Graham's data showed that 99 percent of patients taking Rezulin for longer than four months failed to follow the arduous recommended monitoring schedule.

Warner-Lambert representatives argued to the committee that many of the liver-failure victims may have had other medical conditions that caused their problem, rather than Rezulin. (Nine prominent university diabetes experts who testified at the hearings were later shown to have financial ties to Warner-Lambert.)[24] The committee (three of whom were paid consultants of Warner-Lambert) chose to ignore Graham and voted eleven to one to keep Rezulin on the market. Graham received reprimands from his superiors for his presentation to the committee and was later ordered not to talk with David Willman of the *Los Angeles Times*.[25]

What finally tipped the scale in favor of the Termites and against the higher-ups were, first, the ever-increasing death toll from liver failure, and second, the appearance of two new thiazolidinedione drugs, rosiglitazone (Avandia) and pioglitazone (Actos), which appeared to be less dangerous to the liver. Even as Dr. Woodcock made the final decision to withdraw Rezulin on March 21, 2000, Dr. Lumpkin was still reportedly trying to stall by demanding another meeting of the advisory committee.

An internal audit was carried out by the FDA in the wake of the Rezulin controversy. One-third of the staff of the FDA Center for Drug Evaluation and Review who responded to the survey reported feeling uncomfortable expressing their scientific opinions. Many had felt pressures to favor the manufacturer over any concerns with the public health and had been told by senior FDA officials to alter their opinions when those opinions were against approval of a drug.[26]

SAFETY AND NEED

When the article by FDA leaders appeared in 1999, defending the agency against the charge of releasing unsafe drugs, *JAMA* asked Dr. Alastair J. J. Wood, a pharmacologist at Vanderbilt University, to write a responsive editorial. Wood observed, first, that the five drugs withdrawn for their toxic risks prior to the Rezulin affair had been given to a total of 19.8 million patients, almost 10 percent of the U.S. population. Second, none of the drugs was needed to treat a life-threatening condition, nor were most of them the only drug available to treat that condition. What, Wood asked, justified exposing so many people to possibly dangerous drugs that were arguably not really needed at all?[27]

One drug among the five discussed in the FDA article that especially bore this point home was bromfenac (Duract), which was manufactured by Wyeth-Ayerst and had been on the market only a year when it was withdrawn in 1998. Bromfenac was an NSAID, meaning that there were already at least two dozen similar drugs available for treating musculoskeletal pain, arthritis, and related conditions. The reason it was taken off the market was that it was virtually identical to Rezulin in its toxicity—twenty patients had severe liver failure, four died, and eight needed liver transplants. No patients were reported to have developed overt liver failure in the original, premarketing studies, but some subjects who remained on bromfenac for a little over a month developed the same elevation in liver enzymes that tipped scientists off to the risks associated with Rezulin. When the drug was marketed, the FDA insisted that it be labeled for short-term use only (ideally ten days or less) and that doctors be warned that if for any reason they used the drug for more than four weeks, they should monitor the liver enzymes by blood testing.

As the reports of liver failure rolled in, it became clear to the FDA and to the company that despite the supposedly clear and stern warning, many physicians in practice were *not* restricting the drug to ten days' use and were *not* monitoring the liver enzymes. Finally the FDA prevailed on the company to withdraw the drug because the benefit seemed not worth these continued risks.[28] Dr. Wood asked the reasonable question: Given the plethora of other NSAID drugs, all of which can be used with reasonable safety for months or even years on end, why would one even need to put a drug like bromphenac, which had no documented superiority to any other NSAID, on the market at all, if it could be used safely only under those extremely restricted conditions? What, for that matter, made the company think it would be cost-effective to put such a drug on the market? He then proceeded to answer his own question—during the relatively brief time bromfenac was marketed, 2.5 million people were treated with it.[29] It seems clear in retrospect that Wyeth-Ayerst, having sunk many millions of dollars into doing the research and development on bromfenac, decided it could recoup at least some of its money if the drug were aggressively marketed, even if it was only for a brief period of time. It could rely on its sales force to pitch this "brand-new" NSAID to doctors and to sing its praises. We can never know exactly what was said about bromfenac by Wyeth-Ayerst detail people in the privacy of all those physicians' offices. If other experience is any indication, the side effects and risks were downplayed, and any supposed advantage was talked up. The remaining question, then, is why the FDA allowed itself to play along with that game. Even the minimal arguments available for Rezulin, that it was the first drug in a totally new class of chemical agents for a hard-to-treat and potentially fatal chronic disease, could not be made for bromfenac.

In 2003, the PBS television news program *Frontline* interviewed Dr. Michael Elashoff, a biostatistician who had done drug review at the FDA between 1995 and 2000. Dr. Elashoff had left after being criticized by his superiors for giving negative testimony about Relenza, a flu drug. Dr. Elashoff described a pervasive sense within the FDA that no one could get promoted within the agency unless they supported the interests of the big drug companies: "I mean, it's called the drug approval process. It's not called the drug review process. So that really sets the mindset on what the job is." Dr. Elashoff attributed this mind-set to PDUFA. The influx of company money to hire new FDA staff had begun soon after he joined the agency in 1995, and he judged that the atmosphere when he left in 2000 had become considerably more pro-industry.

The *Frontline* correspondent challenged Dr. Elashoff by quoting loosely from an FDA official who had recently been interviewed for the same show: "No morale problem here at all, everyone is happy, just the weird bird here who is not happy." Dr. Elashoff agreed completely with this characterization:

> Well, the unhappy ones leave, so it's a self-selection process. The people who stay for the long term are those who aren't unduly upset about the fact that drugs are getting approved that shouldn't be, or that reviews are being influenced either by drug companies or by the FDA management.
>
> The whole . . . environment is such that people who raise concerns about drugs don't get promoted. So you have a whole set of people at the top who probably don't have any morale problems, because they didn't see what they were doing as anything different from what they were supposed to be doing.
>
> The ones who had ethical concerns—there's no reason to stay around in an environment such as that for year after year, when it's really so hard to make a difference. So those people would leave, and the ones who stayed might think this is how the drug approval process is supposed to go.[30]

While agency higher-ups insisted that all was well, internal audits and surveys continued to support Dr. Elashoff's assessment of the agency's climate. Yet despite the efforts of the *Los Angeles Times*, *Frontline*, and others, there seemed to be virtually no public outcry—until the twin scandals of 2004 over antidepressants and Vioxx.

THE STORY OF DR. DAVID GRAHAM

By 2004, Dr. David J. Graham had worked in the FDA's Office of Drug Safety for his entire career, thirty years, and had accumulated what some would consider an admirable record. The Johns Hopkins- and Yale-trained physician had recommended that twelve drugs be taken off the market, and had seen his recommendations accepted by the FDA in ten of the twelve cases. Not, it would seem, the record of a person who repeatedly sees smoke where there is no fire.

But this sort of record did not necessarily sit well with the FDA of the 1990s and 2000s. At least in the early to middle 1990s, the entire Office of Drug Safety appeared to be a beleaguered outpost. Both the Office of Drug Safety and the Office of New Drugs, responsible for approval of new drug applications, jockeyed for attention under the Center for Drug Evaluation and Research (CDER). New money flowed into the CDER in the mid-1990s as part of PDUFA. At first all the new funds went to the Office of New Drugs, and the Office of Drug Safety felt itself languishing, understaffed, trying to keep up with an increasing number of reports of adverse drug reactions as many potentially dangerous drugs zipped into the market in record time. It was only toward the end of the decade that some of the PDUFA funds started to show up in the Office of Drug Safety. Moreover, as we saw with Rezulin, it was increasingly clear to staffers that the top leadership of the agency wanted to hear only good news about new drugs. It became harder to make a case that an already-approved drug might have serious problems or might need to be recalled.[31]

In 2004, Dr. Graham was focusing a good deal of his attention on the COX-2 drugs, especially Vioxx and Bextra. Since, as we saw when we reviewed the CLASS study, experts had for several years been calling attention to the possible risks (as well as the much-less-than-expected benefits) of these drugs, Graham found no shortage of data with which to call into question the safety of this drug family. Of particular concern was the apparently increased risk of heart attacks and similar disorders due to excess blood clotting.

In August, Graham and several of his colleagues were due to report the results of their investigation of Vioxx. They had looked at a database of 1.4 million patients enrolled in Kaiser Permanente health plans, and had come to the conclusion that if all the patients taking Vioxx had been taking Celebrex instead, there might have been twenty-seven thousand fewer heart attacks and sudden cardiac deaths (although as we have seen, Celebrex is not completely without risks).

Superiors at the FDA were not pleased with such a forthright statement. John Jenkins, director of the Office of New Drugs, pointed out that the conclusions of Graham's study seemed rather extreme, given that no new warning labeling was at that time being considered for Vioxx. He and Anne Trontell, an official in the Office of Drug Safety, both at various times suggested ways to tone down the implied criticism of Vioxx (as opposed to saying that if the results were true, then perhaps a label warning was indicated).[32]

On September 30, 2004, Merck voluntarily withdrew Vioxx from the market, after a new study it had funded, intended to show Vioxx's value in preventing colon polyps, instead showed a significant increase in coronary problems among those taking the drug.[33] Graham found himself the focus of a good deal of publicity, as Senator Charles Grassley of Iowa began to hold hearings on why the FDA and the company had been so slow to discover Vioxx's dangers. Graham knew he would be called to testify and that he would have to state that not only had the dangers from Vioxx been visible long before anyone took action, but also other drugs now on the market were equally dangerous.[34]

Graham decided that he might need legal representation in case of further harassment from his superiors or threats of loss of his job. He turned to the Government Accountability Project, a nonprofit group dedicated to protecting whistle blowers, and spoke with an attorney, Tom Devine.

Soon, Devine began to get calls from a different group of whistle blowers. These new callers claimed to be colleagues of Graham's at the FDA. They painted him as a demagogue and a bully, who performed unreliable research and who might be trying to hide his own scientific misconduct by blaming the FDA leadership.

The Government Accountability Project were familiar with what they had come to call the smokescreen syndrome, where those against whom a whistle blower is testifying pretend to be whistle blowers themselves and seek to discredit the first whistle-blower. So Devine methodically went about cross-checking all the accusations. He found that when Graham was asked about apparent scientific discrepancies, he had a plausible answer for all the objections. When his accusers were asked to provide more details or documentation, they came up short.

Based both on the telephone numbers they left and on details from the content of their conversation, Devine became convinced that this second group of so-called whistle blowers were actually Graham's superiors at the FDA. He tracked down some of them by phone number and identified them by name in subsequent phone conversations. They acted surprised, but none denied being who Devine claimed that they were.

Because these people had contacted his program claiming to be whistle blowers, Devine told the *Washington Post* that he could not reveal their names. But, he concluded, "It was all a red herring, and it made me believe Dr. Graham far more."[35]

Beside raising questions about whether some highly placed FDA officials have a bit too much time on their hands, the Graham affair would seem to suggest the culture of a government agency that has moved farther and farther away from its core mission of public trust.[36] The FDA had, it seemed, put up a sign, "Frankie Kelsey Doesn't Work Here Anymore." As 2004 drew to a close, newspaper editorials zeroed in on the FDA's alleged failures and hinted that the time might be ripe for another round of reforms.[37]

By the middle of 2005, critics were charging that the agency had responded to the prior year's criticisms in typical regulatory fashion—by a pendulum swing in the other direction. The FDA had issued twice as many black box warnings, and was taking twice as long to approve new drug applications, compared to a year previously. It had warned physicians and the public that ibuprofen—an anti-inflammatory drug chemically unrelated to the COX-2s, and that had been sold over the counter for decades—might possibly cause heart attacks, based on hardly any relevant clinical evidence. Dr. Jerry Avorn of Harvard commented, "They went from comatose to spastic without any rational period in the middle."[38]

With our review of the FDA, we have come to an end of our analysis of the pharmaceutical industry. We have seen at each step of the way that the actual public record does not square with the benign image that the industry has tried to present in its public-relations efforts. But we must also keep in mind why we started down this road in the first place. It was not solely to judge the industry, but rather to determine the most ethical way that the medical profession could relate to the industry. Since we have now identified a long list of problems in this relationship, it is time to turn our attention to possible solutions.

NOTES

1. T. Lieberman, "Bitter Pill," *Columbia Journalism Review* 2005; 44:45–51, quote pp. 50–51.

2. M. Weintraub, "Long-Term Weight Control Study: Conclusions," *Clin Pharmacol Ther* 1992; 51:642–46. For a general history and overview, see R. B. Devereux, "Appetite Suppressants and Valvular Heart Disease," *N Engl J Med* 1998; 339:765–66.

3. For the story of fen-phen generally, see A. Mundy, *Dispensing with the Truth: The Victims, the Drug Companies, and the Dramatic Story behind the Battle over Fen-phen* (New York: St. Martin's Press, 2001).

4. Mundy, *Dispensing with the Truth*, 42.

5. M. A. Khan, C. A. Herzog, J. V. St. Peter, et al., "The Prevalence of Cardiac Valvular Insufficiency Assessed by Transthoracic Echocardiography in Obese Patients Treated with Appetite-Suppressant Drugs," *N Engl J Med* 1998; 339:713–18.

6. H. M. Connolly, J. L. Crary, M. D. McGoon, et al., "Valvular Heart Disease Associated with Fenfluramine-Phentermine," *N Engl J Med* 1997; 337:581–88.

7. S. J. Milloy, "Tort Lawyers Getting Fat off Fen-phen? Blame the FDA," *Wall Street Journal*, August 10, 1999:A24.

8. One company-sponsored study claimed no excess in heart valve disease among fen-phen users; A. J. Burger, H. B. Sherman, M. J. Charlamb, et al., "Low Prevalence of Valvular Heart Disease in 226 Phentermine-fenfluramine Protocol Subjects Prospectively Followed for Up to 30 Months," *J Am Coll Cardiol* 1999; 34:1153–58. A paid consultant to the company added a supportive editorial; N. B. Schiller, "Fen/Phen and Valvular Heart Disease: If It Sounds Too Bad to Be True, Perhaps It Isn't," *J Am Coll Cardiol* 1999; 34:1159–62. It was later shown that these reassuring data were spurious because not corrected for age; L. A. Moye and A. F. Annegers, "Underestimation of the Valvulopathy Effect of Fenfluramine," *J Am Coll Cardiol* 2000; 36:1434–36.

9. For example, Rep. Tom Lantos (D-CA) called FDA officials to his office on February 13, 1997, to argue that a planned open advisory committee meeting, that might reveal discouraging information about the safety of Redux, ought to be closed to the public; Mundy, *Dispensing with the Truth*, 84.

10. L. Abenhaim, Y. Moride, F. Brenot, et al., "Appetite-Suppressant Drugs and the Risk of Primary Pulmonary Hypertension, International Primary Pulmonary Hypertension Study Group," *N Engl J Med* 1996; 335:609–16.

11. J. E. Manson and G. A. Faich, "Pharmacotherapy for Obesity—Do the Benefits Outweigh the Risks?" *N Engl J Med* 1996; 335:659–60; see also J. E. Manson and G. A. Faich, "Conflicts of Interest—Editorialists Respond," *N Engl J Med* 1996; 335:1064–65.

12. A. Liebman, "Producer's Notebook: Spin Doctors," November 13, 2003: PBS *Frontline*, www.pbs.org/wgbh/pages/frontline/shows/prescription/etc/notebook.html. In depositions, Rich has testified to this under oath, while a Wyeth executive has denied the story.

13. M. A. Friedman, J. Woodcock, M. M. Lumpkin, J. E. Shuren, A. E. Hass, and L. J. Thompson, "The Safety of Newly Approved Medicines: Do Recent Market Removals Mean There Is a Problem?" *JAMA* 1999; 281:1728–34; Mundy, *Dispensing with the Truth*, 246, 370–81.

14. Friedman et al., "Safety of Newly Approved Medicines."

15. On the origins of these drugs, see A. R. Saltiel and J. M. Olefsky, "Thiazolidinediones in the Treatment of Insulin Resistance and Type II Diabetes," *Diabetes* 1996; 45:1661–69.

16. E. A. Gale, "Lessons from the Glitazones: A Story of Drug Development," *Lancet* 2001; 357:1870–75.

17. D. Willman, "Waxman Queries NIH on Researcher's Ties," *Los Angeles Times*, December 9, 1998:A26; S. Krimsky, *Science in the Private Interest: Has the Lure of Profits Corrupted Biomedical Research?* (Lanham, MD: Rowman & Littlefield, 2003), 19–22.

18. Gale, "Lessons from the Glitazones."

19. D. Willman, "The Rise and Fall of the Killer Drug Rezulin," *Los Angeles Times*, June 4, 2000:A1.

20. A later review paper strongly supported Gueriguian's contention that this class of drugs had limited usefulness in diabetes treatment; Gale, "Lessons from the Glitazones."

21. Willman, "Rise and Fall of the Killer Drug Rezulin"; D. Willman, "Risk Was Known as FDA Ok'd Fatal Drug Study," *Los Angeles Times*, March 11, 2001:A1.

22. D. Grady, "After Diabetes Drug, New Questions for the FDA" (3 parts), *New York Times*, March 23, 2000:A23.

23. Krimsky, *Science in the Private Interest*, 20.

24. M. Kauffman and A. Julien, "Industry Cash a Potent Habit; Medical Research: Can We Trust It?" *Hartford Courant*, April 11, 2000:A1.

25. Willman, "Rise and Fall of the Killer Drug Rezulin."

26. J. Abraham, "The Pharmaceutical Industry as a Political Player," *Lancet* 2002; 360:1498–1502.

27. A. J. Wood, "The Safety of New Medicines: The Importance of Asking the Right Question," *JAMA* 1999; 281:1753–54.

28. Friedman et al., "Safety of Newly Approved Medicines."

29. Wood, "Safety of New Medicines."

30. Interview: Michael Elashoff, Ph.D., PBS *Frontline*, February 19, 2003. www.pbs.org/wgbh/pages/frontline/shows/prescription/interviews/elashoff.html (accessed November 19, 2003).

31. J. Rehnquist, "FDA's Review Process for New Drug Applications: A Management Review," Washington, D.C.: Office of the Inspector General, Department of Health and Human Services, Report # OEI-01-01-00590, March, 2003; Interview: Michael Elashoff, Ph.D., PBS *Frontline*; M. Kaufman and B. A. Masters, "FDA Is Flexing Less Muscle," *Washington Post*, November 18, 2004:A1.

32. A. W. Mathews, "FDA Officials Tried to Tone Down Report on Vioxx," *Wall Street Journal*, October 8, 2004:B2. Steven Galson, acting director of the CDER, called these ac-

cusations of interference "baloney" and said that the review of Graham's work was nothing more than the routine scientific give-and-take that was standard practice within the FDA; M. Kaufman, "FDA Official Alleges Pressure to Suppress Vioxx Findings," *Washington Post*, October 8, 2004:A23.

33. E. J. Topol, "Failing the Public Health—Rofecoxib, Merck, and the FDA" [perspective], *N Engl J Med* 2004; 351:1707–9.

34. G. Harris, "Study Says Drug's Dangers Were Apparent Years Ago," *New York Times*, November 5, 2004:C1; A. Berenson, G. Harris, B. Meier, and A. Pollack, "Despite Warnings, Drug Giant Took Long Path to Vioxx Recall," *New York Times*, November 14, 2004: A1; D. Kohn and J. Bor, "Scientist's Warnings on Drugs Stir Debate: Some Doctors Question FDA Officer's Assessment of 5 Popular Prescriptions," *Baltimore Sun*, November 19, 2004:1A.

35. M. Kaufman, "Attempt to Discredit Whistler-Blower Alleged: Group Says His FDA Colleagues Made Calls," *Washington Post*, November 24, 2004:A19. Apparently backing down in the face of this negative publicity, Kaufman reported, the FDA issued a statement that it "acknowledges the right of its employees to raise their concerns to oversight groups" and that the FDA "promotes vigorous debate of the tough scientific questions it confronts every day," while denying any knowledge that any employee had contacted the Government Accountability Project.

36. There is a depressing similarity between these alleged attempts by FDA supervisors to discredit Dr. Graham and the poison-pen letters Dr. Gideon Koren eventually admitted to writing about Dr. Nancy Olivieri in the case at the University of Toronto we examined previously.

37. "An Ailing, Failing FDA," *Los Angeles Times*, November 23, 2004:B10; P. B. Fontanarosa, D. Rennie, and C. D. DeAngelis, "Postmarketing Surveillance—Lack of Vigilance, Lack of Trust," *JAMA* 2004; 292:2647–50; "Food and Drug Administration: Safety or Politics?" *St. Louis Post-Dispatch*, November 18, 2004; G. Harris, "F.D.A.'s Drug Safety System Will Get Outside Review," *New York Times*, November 6, 2004:A11.

38. G. Harris, "F.D.A. Responds to Criticism with New Caution," *New York Times*, August 6, 2005:A1.

III

TOWARD SOLUTIONS

16

SOLUTIONS: THE MANAGEMENT
AND DIVESTMENT STRATEGIES

Twisted together like the snake and the staff, doctors and drug companies have
become entangled in a web of interactions as controversial as they are ubiquitous.

—Ray Moynihan[1]

In the final analysis, it is not a patient's responsibility to protect himself against the
medical profession, it is the profession's responsibility to protect the patient.

—Dr. Jerome Kassirer[2]

We have reviewed the many aspects of the relationship between the medical
profession and the pharmaceutical industry. We have seen that this relationship is
quite complex and involves many different institutions and levels of social organization. If the problems are real and require solution, then specific remedies will
have to be implemented at each level and for each institution. Nevertheless, some
strategies cut across multiple levels, and we can begin by looking at those strategies in general terms.

One conceivable strategy is basically to do nothing. The steady worsening of all
the problems we have reviewed, in the face of at least forty years of efforts to "do
something," would at first glance seem to argue in favor of a strategy of laissez-
faire. I will make the assumption here that a do-nothing strategy cannot be ethically justified in the face of the evidence of the severity of the problems that we
have catalogued.

If laissez-faire is excluded, then two other general strategies seem to offer
themselves.

The Management Strategy

This is the strategy that, in one variant or another, comprises the series of "do-somethings" we have seen over the past four decades. The Management Strategy begins with the premise that, like it or not, the pharmaceutical industry and the medical profession will have to relate in more or less the fashion they have been relating through this time period. It is unrealistic to imagine a *fundamental* shift toward a mutually hands-off approach at any level of organization. Realism therefore requires that we manage the relevant concerns and conflicts of interest, using means appropriate to the specific level and institution in question. If previous efforts at management have failed, this strategy merely advises us to learn from those failures and to fine-tune our future efforts to make them more successful.

The Divestment Strategy

This strategy has never been tried in any comprehensive way, though it has sometimes been advocated, during the historical period that we have reviewed. To borrow the metaphor of some Canadian commentators, the Management Strategy begins with the assumption that one has to dance with the porcupine, and then offers suggestions for how to get stuck with as few quills as possible, or for the most painless way to remove the quills, and so forth.[3] The Divestment Strategy starts with the assumption that we do not have to dance with the porcupine in the first place, period. The medical profession can and should simply disconnect from the pharmaceutical industry at most of the levels that we have identified. There is some variation within the Divestment Strategy on matters such as just what divestment means in various contexts, what occasional exceptions might be allowed due to special circumstances, and whether there are at least some levels where divestment is not an option. (For example, I will argue later that it would be poor social policy to reconfigure the FDA so that it acts in a frankly adversarial way toward the industry.) But overall there will be fewer varieties of the Divestment Strategy than of the Management Strategy, since there are many ways to manage the relationship but only a few ways to divest oneself of it.[4]

Let's see now what support can be given for each of the strategies.

IN FAVOR OF THE MANAGEMENT STRATEGY

As we have already noted, perhaps the most common argument made on behalf of the Management Strategy is the apparent, widely accepted inevitability of some form of intertwined relationship of medicine and industry. The vast majority of practitioners visit regularly with reps, accept their gifts, and dispense their samples. Removing the reps would remove one of their principal sources of information about drugs, however flawed that source might be. The industry currently funds more clinical drug trials than do all other sources of research funds combined. Many journals and medical-professional organizations would go out of business without industry largesse. About half of the funding for continuing medical education would disappear. The consequences of trying to remove all industry influence and money from the world of medicine seem too grim to contemplate.

Nor is the relationship merely a matter of money. A university scientist may discover a medical breakthrough, but the university cannot manufacture the products needed to bring that breakthrough to the bedside of the patient, where a cure can be effected. To bring a product to market, the industry must conduct medical research, and a group of physicians will necessarily be involved in planning and conducting this research. Do we wish for that group to be totally under the thumb and within the sphere of the industry, or is it better that they have at least some ties to the broader medical-academic community? When physicians are about to begin to use a novel medication in practice, who can better advise them of its properties than the firm that has been engaged in research into that drug for as much as a decade or more? In each instance there appears to be a natural, organic overlap of function between profession and industry, and trying to pry them apart would seem to do significant violence to the overall medical enterprise.

Second, there is an apparently compelling ethical reason for a Management Strategy, linked to our identification of the underlying ethical challenge as that of conflict of interest. Any analysis of the notion of conflict of interest includes the proviso that calling a state of affairs a conflict of interest *does not* lead to the conclusion that unethical behavior exists. A conflict of interest is a state of affairs in which the *risk or probability* of unethical behavior is increased, assuming that what we believe to be generally true about human psychology holds. If our goal is to eliminate unethical behavior, then banning all conflicts of interest is a very crude tool, which might rule out a good deal of ethically acceptable behavior, even praiseworthy behavior, in order to reduce any risk of unethical behavior. It is much better to devise strategies to deal with or manage conflicts of interest, through means such as disclosure and transparency, to sort out the truly unethical behavior from that which merely provides an appearance of unethical behavior.

For example, no one argues that every single research study funded by the pharmaceutical industry reaches erroneous conclusions. (There is even the rare, praiseworthy study in which a company-sponsored team publishes results that are directly unfavorable to sales of the company's product.) If one banned the publication of all industry-sponsored research trials, one would eliminate a number of flawed studies like CLASS, but at the same time one would exclude a number of perfectly acceptable and valid research reports. It makes much more sense simply to state the sponsorship of studies clearly in the publication, and allow journal editors and reviewers and the readers to draw their own conclusions on a case-by-case basis.

Another argument to be raised in defense of the Management Strategy places the failure of past management attempts in perspective. In hindsight, there are a number of reasons why previous efforts have failed. One reason is that many older efforts were frankly half-hearted; no one really thought the problem was quite as bad as the would-be reformers made it out to be. A second reason is that the industry was popular enough and powerful enough to undermine or evade most attempts at management. Today and in the near future, neither reason is applicable. We now have an enhanced sense of what is at stake. Recent scandals and exposés have made abundantly clear the dangers of half-hearted attempts. The level of opposition to the industry is similarly at an unprecedented high. It seems that we are entering one of those periods, typified by the elixir sulfonilamide and the thalidomide scandals of old, when the industry is on the defensive and when its critics can pretty much have their way for a while. The recent efforts of the Accreditation Council on Continuing Medical Education to tighten their CME requirements, despite loud industry complaints, is only one case in point. In sum, past failures of the Management Strategy must be laid at the door of the specific measures attempted, not used as evidence for the inadequacy of the strategy itself.

IN FAVOR OF THE DIVESTMENT STRATEGY[5]

To discuss the case to be made for the Divestment Strategy, it's helpful to list some of the levels of social organization at which profession-industry relationships occur. The levels we will investigate specifically here—not an exhaustive list of all the levels we have addressed in previous chapters—are:

- The individual medical student and resident accepts sandwiches and educational materials from reps.
- The practitioner accepts fancy dinners and occasional trips to fancy locations to attend conferences from reps.
- The practitioner accepts free drug samples from reps.
- The academic physician accepts research grants, speaker fees, consulting fees, and perhaps stock options from industry.
- The university president accepts large grants and gifts from industry to support scientific work or specific research departments or centers.

The argument for the Divestment Strategy then proceeds roughly as follows:

1. Analogous psychological processes occur at each of these levels.
2. These psychological processes have important ethical consequences.
3. The processes are mutually reinforcing.
4. At none of the levels is a *financial*-exchange relationship *essential* to medical or social ends.
5. Therefore, a financial divestment strategy is both possible and ethically necessary.

Let's now march through the steps of the argument.

1. Analogous psychological processes occur at each of these levels.

The empirical research, as we have seen, has focused on the individual resident or medical practitioner. (We would hardly expect university presidents to volunteer for a double-blind trial in which they will receive or not receive large grants according to random assignment—or even, for that matter, to fill out and return questionnaire forms.) Nonetheless, it is plausible to generalize some of the psychological processes seen at the individual level to the other levels, and previous chapters have summarized evidence to suggest that this is in fact what happens.

The basic psychological process of interest is *denial that one is compromising one's own value commitments by receiving industry benefits, at the same time that one can clearly see that one's peers are influenced in that fashion.* We have noted repeated studies in which residents and practicing physicians attribute susceptibility to industry influence in prescribing to their peer group to a much larger degree than they admit that they themselves could possibly be influenced. Extending this finding to our various levels, we predict that:

- Individual medical students and residents will take lunches and gifts offered by reps, while imagining that once out in practice, they will prescribe only what is needed for their patients' interests, and will be immune from commercial bias.
- Individual practitioners will accept lavish dinners, trips, and so forth while continuing to believe that they prescribe only what is scientifically valid for their patients and that they are immune from commercial influence.
- Practitioners will also accept free samples, convinced that they only do so because of the needs of their indigent patients, and that samples do not influence their choice of drugs to prescribe.
- Academic physicians will accept research grants, and speaker and consulting fees, believing that their scientific judgment is immune from commercial influence and that they will analyze and report their data in an objective way regardless of who pays.
- University administrators accept large grants and gifts while assuring themselves that their institutions remain staunch in defense of the academic freedom of each faculty member to conduct research and to report the truth regardless of industry interests and pressures.

The closely associated psychological process (though much less studied than denial) is a strong feeling of *entitlement* to whatever benefits are offered by industry. Specifically:

- Medical students and residents feel entitled to their sandwiches and occasional free textbooks because they work hard for long hours and often feel a lack of gratitude and appreciation from both patients and their supervisors.
- Practitioners feel similarly beset by the numerous pressures physicians face in today's complex and busy world. They feel that gifts from industry are only their due, especially when so many of their colleagues seem to accept such gifts without qualm and even line up to demand bigger gifts.
- Practitioners justify samples based on perceived patient demand. If the physician down the street gives samples and I do not, I can expect all my patients to go down the street to see her instead. If some of my samples come home in my pocket for my personal and family use, that is simply one more convenience and entitlement of practice to compensate me for all the sacrifices I make.

- Academic physicians view their university pay as less than what they are truly worth—especially since all of them know some private practitioners who are much less academically accomplished but who make two or three times as much money. Moreover, the competition for research grants is cutthroat, and no one on the climb up the academic ladder can afford to ignore a potential source of grant funding. A grant supports graduate students and research staff and pays dividends to the university.
- If individual faculty discover a cutthroat level of competition in securing grants, the university administration is involved in even more stressful competition in trying to secure multimillion-dollar programmatic support, in a climate where all elected officials are trying to cut taxes and reduce government spending.

Another aspect of the psychological process of denial that we first discussed is that each party at each level can clearly see how the *other parties at other levels* are influenced, and yet feel secure that they personally are not open to similar influence. The same university administrators that are happy to accept large gifts from industry, for instance, may be busy trying to implement stringent conflict-of-interest guidelines to govern their individual faculty relationships with commercial sponsors. (It is relatively rare to see a U.S. university conflict-of-interest policy that even mentions the possibility that the university as a whole, as opposed to individual faculty, might have a conflict of interest.) The same academic physician who freely accepts stock options from a drug company might never allow a member of her family to be seen by a private practitioner if she knew that that practitioner received his drug information mostly from reps rather than from journals. Residents who happily chow down on drug company lunches might be contemptuous of one of their faculty who is always off giving drug-company-sponsored lectures and who lets the company supply him with all his slides and notes.

The extent to which physicians have accommodated themselves to an attitude of denial and entitlement seems all the more evident when we compare medicine with other fields in which a more robust sense of the ethics of conflicts of interest seems to have become ingrained. Reporter Shannon Brownlee was shocked to realize what we have already described at length—that you can no longer trust what is published in medical journals. She reflected on the issue from her perspective as a journalist:

> Here's a little thought experiment. Imagine that a medical journalist—me, for instance—makes a tidy sum writing press releases for, say Pfizer, the manufacturer of Viagra. I don't make a fortune, maybe just enough to cover a year's tuition for my son's private high school. And let's say for the sake of argument that I also buy a few dozen Pfizer shares. Then I turn around and write a story for *The New York Times* about several new drugs for treating erectile dysfunction.
>
> What would you think, dear reader, should my financial relationship with the pharmaceutical company that makes one of the drugs featured in my story come to light? Would you have reason to doubt its objectivity and accuracy? Of course you would. Not only that, I would be ashamed to show my face in any newsroom, and I would not be writing for the *Times* again. I'm not trying to claim that journalists are paragons of

virtue, but we have no illusions about our ability to withstand temptation and avoid shading what we say when faced with a wad of cash.[6]

Brownlee contrasts these journalist's reactions with the medical perspective:

"Lots of eminent people took great offense at being accused of being influenced," [Dr. Arnold] Relman told me recently. "'What an insulting thing to say. I value my reputation; doctors and scientists know best. Trust us.' I spent the first 25 years of my career doing clinical research and being one of them, and I know the feeling." As Harvey Lodish, professor of biology at MIT, huffed to *Technology Review* in 1984, when Relman first required disclosure at the [*New England*] *Journal* [*of Medicine*], "Scientists have all kinds of private consulting arrangements with biotechnology companies and many own stocks in these companies, but that's nobody's business. It has nothing to do with the quality of their research."[7]

Brownlee added an anecdote about a journalist friend whose former girlfriend was a neurosurgeon. She received an unsolicited check for several hundred dollars from a drug rep. It seems she had given a lecture and had made favorable mention of one of the company's drugs, and the company wanted to show appreciation. "When my friend told her she could not in good conscience cash the check—that it was a conflict of interest—she looked at him, he said, as if he were speaking in some unintelligible language."[8]

Brownlee did not explain exactly what, if anything, this had to do with the fact that the neurosurgeon was a former and not a current girlfriend of the journalist. But it does drive home the point that calling for a Divestment Strategy for medicine could be construed merely as calling physicians to rise up to the ethical level of journalists—or at least to come up equal with journalists in the lack-of-denial department.[9]

2. These psychological processes have important ethical consequences.

Some psychological states have few or no ethical implications. If I violate a person's basic human rights, it does not matter whether that person is angry at me or not when I come to assess the ethical meaning of my actions. Other psychological facts, however, have much greater ethical significance. This would be especially true when one is proposing rational guidelines to resolve a problem, and the psychological data point strongly to an essentially irrational thought process that creates and perpetuates the problem.

Philosopher Sissela Bok, in a classic work on the ethical implications of lying, based an important part of her argument on a psychological analysis. She argued that human history, as well as specific psychological research studies, shows a consistent pattern—how people start to think when they contemplate solving a particular dilemma by telling a lie. Unconsciously they begin to imagine that their own motives are purely altruistic, that the consequences of lying will be minimal and easily contained, and that there is no other way to resolve the problem that does not involve deception. If they could, at the outset, have adopted the psychological perspective of the *person being lied to* rather than the person telling the lie, they would, by contrast, have realized that the lie is basically self-serving; that the lie will have profound ripple effects that will go on plaguing the teller for a long time; and that there were several alternative, candid approaches to the problem that could have avoided all the consequences created by the lie. Bok claimed that whatever ethical rules we develop to deal with lying have to take into account the pervasive nature of this psychological process.[10]

Similarly, the argument for the Divestment Strategy claims that we now have ample evidence that whenever we assume that the profession-industry relationship can be adequately "managed," we have failed to take into account the irrational forces at work. We have failed to appreciate that physicians and other players who are in the throes of denial and the associated sense of entitlement are not going to apply, or to understand the need for, various guidelines designed to manage this relationship. They will see the guidelines as intended for others and not *really* for themselves. In the face of this pervasive denial and sense of irrational entitlement, the only rules that will have any force at all are rules that shake us by the scruff of the neck and force us to look squarely in the cold light of dawn at what we have systematically avoided seeing.

The argument for the Divestment Strategy could be framed at an even deeper and more radical level—*the Management Strategy itself, and the arguments (read: rationalizations) that support it, are nothing but a part of this pervasive psychology of denial and entitlement.*

3. The processes are mutually reinforcing.

We might next look over our list of organizational levels and ask whether ethical reform at one level would be effective if activities at the other levels did not change. There are two answers to that question. First, reform at one level would leave serious social problems in place at other levels. Just to mention one example, it is a serious problem that practitioners rely on biased sources of information when selecting drugs to treat patients. We could imagine a system in which all practitioners refuse to visit with drug reps, and all academic medical centers have evidence-based medicine units that keep practitioners in their region continuously supplied with updated hand-held computer programs, easily accessed in a minute or two during a busy day of seeing patients, that are based on syntheses of the best available randomized controlled studies. If the randomized studies themselves are hopelessly contaminated by commercial bias—if, for instance, four negative studies have been suppressed and only the single positive study has been published—then we have hardly arrived at the point where we wish to be.[11]

The second answer to this question is that, while we here again go beyond the published empirical literature, it is plausible to see activities at each level of organization and the psychological habits exemplified at each level feeding off of the activities and attitudes at the other levels. The academic physician at the university feeling entitled to stock options and consulting fees from the industry did not spring fully formed from the brain of Zeus. She first was a medical student, then was a resident, and all that time had regular encounters with practitioners who eagerly lapped up rep-supplied goodies, even if she never herself worked in a practice setting before entering academic research. It seems unlikely that that earlier accul-turation process did not influence her present system of beliefs and her ethical code. University administrators commonly begin their careers as research scientists; and indeed those who choose academic administration over science may be precisely those who find that they enjoy working at the interface with outside agencies and industry more than they enjoy the day-to-day grunt work in the lab. So it appears unlikely that one set of players will suddenly sprout ideally ethical behavior unless something changes at all different levels of organization. A fully developed ethical solution will have to take into account the linkages among the levels and not merely the multiplicity of levels.

4. At none of the levels is a *financial*-exchange relationship *essential* to medical or social ends.

This provides further indication of how deeply the denial-entitlement mentality has become ingrained. We imagine that just because *some sort of contact* must be made between the profession and industry at each level, in order for patients to be treated with up-to-date, effective drugs, that it is equally inevitable that *financial benefits* must be exchanged at each level. Let's instead take a step back and ask whether we could not imagine divestment occurring at each level of organization—without necessarily arguing that this would be either easy or cheap:

- Medical students and residents need have no contact whatsoever with the industry. They can afford to buy their own lunch; or medical schools and hospitals could afford to buy them occasional free lunches to show appreciation for their hard work. Medical schools and hospitals could also supply them with all the education that they require.
- Even if practitioners felt the need to accept information from reps about new drug products, there is no need whatsoever for them to accept branded re-minder items, much less lavish dinners and gifts of higher value. Certainly physicians are paid well enough in our society so as not to *need* free gifts of this nature.
- Various programs could be created to ensure that indigent patients receive basic, necessary drugs. The industry has already commendably taken action to ensure that its charitable drug giveaways are more user-friendly for physicians' staff.[12] Some form of universal access to health coverage including prescription drugs would be the ideal way from a standpoint of social justice to end the only legitimate social need that free samples fill. Even without national reform, programs to supply indigent patients with the most appropriate as well as cheapest generic drugs for most common illnesses would be relatively inexpensive to launch, and would lead to more appropriate later pre-scribing than commonly occurs when patients are started on samples.[13]
- Society could presumably decide that the inability to trust what is published in medical journals due to commercial sponsorship of research is a sufficiently serious problem, that our tax-cutting fervor must be tempered in favor of in-creasing public support for academic medical centers and the research they

conduct. In the process, we could fund many more so-called head-to-head drug trials that truly inform practitioners, rather than studies designed solely for marketing purposes without concern for the practical clinical questions that need to be answered.[14]

Arthur Schafer, a professor of philosophy at the University of Manitoba, has been particularly helpful in demonstrating that the undoubted need to translate new research findings into commercially available products need not imply a corresponding need for money to change hands during the process. But the price, in an era in which the U.S. Congress and the American public have apparently never seen a tax cut that they didn't like, could be high: "If the community values public science in the public interest then it will have to be paid for by public tax dollars."[15] The cost would be that of setting up firewalls. Industry could still pay for the lion's share of the research they now pay for. And universities and their scientists could still get generous grants to do their research on pharmaceuticals. The trick would be to create a public entity that would collect money from industry on one hand, and disburse funds to academia on the other, while in the meantime cutting all the strings that now produce the conflicts of interest. When we consider regulatory solutions in a later chapter, we will explore this proposal in more detail.

The firewall proposal takes very seriously the argument that universities may discover exciting new things but cannot deliver any products to the bedside of a sick patient. There must be an ongoing partnership between academia and industry to ensure that new discoveries in the laboratory are brought quickly into public use. But academia and industry do not have to be in financial bed with each other for this to happen. Indeed, the process can work much better, in the public interest, when they are not in bed with each other.

5. Therefore, a financial divestment strategy is both possible and ethically necessary.

In sum, the argument that various forms of contact must persist between the medical profession and the pharmaceutical industry need not imply a corresponding argument that *financial* conflicts of interest are inevitable and therefore must be managed as best as possible. And the observations about the deep-seated nature of the denial-entitlement psychology in medicine supports the conclusion that the usual means of trying to manage financial conflicts of interest will predictably work very poorly in this setting.

We have seen in our historical surveys how a medical culture of entanglement with the interests of the pharmaceutical industry has grown up gradually, and in some cases imperceptibly, over more than a half century. In hindsight we can see that the popularity of the Management Strategy, and the arguments raised in its favor, are really a part of that culture. But the totality of that culture and its implications for both medicine and society dictate in the end that the Management Strategy is inadequate.

I will, therefore, devote the rest of the discussion of solutions primarily to the task of assessing what the Divestment Strategy would require of us at each level of organization, and how one might practically move from where we are now to where we wish to go. For completeness, I will continue to list and assess arguments that favor more of a Management Strategy. I will do so for several reasons. Some readers will be unconvinced by the arguments I have just reviewed, and so will be loath to abandon the Management Strategy completely. Also, as we said initially, there may be exceptional nooks and crannies in the overall relationship between medicine and industry where for specific reasons the Divestment Strategy will not work, and only some version of the Management Strategy will bring needed reform. Finally, I wish to be as thorough as possible in assessing the existing literature that proposes possible solutions.

The solutions we must consider fall under two major headings. First, physicians must have a reawakened sense of our own professionalism. We must learn to see that having our fingers in the pockets of industry does not lead to the sort of professional behavior that our patients and the general public will or ought to find trustworthy.[16] Our professional associations should set examples of divestment rather than entanglement as individual physicians try to reset their moral compasses. We must also, in the end, reexamine the ethics of ostracism, when we address how to treat our fellow physicians and academic scientists who are slow to forgo the benefits of industry gifts.

Next, we must address those activities that fall outside the purview of professional behavior and that require specific legislative or regulatory actions before reform can be instituted. Ideally we should anticipate a synergy between the intraprofessional and the regulatory aspects of reform.

NOTES

1. R. Moynihan, "Who Pays for the Pizza? Redefining the Relationships between Doctors and Drug Companies, 1: Entanglement," *BMJ* 2003; 326:1189–92.

2. J. P. Kassirer, *On the Take: How Medicine's Complicity with Big Business Can Endanger Your Health* (New York: Oxford University Press, 2005), 153.

3. S. Lewis, P. Baird, R. G. Evans, et al., "Dancing with the Porcupine: Rules for Governing the University-Industry Relationship," *CMAJ* 2001; 165:783–85.

4. On these general points I have benefited from discussions with Jerome R. Hoffman.

5. Here I largely follow Arthur Schafer, a philosopher at the University of Manitoba, who has published one of the most thorough and thoughtful defenses of the Divestment Strategy; A. Schafer, "Biomedical Conflicts of Interest: A Defence of the Sequestration Thesis—Learning from the Cases of Nancy Olivieri and David Healy," *J Med Ethics* 2004; 30:8–24. Schafer is primarily concerned to urge divestment at the level of the academic medical center refusing to accept industry grants and gifts. In the process of arguing his case, however, he indicates reasons to think that the Divestment Strategy is pertinent at other levels as well. Indeed, it is precisely because of the interconnections among the levels that he depicts, that the Divestment Strategy is essential at multiple levels at once.

6. S. Brownlee, "Doctors without Borders: Why You Can't Trust Medical Journals Anymore," *Washington Monthly* April, 2004, 38–43, quote p. 43.

7. Brownlee, "Doctors without Borders," 42.

8. Brownlee, "Doctors without Borders," 42.

9. "It should be mentioned that bioethicists—who are latecomers to the drug industry gravy train—seem equally confident that their judgment is not prejudicially affected by the acceptance of money and other benefits from industry." Schafer, "Biomedical Conflicts of Interest," 20.

10. S. Bok, *Lying: Moral Choice in Public and Private Life* (New York: Pantheon, 1978), 17–31.

11. B. A. Masters, "N.Y. Sues Paxil Maker over Studies on Children," *Washington Post*, June 2, 2004:E1.

12. B. Taylor, "Giveaway Drugs: Good Intentions, Bad Design," *Health Aff (Millwood)* 2004; 23:213–17; "Record Number of Patients Receive Assistance from America's Pharmaceutical Companies," PhRMA, February 22, 2005, www.phrma.org/mediaroom/press/releases/22.02.2005.1129.cfm (accessed March 12, 2005).

13. S. Erickson and S. Cullison, "Closing the Sample Closet: How Well Could You Get Along without Medication Samples—and without Drug Reps?" *Family Practice Management* 1995 (October): 43–47. A commercial firm, MedVantx, has reportedly been able to secure funding from insurers to place generic sample cupboards, along with patient and physician educational material, in physicians' offices, based on the savings to the insurance plans when patients are begun on more rational, generic medications at the outset; www.medvantx.com (accessed March 12, 2005).

14. R. Pear, "Congress Weighs Drug Comparisons," *New York Times*, August 24, 2003:18; "Comparing Prescription Drugs" [editorial], *New York Times*, August 27, 2003:A20; "Let Drugs Duke It Out" [editorial], *Los Angeles Times*, September 7, 2003:4; U. E. Reinhardt, "An Information Infrastructure for the Pharmaceutical Market," *Health Aff (Millwood)* 2004; 23:107–12.

15. Schafer, "Biomedical Conflicts of Interest," 23.

16. J. Andre, "Learning to See: Moral Growth during Medical School," *J Med Ethics* 1992; 18:148–52.

17

SOLUTIONS REQUIRING ENHANCED PROFESSIONALISM IN MEDICINE

It is clear that our efforts to establish a scientific basis for this treatment of childhood depression are severely compromised by both unpublished research and uncritical acceptance of published data. It is disturbing to note that there has been no formal response to this crisis from opinion leaders in child psychiatry, many of whom were investigators in both published and unpublished trials.

—Dr. E. Jane Garland[1]

Is Academic Medicine for Sale? [title of editorial in *New England Journal of Medicine*]

—Dr. Marcia Angell[2]

No. The current owner is very happy with it.

—Dr. Thomas J. Ruane[3]

Medicine's Divestment Strategy toward the pharmaceutical industry will require both a heightened sense of professional responsibility, and changes in administrative regulation. In this chapter I will discuss the professional side of this strategy.[4]

Professional responsibility is important in the strategy for two reasons, one dealing with consequences, the other with principles. First, it is difficult if not impossible for regulators to correct the problems if the physicians themselves are not motivated to do so. Bureaucrats cannot police what drug reps say to physicians, one on one, in the physicians' offices. It is much more difficult to detect falsification or spin of research results to suit a company's commercial interests, than for the scientists conducting the research to avoid spin and falsification in the first place.

Second, no group can call itself a *profession* if it does not espouse a moral code, and instead relies totally on external policing to correct misbehavior among its members. Adopting a moral stance toward its own responsibilities to clients and to the public, and insisting that its members place dedication to that moral code ahead of personal gain, is one of the characteristics that ought to define a profession in modern society.[5]

I will address two places where professionalism is most often called into question—the practicing physician's relationship with drug reps, and the physician-investigator's relationship with industry sponsors of research. I will then briefly discuss professionalism in the behavior of medical societies.

PHYSICIANS AND DRUG REPS: JUST SAY NO

A Divestment Strategy would require that physicians refuse to have interactions with drug reps, except for some unusual exceptions. In the language of the activist website "No Free Lunch," the response to any offer from drug reps of gifts, samples, or information is "Just Say No."[6]

The first step in defending such a strategy as an ethical position is to show that nothing of value to patient care, or to any other of the physician's professional responsibilities, is lost as a result of "Just Say No." This case seems hard to argue to the average practitioner, since relying on reps for many things has become so commonplace for so long that it is simply never questioned. There seems no realistic possibility that the world could turn on its axis in any other fashion. But despite the common wisdom, the case seems very strong.

Information

The standard defense of interacting with reps, even before Charles May wrote his critique in 1961, is "education." It seems obvious that patients want their physicians to prescribe the most up-to-date drugs. It also seems obvious that when a drug is first introduced, the company that has manufactured it and has shepherded it through the complex FDA approval process has more information at its disposal about the drug than anyone else. It therefore seems evident that only by interacting with reps or other industry spokespersons can the physician stay up to date and prescribe what the patient most needs. True, the well-educated physician should never rely only on reps; she should use many other sources of information as well. Those other information sources ensure that she will never be misled by any commercially biased information from the industry.

We have seen that this standard defense made some sense in the 1940s and 1950s, when academic and organized medicine largely abandoned its responsibility for the continuing education of the practitioner in pharmaceutical matters. Does this defense make any sense today? Even by 1961, May was able to point to *The Medical Letter* as a cheap, easy-to-read, and quite up-to-date source of information on the newest drugs that was free of commercial bias. *The Medical Letter* is still published today, and is still useful. Recently it has been joined by a number of other information technologies that were unavailable in the mid-twentieth century. However belatedly, academic medicine has begun to realize that articles in medical journals are simply not a usable source of information for busy practitioners in the field. New forms of evidence-based synthesis are being produced both in print and electronically, one popular modality being downloads for the physician's personal digital assistant (PDA).[7] These summaries of evidence are produced by organizations that do not rely on any pharmaceutical industry funding.[8] There are now so many ways for the physician to get unbiased information that the drug rep no longer fulfills any *essential* function.

What of the stipulation that the physician should never rely only on the rep but should use other sources? Does this not suggest that the best way to stay informed is to *add* these evidence-based tools to rep visits, rather than to abolish the rep visits? The literature we have reviewed suggests two replies. First, however much the "ideal" physician uses other sources to amplify what the reps tell him, far too many physicians take the easy way out and come to rely on the reps as their *chief* source of drug information. Other sources of information don't give out nice gifts, and other sources of information don't show up at the door in person. Once again, the notion that the average physician can be relied upon to "manage" the relationship with industry, so that total divestment is too harsh a remedy, turns out to be largely a self-serving rationalization.

Second, research has shown that physicians tend to be poor screeners of commercial information. When biased and scientifically accurate information are both presented, individual clinicians often cannot discern which is which. This is especially true when the industry has at its beck and call the most expensive and most talented advertising firms and consultants, eager to help them find the most seductive way to transmit any information they wish. So merely adding better information is no guarantee that physicians will ignore the misinformation that reps might promulgate.

Another flawed assumption feeds physicians' reliance on reps as "educators"— the very American view that the *best* physicians always prescribe the *latest* drugs. This may have often been true in the 1950s, and is still occasionally true today. An AIDS specialist who was too slow in adopting protease inhibitors when that class of drugs first appeared would have had dead patients on her conscience. The "latest equals best" equation, however, is true far less often than many believe.

We have seen that most of the "new" drugs introduced by the industry fall into either the "me-too" or the "evergreen" category, and do not constitute significant therapeutic advances over existing drugs. In the average year, unbiased U.S. observers would judge that only one or two new drugs fall into the "advance" category. And a certain number of these undeniable advances affect only a narrow slice of physicians and patients, being perhaps good only for one particular disease and being appropriately prescribed only by one specialty group (for example, a new drug for severe psoriasis which in all likelihood would be used primarily by dermatologists). The average physician does not need a rep coming to her door weekly to be sure that she does not miss a major new drug breakthrough.

The complementary reason why latest is not always best is the relatively small number of patients that must be included in therapeutic trials before gaining FDA approval. (This assumes that the company discloses to the medical community all the risks and adverse effects, which we have seen all too often does not occur.) Proverbial wisdom states that the prime time for discovering a side effect of a drug is about two years after its introduction into the market, based on how many patients need to be taking a drug before a relatively unusual but still serious side effect makes itself known. Our recent experience with the COX-2 drugs tends to confirm this rule of thumb. It could be argued that any physician who prescribes a drug that has been less than two or three years on the market is playing a roulette game. The roulette game may be worth the stakes if the drug is the only one that can give this patient an important health benefit. It is hardly worth the risk if the drug is the twentieth new drug on the market for diabetes or the fortieth for hypertension.

Samples

Beside the information provided by reps, the next "disinterested" reason physicians commonly give for maintaining contact is the desire to have free samples, especially to help one's indigent patients. As we saw previously, patients have bought into this rationale; they judge this sort of gift from drug reps much more acceptable than anything else the physician might receive.[9]

The "sample" rationale can be peeled away a bit at a time. First, we should note frankly what the presumed problem is—indigent patients who cannot afford to buy drugs and who have no insurance coverage with prescription benefits. We might next ask whether providing free samples left by reps—so that the samples made available depend on the discretion of the rep rather than the needs of the patients—is a lasting and appropriate solution to that problem. Instead, as virtually everyone now agrees, the United States needs some system of guaranteeing access to a decent set of health care services—prescription drugs included—to all citizens. There are deep divisions about how to accomplish this, whether by a single-payer government-administered system, by some form of free market system, or some combination of both. But that it should be done in some way or other is becoming harder and harder to deny. The pharmaceutical industry strongly favors such a system, as long as it would provide every American with generous drug benefits, and avoid any centralization of buying power that would force the industry to lower prices.

Reform of the entire system will not happen soon, and indigent patients need medications today. But it is at least worth noting that the full sample cupboard might tempt many physicians, who otherwise could be lobbying on behalf of universal access, to avoid the hard work of advocating basic systems change.

Next, we might ask whether, in the absence of a reformed health care system, samples are the only way to secure drugs for the indigent. The answer, again, is no. The majority of drug companies offer charitable programs that will supply a patient who meets their criteria for need with a three-month supply of many medications. Not all medications are available in this way; and until recently the programs were extremely cumbersome. Clinics with a heavy load of indigent care reported keeping several volunteer staff members busy full time, just tracking down and filling out all the different forms.[10] Fortunately, PhRMA, in a genuinely helpful and public-spirited move, announced in 2004 that it would centralize and coordinate the charity programs and make it much easier for physicians and patients to track down and apply for the benefits.[11] So ironically, even the industry itself has made it easier for physicians to use the charitable drug giveaway programs and therefore not to have to rely on samples.

The next stage in peeling away the rationale is to ask where samples actually go. Data are limited, but studies strongly suggest that the minority of sample drugs end up serving the needy. Instead it seems that at least a third of the samples end up as gifts to the clinic's staff and their families, taken home before any patients can get to them.[12] Many other samples are used as convenience items for patients who are well able to afford medication, to save a trip to the pharmacy over the weekend, or to try several different drugs to see which has the fewest side effects before writing a long-term prescription.

This point suggests a possible exception to my negative judgment of a physician who regularly sees drug reps just to get free samples. I have met a few physicians who serve a particularly high number of indigents, and who work in specialties where a small number of very expensive drugs are used commonly. They claim to have found that the only way they can serve the needs of these patients is to rely upon a steady flow of samples from reps, and they basically have to welcome the reps as allies and friends in order to ensure an adequate flow of samples. As we saw in our account of the typical drug rep, "Stan," a rep can get away with supplying a large number of expensive samples to a few offices, as long as his territory includes many better-off neighborhoods to balance things out. The reps themselves, not surprisingly, often enjoy playing Santa Claus to these few, needy offices. A physician who works long hours and probably foregoes a comfortable income to serve these patients is not one that I am about to attack as unprofessional just because he makes extensive use of samples.

Unfortunately for these few physicians, if the reforms in professional behavior that I am calling for come to pass, the majority of physicians will refuse to see reps at all and refuse also to accept any samples. That means that the only offices left asking for samples will be these few that serve primarily the indigent population—the least desirable market for the firm. It is then most unlikely that the companies would continue to supply free samples as a marketing tool. (We would hope that they would continue their charitable programs, which are presumably funded by a different pool of company money.) So if the rest of medicine got its ethical act together, these few physicians who serve primarily the poor would have to make other arrangements to get needed medications for their patients—unless we managed to move toward wider system reform quickly.

To peel away the rationale further, we must ask how much free samples contribute to the health of the poor patients who rely on them. Again evidence is limited, but at least one study showed that patients with hypertension treated by means of samples had poorer control of their hypertension than those treated by prescription.[13] It has been noted in other studies that physicians who rely on samples to treat a patient commonly find themselves giving out a medication that they regard as less than ideal or even less than rational.[14] Inertia being what it is, when the patient who had originally had samples comes to be treated later with a prescription, it is easy merely to continue the same irrational drug than to try to switch the patient over to the more rational choice.

The rejoinder, of course, is that a less rational choice of drug may still be far better than no drug at all. And this appears to be true in many cases. This leads then to the next item in our list of arguments against the common rationale.

Finally, the question may be asked: if one's goal is both to practice good quality medicine and also to have free drugs available for one's neediest patients, have we really explored all alternatives before deciding that samples are the superior strategy? The following story shows what happened when one group of physicians decided, along with Harry and Louise in the TV ads, that "there had to be a better way."

A Drug Sample Story

Dr. Sam Cullison wrote this story for the magazine *Family Practice Management* in 1995. He practiced in a twelve-physician group in a rural area in Washington State. It simplified a part of their story that there was one large pharmacy that served their community, and virtually all their patients went to that pharmacy, which was conveniently located next door to the medical clinic.

The group got together and discussed a set of interconnected problems. Drug reps showed up at odd hours wanting some of their time to present them with questionable or biased information. They would rather have had reliable, commercially unbiased information but were unsure where to get it. They used the samples left by the reps for their needy patients, but often ended up giving out an expensive drug that was not what they would have preferred. The patients were often upset when the samples ran out and they had to pay for the medication. Nothing seemed to be working to their benefit or that of their patients. (Fortunately, this group of physicians apparently was not much impressed by whatever gifts these reps gave out.)

They turned to the local pharmacists for advice and eventually came up with a solution. One of the pharmacists, Steven H. Erickson, coauthored the article with Dr. Cullison.

The office closed its sample closet and refused to see any more drug reps. Once a month, one of the pharmacists came over during the lunch hour and presented the entire staff with a drug treatment update, drawn from pharmacy data sources and independent of any commercial bias. They discussed the pros and cons of any new drug just on the market.

The pharmacy then stocked its own closet with a variety of the most commonly prescribed generic drugs for the most common medical problems. Since they selected the cheapest generics instead of the most expensive new brand-name products, the out-of-pocket cost of the stock in this closet was minimal. If the physicians wanted a patient to have a drug out of this closet, they simply marked it on the script and sent the patient with the prescription to the pharmacy.

For this service the pharmacy charged each physician in the group $100 per year. The group was happy to pay this sum as an ideal solution to their set of problems, as a way to stay educated, and as a service to their indigent patients.[15]

Let's update this story a bit. Given inflation, the charge today would probably be more like $300 annually. It might also be more because when the article was written, some of the most expensive new classes of drugs, notably the statins for cholesterol and the proton-pump inhibitors for acid reflux and ulcers, were only just coming into widespread use. Today it would cost that much more to stock the sample closet with the most widely used medications that the majority of the indigent patients need, because no generic equivalents are as yet available for many of these drugs. Despite all that, I would argue that the average physician can still easily afford a $300 or $400 annual payment in exchange for both high-quality education and better services for her needy patients.

The skeptic can immediately point out many ways in which this model would not work in the skeptic's own community. Perhaps there are many small, competing pharmacies rather than one big one. Such arguments show that the skeptic has missed the anecdote's take-home message: once a group of physicians found themselves sufficiently motivated to seek a solution that did not involve seeing reps and accepting samples, they rather quickly hit upon a workable program. They did not need a big federal grant, or a bevy of outside consultants, or a detailed needs assessment. They just needed motivation and a little creativity. There are probably many more solutions that would work in different settings.[16] The skeptic's objections merely show how paralyzing to thought the medical status quo can be.

Gifts

The last reason to see reps is to collect their gifts. As we have seen, these run the gamut, both in nature and in value. We are led to believe that these have greatly declined, at least at the high-value end, since PhRMA put into place its new code of ethics in 2002.[17] At the time that I write this there are no clear data on whether the code of ethics has made any practical difference. Anecdotal reports from "Stan" and others suggest that the code did not diminish the number and value of gifts so much as change their type—fewer golf outings, more lavish dinners. I remain to be convinced that anything has changed much.

It is also probably a mistake to focus on the most expensive or the most outrageous gifts. The less expensive gifts may be a greater threat to medical professionalism, for two reasons.[18] First, the gift-giving act relies on a bit of human psychology that was programmed into our brains at a preconscious stage, and that few of us are able consciously to resist—a person who gives us a gift is owed our gratitude, and we owe that person in return a suitable display of our gratitude. The mere fact that the industry has never tried in any serious way since the 1940s to send out a bevy of reps *without* armloads of freebies speaks to the central role that the industry assumes that gifts occupy in cementing the physician-rep relationship.[19] Similarly, the relative disregard "Stan" encountered among his superiors for exactly how much he was spending on gifts to physicians in his region testifies that the companies believe that almost any sum spent on gifts is a worthwhile investment.

Second, our analysis of the development of the physician-rep relationship as the physician progresses from medical student to resident to practitioner highlights how, at the earliest stages, the cheaper gifts are the ones that most influence the progress of the interaction. The more expensive gifts are likely to set off ethical alarm bells; the least expensive gifts are unlikely to arouse any sort of ethical scrutiny, or indeed any thoughtful reflection of any sort. The basic relationship between rep and physician is built on the innumerable small gifts that are passed along day by day, and not on the occasional large gift. If I treated my wife badly on a day-to-day basis in all the little things that make up a marriage, and tried to compensate by buying her something really splendid for her birthday, it is unlikely that our relationship would be a strong one.

So a Divestment Strategy requires no gifts of any sort, rather than merely no expensive gifts. Since gifts are by definition the least patient-centered of all the things drug reps provide, physicians should not *need* any of the gifts. As beleaguered as physicians might feel themselves to be, and indeed as underpaid as residents might feel themselves to be, one cannot argue on any objective grounds that physicians cannot afford to buy their own lunches or notepads or reflex hammers.

Instead of employing the stock rationalizations that physicians have been prone to use (and that the industry is happy to supply and reinforce), it is worth asking for the *real* reasons why physicians would feel unfairly deprived if they were made to stop accepting the gifts from reps. I think those answers were well identified by the Dichter study back in 1955. What the physician would most lose, if reps and their gifts disappeared suddenly, is the basic sense that somebody cares about and appreciates them. Patients are more prone to whine about their symptoms than express overt appreciation for the physician's care, and certainly today the physician cannot expect much of a display of affection from insurance companies, hospital executives, and malpractice attorneys.[20] The rep is often the friendliest face one sees all day, and the giving of gifts is one manifestation of that friendliness.

The medical profession should be concerned that so many of its members are so susceptible to the blandishments of the reps. It seems that a form of demoralization is quite widespread within medicine. Physicians who feel that demoralized are hardly likely to perform at the highest possible level on behalf of their patients, and are certainly not a good advertisement for the best and brightest of today's college students to seek out a career in medicine. Instead of abandoning this field to the pharmaceutical industry, the profession should look at itself and ask what more it should be doing to secure the psychological well-being of all of its members.

Counter-detailing, or academic detailing, has been proposed as the profession's best answer to the rep problem. Use the same sales techniques that reps employ so effectively, but do so to send out a message that is scientific and evidence-based, rather than a message that sells a particular drug.[21] At one level, if the Divestment Strategy takes hold, there will be no need for counter-detailing. Physicians will stop seeing reps and hearing the wrong message, so there is nothing left to counter.

At another level, however, the need for the right sort of academic detailing will only become more acute if the reps disappear and the psychological needs of the physicians are now unmet. For example, a medical school might send a representative to visit briefly with each of its graduates each month or so. Ask how the graduate is getting along, what practice is like, how she is handling the stresses and strains. Briefly mention new developments back at the campus. Pass along a handy reminder item, with the school's logo, that embodies a clinical tip based on the best recent evidence. What clinical problems is the practitioner seeing that would make a good topic for a future visit? What problems does the practitioner face that should be more intensively investigated by the research teams back at the medical school? Perhaps the academic detail reps could be today's medical students; they might as part of their course work do the research on the clinical tips and design the reminder items. Having a friendly visit and a genuinely concerned inquiry from a future physician at one's alma mater could easily become the high point of the practitioner's day.[22]

Going back down the developmental ladder, why should not a hospital that employs residents commit itself to providing a nice catered lunch once a week, of the sort now provided routinely by reps? What would the cost of this be, compared to the tangible display of gratitude for the labors provided by these young doctors working long hours? Why rely on commercial sources to do something that a healthy, vibrant profession might better do on its own?

Gifts to physicians from drug reps challenge professional integrity by creating a conflict of interest (or rather duty), in which physicians are tempted to put their own interest in receiving gifts and their own sense of gratitude to the giver ahead of the medical needs of their patients. So gifts to physicians from industry should be eliminated, as part of our Divestment Strategy. But the psychological vulnerabilities that have traditionally made physicians such ready recipients of gifts—to be blunt, that have made us so much putty in the industry's hands—are worth studying for their own sake. And it might turn out that a truly compassionate and humane profession could do a lot more than it does today to address these psychological vulnerabilities. Getting the industry out of the way would allow the right people to take this over, if all of us within the profession are willing to expend the resources of time and money.

PHYSICIAN-INVESTIGATORS AND THE ETHICAL IMPORTANCE OF OSTRACISM

We saw in the last chapter that the benefits of collaboration between academia and industry could in theory be maintained, while cutting all financial ties between academic institutions and individual investigators on the one hand, and drug companies on the other. With the right sort of institutional reform (to be discussed in the next chapter), most physician-investigators who are now the captives of industry would be set free, and would be able to do good science and report the results truthfully.

But we would not expect the system that has been so pervasive for so long to die overnight. Many investigators have become used to the additional perks provided by industry—consultant contracts, speaker fees, first-class travel, and stock options. These could not be prohibited by academic regulations, in many cases, without inappropriate curtailment of academic freedom. One cannot, for example, prohibit a university physician from giving a speech in which she praises a certain drug.

The Management Strategy tries to handle all such problems by disclosure of payments over a certain sum. Disclosure requires voluntary compliance; few institutions can snoop on their faculty and detect any but the most egregious reporting violations. The Divestment Strategy says that one should put an end to these contacts. This too would require voluntary compliance. The Divestment Strategy would be greatly aided if there were some professional price to be paid for violations, a point to which we shall return.

As a matter of professional integrity, we have asked practitioners to forego all the personal benefits of drug company gifts. Also as a matter of professional integrity, we similarly ask physician-investigators to forego such benefits. We are asking these investigators to rise to the ethical level of journalists and judges, and admit that reasonable onlookers could question the objectivity of their "scientific" judgments if they are known to be accepting cash payments from an interested party. Once the layers of denial are peeled away, questioning one's objectivity under such circumstances is not the personal insult that it is often taken to be; it is simply an acknowledgment of human psychology. Even if the individual had the capacity to remain totally objective in the face of cash or other gifts, professional integrity demands more than this. It demands *trustworthiness*. And trustworthiness demands that one behave in ways that would convince even skeptical onlookers of one's good faith.

One objection to this account is that it is all very well to say that *in theory*, we have maintained the benefits of collaboration between industry and academia. In actuality, however, we have seriously compromised the collaboration. Today, with academics regularly consulting with industry, there is a free flow of information back and forth. This has to work to the advantage of both parties. If no university physician-scientist was willing to be hired as an industry consultant, this vital avenue of information exchange would be eliminated.

There is some weight to this objection. One would ideally like to maintain the sorts of information flow that allow industry to create better products for human health and that allow academics to design better and more useful research projects. Under a Divestment Strategy, at least as I envision it, there would be no objection to a physician-investigator taking a leave from the university and working during that time as a paid employee of the industry.[23] It would also be acceptable for a physician-investigator to go to a reduced-time position at the university and work part-time for industry.

Yet we must, once again, separate the need for *information* to flow from the need for *money* to flow. Suppose that we accepted two propositions: (1) it is desirable that information be exchanged between industry and academia, and (2) it is equally desirable that no money change hands between the companies and individual physicians. Is it all that difficult to figure out ways for information to be exchanged? Could we not imagine regular conferences and briefings (with appropriate confidentiality assurances) by which academic physician-investigators could meet with industry personnel? The goal of information exchange hardly implies that we must maintain the financial status quo.

Imagine that physicians generally come to understand the requirements of professionalism as we have laid them out. The majority of physicians would then, over time, cease to accept gifts from the industry. If the momentum could start to flow in that direction, many reforms would then become easier to accomplish. At some point, for instance, the industry would probably simply dismantle some of its marketing structures, as the diminishing numbers of physicians potentially reachable by those efforts fell below some threshold of cost-effectiveness. Why spend about $40,000 training a successor to Stan, and pay him $50,000 or more a year plus fringes, if most physicians will refuse to see him? The few physicians remaining who are eager to accept company gifts would find those gifts drying up regardless.

The change in momentum could produce an important shift in values within the academic workplace. The shift would in some ways turn the calendar back to the era between 1950 and 1970, when academics proudly held themselves above such practices as profiting from discoveries. In discussing these issues with various colleagues and informants, I was unable to learn of any specific recent instance in which a university physician's willingness to accept numerous gifts from industry, or even to spin research results, was detrimental to that individual's career.[24] The shift in our perception of professionalism would mean that the rare physician, in the future, who is tempted to stray in the direction of accepting company largesse would be faced with the countervailing threat of professional ostracism. He would be worried that if he gave in to temptation, he could *no longer show his face* in places where his academic colleagues gathered.

Ostracism or shunning has gotten a bad name. I could not find, in philosophical databases, any recent articles in which ostracism was discussed as a potential solution to an ethical problem. The shunning of ostracism, as it were, is hardly surprising, given its potential for misuse and cruelty. A rigid, puritanical society might ostracize individuals for presumed moral lapses that the rest of us would judge minimal or nonexistent. Moreover, self-esteem is enjoying a bull market in today's pop psychology. It sometimes seems that threatening another person's self-esteem by frankly pointing out her moral lapses is judged a worse offense than the moral lapses themselves.

We have nevertheless seen a highly positive and creative use of ostracism as a tool of social reform in the campaign of Mothers Against Drunk Drivers (MADD). People who had lost relatives to accidents caused by drunk drivers were enraged when these drivers were given very light penalties, often returning to the road to cause more accidents. It seemed that police, judges, and other authorities were unconsciously entangled in a near-conspiracy to belittle the importance of driving while drunk. The message conveyed seemed to be, "We can all relate to the fellow who has had a momentary lapse in judgment after taking a little too much; the best thing to do is to slap his hand and let him to get back about his business with the minimum of inconvenience." When the MADD campaign first began, most "realists" would have said that these attitudes were firmly ingrained and that no reform movement would be able to budge them.

MADD attacked these attitudes head on, very effectively, using a combined strategy. On the one hand, MADD demonstrated that one could behave in new ways. Previously unthinkable acts like confiscating the car keys of a drunken fellow-party-goer suddenly received a social imprimatur. On the other hand, MADD argued forcefully that the supposedly minor moral lapse had such horrific consequences that we had no choice but to reclassify it as a much more serious matter than we had first thought. A negative moral judgment about a particular, avoidable behavior— driving while under the influence of alcohol—was successfully separated in public opinion from moralistic disapproval of alcohol consumption per se. So legislatures passed more stringent penalties for drunk driving. And judges who gave out light sentences to drunk drivers found themselves facing social disapproval.

I doubt that MADD explicitly said that its goal was to ostracize drunk drivers and those who defended or enabled them; but that was one result of their campaign. Most of us would judge this social change to be positive. Our society does not seem more inclined to ostracize other people for minor offenses; and it is a good thing that people now think twice before getting into a car after drinking.

The *primary* goal of the professional reform I call for is *not* to ostracize physicians, especially academic investigators, who get too cozy with the pharmaceutical industry. The intent is rather to bring about a heightened professional sensitivity, in which a behavior that previously was seen in terms of "who cares" and "everyone does it" is now revealed more clearly as a true threat to basic professional values. The end result would be that physicians who continue to engage in that behavior would be subject to professional ostracism; but the preferred outcome would be that physicians would stop behaving that way, leaving no one to ostracize. We seek to eliminate the problematic behavior, not to look for an excuse to punish someone.

REFORMING PROFESSIONAL ORGANIZATIONS

Because medical professional societies are aggregates rather than individuals, one might imagine that their activities need to be regulated in the ways we will be discussing in the next chapter. But because these are *professional* organizations, there is a more direct link between how a medical organization behaves and how individual physicians behave. After all, medical societies commonly promulgate codes of ethics for their members. One could reasonably ask whether the society itself is acting in ways that seem to violate the spirit (if not the letter) of its code of ethics. This is one way to understand the meaning of the AMA's Sunbeam scandal, in which the organization's leadership negotiated a multimillion-dollar royalty deal with a private corporation in exchange for product endorsements.[25] It did not seem right that an organization whose code of ethics required individual physicians to beware lavish gifts from corporate interests should itself be so ready to sell its reputation.[26]

The behavior of medical societies is a part of the overall professionalism of medicine. Individual physicians look to the societies they belong to for examples and indications of proper professional behavior. Even if other considerations do not require that these societies divest from pharmaceutical cash as much as possible, divestment may still be the correct action because of the example this sets for the society's membership.

We saw that in the wake of Sunbeam, the distinguished physician-ethicist Edmund Pellegrino and Dr. Arnold Relman proposed a new code of ethics for professional organizations. They began with the assumption that just as a physician, morally, should "profess" to be something more than a mere businessperson, medical societies should "profess" to be more than "self-serving trade associations, lobbies, or unions."[27] Public trustworthiness is as important at the organizational as on the individual level. They proposed the following specific guidelines, which are consistent with a very strict Divestment Strategy:

- Promoting the economic interests of members should be secondary to serving the public interest and promoting public health.
- Societies should not attempt to become physicians' unions.
- Societies should be supported by dues and largely avoid for-profit ventures; they "should not seek or accept support from companies that sell health care products or services."
- Editorship of society journals should be independent of the organization; strict limits should be placed on the amount and type of revenues gained from advertising.
- Commercial sponsorship of society meetings should be avoided.[28]

What, on balance, does professional integrity require of medical societies? First, it is important to note that the category itself is very heterogeneous. Some societies are large national entities, some have only a few hundred members. Some have huge budgets and fill large office buildings with their staffs; others are shoestring, largely voluntary operations. Some deal with the pharmaceutical industry as virtually their only source of commercial funds; others have little or nothing to do with the pharmaceutical industry, but may be heavily involved with the medical-device industry or other for-profit concerns. It will be difficult to come up with simple rules suitable for all of them.

Next, we saw that a "typical" medical society receives pharmaceutical money under three general headings—journal ads, CME support, or special-project grants. I regard the purchase of journal ads as an activity immune from the Divestment Strategy for several reasons. In a capitalist society, the right of a company to advertise its products amounts to a free-speech right, so that any inhibition of that right is legally as well as ethically questionable. Physicians can ignore journal ads more easily than most other forms of pharmaceutical marketing. There is little evidence that journal ads alone influence physician prescribing practices in a deleterious way.[29] And mechanisms now exist for the FDA to police misleading ads, though there are a number of weaknesses in that system.

Even if selling ads in a society's journal is a relatively innocuous proceeding, professionalism should still place limits. While it might be hard to specify a cut-off point, it is reasonable to imagine that once the total dependence of a society on industry crosses a certain threshold, it will become much more difficult for the society to take actions that might jeopardize industry's continued monetary support. One analysis of the ethics of financial arrangements between physicians and managed care plans concluded that once more than 20 percent of a physician's "bonus" is considered "at risk," the physician is more prone to start thinking about his own financial interests rather than the well-being of the patient when he is considering ordering a potentially beneficial but expensive intervention.[30] The authors recommended the 20 percent figure as a rough cut-off for an allowable financial incentive. Using the same rough rule of thumb, one might suggest that whenever a medical society's *total* dependence on industry exceeds 20 percent of its annual budget, its leadership might be inappropriately tempted to view the society's and the industry's interests as overlapping. While journal ads per se might be relatively innocuous, they could contribute to undue dependence.

We will address CME in detail in the next chapter and the guidelines suggested there could apply to medical societies as well as to any other CME-sponsoring organization—with the same proviso that one must look out for the total level of dependence as well as the details of any individual transaction.

Finally, gifts and grants directly from the industry to the society would seem ethically to be most problematic and would call for the most stringent safeguards. The best rule might be not to accept any such money unless there are especially compelling reasons why a particular project must be carried out for the good of the society, its members, and the public health, and no other funding source can be identified.

As important as the financial transactions between industry and medical societies is the need for greater transparency. When some colleagues and I tried to calculate the total financial reliance of the U.S. medical profession on the pharmaceutical industry, we found that data about journal publishing costs and revenues were the hardest data to obtain, with professional society revenues and budgets running a close second.[31] Since many societies publish journals, these are overlapping categories, and it raises questions about how well a medical society can set an ideal professional example for its members when its own reliance on industrial funding is kept secret.

In a world where professional integrity is highly valued, medical societies would be very open about the extent to which they receive funding from the pharmaceutical industry, and would take pride in reducing this sum. A society would be quicker to go to its members to seek a dues increase, than to turn to industry largesse. A physician who would resign from a medical society simply because it raised its dues, when she knew that the alternative would make the society even more dependent on funding from industry, would be the sort of member that a society would least miss. A medical society modeling an ideal level of integrity would refuse to pander to that sort of member at the price of allowing the industry to gain more influence over the society's operations.

We can accomplish a great deal solely through enhanced professionalism, at both the individual and the organizational levels. Still, in other areas, reform can come only via changes in regulatory guidelines or rules. That leads us to the discussion in the next chapter.

NOTES

1. E. J. Garland, "Facing the Evidence: Antidepressant Treatment in Children and Adolescents," *CMAJ* 2004; 170:489–91.

2. M. Angell, "Is Academic Medicine for Sale?" [editorial], *N Engl J Med* 2000; 342:1516–18.

3. T. J. Ruane, "Is Academic Medicine for Sale?" [letter], *N Engl J Med* 2000; 343:510.

4. "Doctors and leaders of drug companies are mature, consenting parties in relationships that both are highly motivated to maintain. . . . One can predict, therefore, that there

will be ongoing cycles of scandal and reform for the foreseeable future. . . . In many ways, the ultimate arbiter of the nature, extent and consequences of interactions between drug companies and physicians is the medical profession itself"; D. Blumenthal, "Doctors and Drug Companies," *N Engl J Med* 2004; 351:1885–90, quote p. 1889.

5. E. Freidson, *Profession of Medicine: A Study of the Sociology of Applied Knowledge* (New York: Harper and Row, 1970); D. J. Rothman, "Medical Professionalism—Focusing on the Real Issues," *N Engl J Med* 2000; 342:1283–86. There is at present a good deal of debate over what counts as "professionalism" in medicine, and especially what sorts of things should be included in a professionalism curriculum for medical trainees; see, for example, D. Wear and M. G. Kuczewski, "The Professionalism Movement: Can We Pause?" *Am J Bioeth* 2004; 4(2): 1–10, and the commentaries that followed in the same issue of the journal. I believe that what I will propose in this chapter relies on the least controversial aspects of professionalism, even if the specific steps I propose will be controversial. See also the previous chapter on ethical foundations.

6. www.nofreelunch.org (accessed March 13, 2005).

7. See, for example, M. H. Ebell and H. C. Barry, "InfoRetriever: Rapid Access to Evidence-Based Information on a Handheld Computer," *MD Comput* 1998; 15:287–97; T. Greenhalgh, J. Hughes, C. Humphrey, et al., "A Comparative Case Study of Two Methods of a Clinical Informaticist Service," *BMJ* 2002; 324:524–29. It is now becoming much more common for electronic medical records to include evidence-based guidelines and clinical prompts as part of the system, to guide physician decision making at the point of care; see, for example, V. J. Mikulich, Y. C. Liu, J. Steinfeldt, D. L. Schriger, "Implementation of Clinical Guidelines through an Electronic Medical Record: Physician Usage, Satisfaction, and Assessment," *Int J Med Inform* 2001; 63:169–78.

8. Even here it can be hard to detect commercial influence, and the same reasons thoughtful physicians might be drawn to such PDA information services tempt the industry to find ways to sneak in their commercial messages. For example, *Advertising Age* reported that pharmaceutical companies were quietly investing in Epocrates, a popular software information product; R. Thomaselli, "Big Pharma Finds Way into Doctors' Pockets; in Wake of DTC Storms, Epocrates Mobile-device Software Lures Sponsors," *Advertising Age* 76 (September 19, 2005): 4. My colleagues better trained than I in medical informatics tell me that the commercially biased features within Epocrates can be very difficult to distinguish from those portions that supply straightforward, unbiased material.

9. R. L. Blake Jr. and E. K. Early, "Patients' Attitudes about Gifts to Physicians from Pharmaceutical Companies," *J Am Board Fam Pract* 1995; 8:457–64.

10. K. Montemayor, "How to Help Your Low-Income Patients Get Prescription Drugs," *Family Practice Management* 2002; 9 (Nov–Dec): 51–56; B. Taylor, "Giveaway Drugs: Good Intentions, Bad Design," *Health Aff (Millwood)* 2004; 23:213–217.

11. "Record Number of Patients Receive Assistance from America's Pharmaceutical Companies," PhRMA, February 22, 2005, www.phrma.org/mediaroom/press/releases/ 22.02.2005.1129.cfm (accessed March 12, 2005). Unfortunately, as of the spring of 2006, I was unable to see signs that anything substantially had changed with the difficulties of securing charitable drug supplies for indigent patients; it may have been that the announcements of progress from PhRMA preceded tangible action.

12. D. Morelli and M. R. Koenigsberg, "Sample Medication Dispensing in a Residency Practice," *J Fam Pract* 1992; 34:42–8; J. M. Westfall, J. McCabe, and R. A. Nicholas, "Personal Use of Drug Samples by Physicians and Office Staff," *JAMA* 1997; 278:141–43.

13. J. Zweifler, S. Hughes, S. Schafer, B. Garcia, A. Grasser, and L. Salazar, "Are Sample Medicines Hurting the Uninsured?" *J Am Board Fam Pract* 2002; 15:361–66.

14. J. M. Boltri, E. R. Gordon, and R. L. Vogel, "Effect of Antihypertensive Samples on Physician Prescribing Patterns," *Fam Med* 2002; 34:729–31; L. Page, "More Clinics Ban Drug Samples, Citing Cost, Safety Concerns," *Am Med News*, October 16, 2000.

15. S. Erickson and S. Cullison, "Closing the Sample Closet: How Well Could You Get Along without Medication Samples—and without Drug Reps?" *Family Practice Management* 1995; (October): 43–47.

16. See www.medvantx.com/ (accessed March 12, 2005) for an example of a commercial enterprise that has sought in its own way to emulate Dr. Cullison's solution in a way that is applicable to a wide variety of office settings.

17. PhRMA, *Code on Interactions with Health Professionals*, PhRMA, July 1, 2002, www.phrma.org/publications/policy//2004-01-19.391.pdf (accessed January 31, 2005).

18. D. Katz, A. L. Caplan, and J. F. Merz, "All Gifts Large and Small," *Am J Bioeth* 2003; 3(3): 39–46.

19. R. Pear, "Drug Makers Battle Plan to Curb Rewards for Doctors," *New York Times*, December 26, 2002.

20. My comment about "whining" patients is not intended to be patient-bashing or to feed into the physicians' self-serving stereotypes. Rather it tries to recognize that when I am sick and in need of care, I am at my most self-absorbed and least likely to be mindful of others' feelings.

21. S. B. Soumerai and J. Avorn, "Principles of Educational Outreach ('Academic Detailing') to Improve Clinical Decision Making," *JAMA* 1990; 263:549–56; D. Berings, L. Blondeel, and H. Habraken, "The Effect of Industry-Independent Drug Information on the Prescribing of Benzodiazepines in General Practice," *Eur J Clin Pharmacol* 1994; 46:501–5; A. Figueiras, I. Sastre, F. Tato, et al., "One-to-One versus Group Sessions to Improve Prescription in Primary Care: A Pragmatic Randomized Controlled Trial," *Med Care* 2001; 39:158–67; M. Kaufman, "Doctors Hear Alternatives to Drug-Firm Sales Pitches," *Washington Post*, August 5, 2002:A01.

22. Another development that might address demoralization among practitioners, especially those relatively early in their careers, is an increased interest in providing mentor support from more senior physicians by state and local medical societies.

23. We have not yet addressed the question of what it means for a physician to adhere to optimal professional values while employed full-time by industry—a code of ethics for physician-pharmaceutical employees. There is indeed a code of ethics and an organization for such physicians; American Academy of Pharmaceutical Physicians, *Code of Ethics for the Practice of Pharmaceutical Medicine* (Apex, NC: American Academy of Pharmaceutical Physicians, 2001); http://aapp.org/ethics.php (accessed March 13, 2005). Sadly, it would appear from the available record that the code is today honored more in the breach than in the observance.

24. In March 2005, two high-level NIH staff scientists left under a cloud. Drs. Lance A. Liotta and Emanuel F. Petricoin III, while at the National Cancer Institute, accepted consulting fees from competing firms in arrangements that could have slowed down the development of a new test for ovarian cancer; D. Willman, "Case Study: Dr. Lance A. Liotta and Emanuel F. 'Chip' Petricoin III, Firm's Research Stalls as Cancer Experts Work for Rival," *Los Angeles Times*, December 22, 2004:A28. Both had received permission from NIH leadership to engage in these consulting arrangements. Their case was one of a handful that, when exposed by the *Los Angeles Times* late in 2004, led the new NIH director, Elias Zerhouni, to conclude that extremely strict new conflict-of-interest guidelines were needed at his agency. When Liotta and Petricoin left NIH, they were immediately snapped up by George Mason University's College of Arts and Sciences in Manassas, Virginia; the university president stated, "We are excited that Drs. Liotta and Petricoin are joining us in our mission to build a

research program of national prominence"; D. Willman, "Three Researchers in NIH Controversy Are Leaving: Their Paid Consulting for the Drug Industry Is Central to the Issue of Professional Conflicts at the Agency, Which Is Banning Such Income," *Los Angeles Times*, March 10, 2005:A14. If any conditions about avoiding conflicts of interest, or any concerns about previous commitments to professional ethics, were part of the university's hiring of these scientists, the news release was silent on the subject; http://gazette.gmu.edu/articles/index.php?id=6580 (accessed March 13, 2005).

25. J. Kaiser, "Furor over Company Deal Roils AMA," *Science* 1997; 278:26; J. P. Kassirer and M. Angell, "The High Price of Product Endorsement," *N Engl J Med* 1997; 337:700.

26. As we noted, it did not help the AMA's ethical status any when it later had to announce that it had accepted gifts from the pharmaceutical industry to help fund its project to better educate physicians about its ethical code on accepting gifts from the industry; M. McCarthy, "Drug Firm Support of American Medical Association Ethics Effort Draws Fire," *Lancet* 2001; 358:821; S. Okie, "AMA Blasted for Letting Drug Firms Pay for Ethics Campaign," *Washington Post*, August 30, 2001:A3. The American Medical Student Association (AMSA) provides an interesting contrast in professional ethics to the AMA; it has taken leadership in urging its members to declare medical practice a "pharmfree zone"; www.amsa.org/prof/pharmfree.cfm (accessed May 30, 2005).

27. E. D. Pellegrino and A. S. Relman, "Professional Medical Associations: Ethical and Practical Guidelines," *JAMA* 1999; 282:984–86; quote p. 984.

28. Pellegrino and Relman, "Professional Medical Associations," 986.

29. One would not expect there to be any such evidence since the companies do not consider journal ads a separate route for marketing. The typical company marketing strategy calls for journal ads to reinforce personal detailing and vice versa. However, for an opposing point of view, that perhaps journal ads are more influential than I have stated, see D. K. Scott and R. E. Ferner, "'The Strategy of Desire' and Rational Prescribing," *Br J Clin Pharmacol* 1994; 37:217–19; and T. Scott, N. Stanford, and D. R. Thompson, "Killing Me Softly: Myth in Pharmaceutical Advertising," *BMJ* 2004; 329:1484–87.

30. S. D. Pearson, J. E. Sabin, and E. J. Emanuel, "Ethical Guidelines for Physician Compensation Based on Capitation," *N Engl J Med* 1998; 339:689–93.

31. I am grateful to John Goddeeris and Andrew Hogan for assistance with this unpublished work.

SOLUTIONS REQUIRING REGULATORY REFORM

Courageous leadership is urgently needed to redirect American health care—not unlike the leadership provided by President Teddy Roosevelt a century ago when the enormously concentrated power of the railroad, steel, and oil "combines" similarly threatened the public's interests. Government needs to be re-empowered, and a good place to start might be public hearings that investigate the commercial distortion of our medical knowledge.

—Dr. John Abramson[1]

We have seen that much can be done to remedy the present situation if medicine simply puts its own house in order and acts more professionally. But other important aspects of the dysfunctional relationship between medicine and the pharmaceutical industry are relatively immune to unilateral action without substantial changes in public policy and legal regulation of the industry. In this chapter we must address that part of the equation.

SOME PRO-INDUSTRY REFORMS

Early on, we looked at the pharmaceutical industry's view of the issues addressed in this book, before we began to state the contrary case. In a similar vein, I want to start by suggesting a few reform measures that might be interpreted as favoring the industry. The goal of reform is not to punish the industry. If the industry can continue to make record profits while at the same time nurturing an environment in which medicine can be practiced with the highest level of professional integrity, so much the better. Let's look, then, at a few possible reforms that might favor industry.

Patent Life Equal to Marketing Life

One complaint used to justify undesirable industry behavior is the limited lifetime of drug patents once a drug comes to market. Companies have negotiated a twenty-year patent length, with some possible extensions, because it typically takes at least eight years of a drug's patent lifetime to complete the research needed for FDA approval. The revenues to make up for the high costs of research and development must all be wrung out of the remaining years of patent protection before the drug loses as much as 80 percent of its value when it becomes available generically.

A patent, as we have seen, is a form of government interference in the working of the "free" market, to promote a certain sort of public good. Ideally, the public always has the prerogative to stand back and to decide that the same good could be purchased at lower cost by modifying or even eliminating the patent system. It has been argued with some cogency that the U.S. patent system for pharmaceuticals is a bad bargain. The gains come in the form of new drugs resulting from the companies' expenditures on research and development. The costs come from the higher prices U.S. patients have to pay for their drugs because they are protected by patent. What would happen if the U.S. government assumed the entire cost of research and development, in effect making all drug companies into generic manufacturers? Publicly funded labs would discover and test the drugs, which on FDA approval would then be licensed to multiple firms to manufacture and sell at generic prices.

Dean Baker and Noriko Chatani of the Center for Economic and Policy Research calculated these costs and concluded that even if we look only at the roughly half of health care in the United States that is paid for with federal dollars, it would be worth it to do away with patents and to fund research and development out of public funds. The amount saved in the federal drug budget alone, in Medicare, Medicaid, the Veterans Administration, and so forth, would pay for all the research costs.[2]

I am not about to propose doing away with all industry-funded research and development, except as an extreme backup measure if two earlier stages of reforms in pharmaceutical research, to be described below, fail to solve the problems. Therefore, I do not propose to do away with patents on new drugs. As long as this is so, it makes little sense to grant a patent that begins to tick away as soon as a drug is put into development, and not when the drug reaches the market. If companies dragged their feet in bringing new drugs to market, we could see the value in creating a financial incentive to speed up the process. But we have seen no evidence of that problem, and far too much evidence of drugs being rushed to market with all sorts of corners being cut in the research process. If we wish the active patent life of a new drug to be twelve years, then make it twelve years, but start it whenever the drug can be sold. Let the company have the security of knowing exactly how long the real patent-protection period is going to be.[3]

Exclude Trial Results from Mandatory Registry

I will argue below that a mandatory clinical trials registry is a critical first step in returning integrity to the system of pharmaceutical research. Companies are naturally fearful of being forced to post what they see as proprietary information, that can be used by competitors, on public websites. I will argue that for these registries to work, a good deal of information about the inception of a clinical trial must be posted. But these rich data about trial design from the inception make it less important that the *results* of the trial also be posted. Quite naturally, patient advocates want results so that people will know about promising new treatments and can lobby to be included in new drug trials. Drug companies may decide that the public relations benefits of assisting with these legitimate public desires, as happened with Gleevec, make losing some control over proprietary information worthwhile. But full disclosure of results in this particular form and venue is not absolutely necessary to ensure the ethical integrity of the research process. My proposals will therefore allow firms to continue to treat trial results as proprietary information, except as required by the FDA approval process and other considerations, such as contracts signed with universities demanding rights to publish.[4]

Limit Regulation Aimed at "Me-Too" Drugs

Dr. Marcia Angell, in her widely quoted book attacking the industry, focuses on me-too drugs, and would redo the entire FDA drug approval process in order to limit them.[5] She urges that the FDA consider improved efficacy compared to existing drugs as a necessary criterion for approval. I have argued that me-too drugs are more complicated than Angell admits, and that me-too drugs sometimes turn out to have unexpected therapeutic advantages.

If all the reforms I list below are implemented, the remaining problems around me-too drugs would be minimized, and further regulation aimed specifically at that class of drugs would not be required. For example, if an NIH institute independent of industry were adequately funded to do head-to-head studies of drug efficacy, and if physicians got their drug information from evidence-based sources instead of reps, much of the financial incentive that now pushes the companies toward more me-too drugs would be eliminated.

REFORMING RESEARCH: THE INITIAL STAGE

We have seen how the present profit-driven environment has threatened basic scientific values by tempting companies to view research as subservient to marketing. This undermines medicine at its core—the basic building blocks of scientific knowledge. A great deal can be done simply by calling upon individual research investigators to assume a higher standard of personal ethical integrity, and seeking through collective action to attach social consequences to the continued lack of integrity in science. But we can also speed up that process of ethical reform by creating the right research environment with the right sorts of financial incentives.

The Divestment Strategy would argue that ultimately, we must drive a wedge between industry financial support of research and the outcomes of the research. The current research system is so dependent upon industry funding, and is characterized by such a striking lack of firewalls, that it will necessarily be a slow process to make the required transition. The full transition, therefore, is what I call the second stage of research reform.

Mandatory Registry of Clinical Trials

A great deal can be done in the interim by adopting a reform measure that can be implemented quickly and that has already received votes of approval from key players. In the summer of 2004, in the wake of the scandal involving antidepressants in children, there were calls in the press and in Congress for mandatory trial registries.[6] The drug firms, feeling the pressure, started to bow to the registry movement.[7] Perhaps most importantly, the editors of a group of the world's leading medical journals announced their intention of rejecting papers for publication in the future if the clinical trial had not been openly registered.[8] The editors' stance is particularly important because that group, above all others, has the authority to make the change happen.

What does a mandatory registry entail? We can perhaps best see its necessary scope if we use CLASS as an example. Suppose that the CLASS investigators had known that no journal would publish their findings unless they registered the trial at its inception. What would journal editors later need to know? In mid-2005, the International Committee of Medical Journal Editors suggested the following "minimal registration data set":[9]

- unique trial number
- trial registration date
- funding sources
- primary and secondary sponsor(s)
- title of study
- research ethics review
- medical condition being studied
- description of study interventions, including comparison or control, and duration
- key inclusion and exclusion criteria
- study design (randomized, crossover, etc.)
- start date
- target size of subject sample
- primary and key secondary outcomes

Would such a registry have prevented the CLASS debacle? On receiving the manuscript, the editors of *JAMA* would have looked up the trial in the registry, using the unique identifier number. Would they have been able to see that they had been sent only six months' worth of data from a study designed to run for twelve months? As the precise duration of the intervention is one of the required data, the cat presumably would have been out of the bag.

The same would be true for most of the baldest ways that data are manipulated upon publication to misrepresent findings unfavorable to the company. Suppose, for instance, that a drug is intended to increase survival following cardiac surgery.

A group of subjects are studied and the survival after surgery turns out to be no better; but the subjects turn out by chance to show lower cholesterol. Today, the common way to handle this is to publish a paper on how the drug is a great success in lowering cholesterol in a group of high-risk patients. Under the registry system, the journal editor (or reviewer) would immediately be aware of the substitution of study endpoints, and could demand that the authors account for the missing or downplayed data.

It would be harder to use the registry to detect the problem that led to the widespread demand for its use—suppression of trials that show unfavorable data. Since the relevant manuscript is never submitted for publication, no journal editor is in a position to take any remedial measures. Correction would instead come during regulatory actions, such as FDA advisory boards, or could be triggered by inquiries from advocacy or public interest groups. When a claim is made that a certain drug is safe or effective, doubters could consult the registry and track all trials involving that drug. If one or more studies are well past the scheduled completion date, but results have never been published, the company can be asked to account for the missing data. At any rate, the fact that the trials were conducted but the results never published would not remain a secret within the company.

The worst sorts of abuses could therefore be prevented or rendered much more difficult through a mandatory trials registry, even if the trial *results* were not part of the mandatory disclosure. Excluding results while recording almost all aspects of trial design and methods seems to be a reasonable way of allowing the company to protect some proprietary interests while ensuring the integrity of research.

Who should manage the registry? An existing NIH registry, currently voluntary, has been promoted as a model, and could be expanded to require all the elements we have listed.[10] Registry of all drug trials should be required. This could be enforced by requiring prior registry before any trial data would be accepted by the FDA for purposes of drug approval or review, and also by insisting upon registry as a condition to enroll human subjects in a trial. The latter requirement follows from the ethical conclusion we discussed, that it is unethical to expose human subjects to the risks and inconvenience of trial participation, unless the data obtained from the trial will advance medical science; and the advancement of science can only be assured through some mechanism such as mandatory registration.

Strict Enforcement of Informed-Consent Requirements

We saw in chapter 2 that a good deal of today's pharmaceutical research is unethical because subjects do not give an adequately informed consent. Most subjects in human research studies assume that they are contributing to science. Studies that are designed with marketing as a top priority—especially studies that might never be published if the data do not turn out favorably for the sponsor—hardly count as advancing science. If subjects are put to any risk at all—even a minor inconvenience—as a result of participating in such a research study, they have a right to be informed frankly of the real purposes. Moreover, if their personal physicians are pocketing hefty finder's fees for recruiting subjects, the patients deserve to know this so that they can demand their fair shares. Strict enforcement of informed-consent requirements would start to dry up the subject pool for studies that today constitute the worst offenses against good science.

REFORMING RESEARCH: THE SECOND STAGE

As important as it is, a mandatory trials registry does not eliminate the conflicts of interest in the present system of industry-funded research. It remains the case that the company decides which investigators, working for which organizations, receive the grants to do the research, plus any other perks the company wishes to bestow; and both investigator and organization know that producing results that please the company increases the chance of future largesse.

National Institute of Pharmaceutical Development

Accordingly, several authors who have looked at this problem favor some arrangement whereby funding for drug trials is channeled through an independent research body not controlled by industry. The model that has the most adherents imagines this entity to be something like a new Institute within the structure of the NIH.[11] Sheldon Krimsky suggests calling this new entity the National Institute of Drug Testing. For reasons that will be clear later, I would modify this to the National Institute of Pharmaceutical Development (NIPD).

Krimsky imagines that companies would develop molecules worthy of clinical testing by current methods. They might discover the molecule in their in-house laboratories; they might obtain promising ideas from basic science labs in universities or at other NIH institutes; or they might buy rights from biotech companies. Whenever the molecule had passed the necessary animal tests and seemed ripe for human testing, the company would send a proposal to the NIPD. The NIPD would then send back a general protocol for a sequence of clinical trials. Negotiation could occur between the company and the NIPD until both a general approach to research trials and a funding amount had been agreed on. The NIPD would then put out calls for proposals, giving an outline of the sort of trial needed but protecting the most detailed information about the molecule and its properties as proprietary information. University and other scientists could apply for these grants just as they now apply for research funding from NIH.[12] The scientists, once their initial approval had been accepted, would be able to learn full details about the molecule to be tested (under pledges of confidentiality) and would negotiate with the NIPD the final details of the research design. Funding would come from the company to the NIPD and then be disbursed to the scientists and their institution. Direct payment of any benefits from the company to the scientists would be prohibited. Universities would be required to have strong conflict-of-interest policing policies as a condition for being awarded NIPD grants.[13]

As the first trials were completed, there would naturally be a need to reconsider both the design and the cost of later trials in light of any unexpected results. At each stage the NIPD would act as an intermediary between the firm and the scientists conducting the research. The company would still be free to do whatever research it wanted to with its own scientists and its own funds. But it would be a condition of later FDA approval that all clinical trial data submitted as part of the approval process would have to have been certified as following a protocol stipulated by the NIPD. The NIPD would assure the scientists the right to publish all trial results, with brief delays (on the order of three to six months) to allow the company to file for new patents or to make appropriate commercial use of any trial findings.

Drug Research Lacking Commercial Incentive

I have proposed calling this new National Institute "Pharmaceutical Development" rather than "Drug Testing" because the latter title suggests a narrower mission. Critics of the drug industry frequently point out how little research is conducted in areas critical to the public health, but lacking in potential profitability. The studies *not* being conducted often enough include:

- Head-to-head comparisons of existing drugs to determine which are most effective, or cost-effective, for common conditions
- Development trials for drugs needed in developed countries, but for which sales are projected to be low (including, today, most new antibiotics)
- Development trials for drugs needed primarily in developing countries for epidemic diseases

The NIPD would either conduct these trials directly under their external grant programs, or coordinate basic laboratory efforts to identify promising new drug entities with other NIH Institutes. (As we have seen, a large proportion of the basic research leading to important new drugs, for which credit is often claimed by the industry, is performed already in NIH and university labs.) The NIPD would receive substantial funding from the federal government for the important public health mission of obtaining unbiased scientific data on how drugs perform.[14] The government funding would also recognize the financial benefits of head-to-head drug trials, which could easily save Medicare and Medicaid billions of dollars if they show that cheaper generic drugs are as effective for some common conditions as newer brand-name drugs.[15] Money received from the industry to conduct new drug approval trials on a contractual basis would therefore be only one portion of the NIPD's total budget.

What are the implications for the American taxpayer? Critics of the NIPD proposal would object that we would have to raise taxes substantially in order to fund these new federal initiatives. But the present way that we fund medical research, professional societies, and CME is all geared to keeping drug expenditures in the United States at the highest possible level. The total contribution of the pharmaceutical industry to research, CME, and medical organizations is in the range of $28 billion annually.[16] This amounts to about 5.6 percent of the $500 billion annual revenues of the American pharmaceutical industry.[17] That means that if we could, through improved approaches to research and physician education, reduce current drug expenditures by only 10 percent, we could replace all the funding that the industry now plows into research, CME, and professional societies, and have money left over.[18]

Creation of the NIPD in the second stage of reform would largely eliminate the financial incentives for the abuses that have led to calls for a mandatory trials registry. There is no reason, however, simply to ditch the registry. The NIPD can take over management of the registry and also ensure that all trials that it conducts or sponsors are registered at inception.

Tough Academic Policies on Conflicts of Interest

The NIPD would be in an excellent position to require universities and independent laboratories to have policies in place as a condition of receiving grant funds. This assumes, if the NIPD is to be part of NIH, that the NIH has already cleaned up its own mess on conflict-of-interest policies. David Willman, investigative reporter for the *Los Angeles Times*, deserves credit for almost single-handedly shining the light of publicity on how NIH leadership looked the other way while many of its top scientists pocketed tens of thousands of dollars in pharmaceutical consulting fees.[19]

As part of professional reform, the NIH, academic medical centers, medical journals, and FDA need explicitly and loudly to reject the defeatist attitude, "They all do it." The rationalization for the status quo says that if one stopped allowing lucrative industry consulting and speakers' fees, "the best" scientists would simply pack up and go elsewhere, leaving one to do research with the dregs.

One of the assumptions that must be challenged as part of this rationalization is whether the scientists who act that way deserve the title of "the best." It is logical here to recall David Healy's observation in connection with ghostwriting. The flow of industry cash into medical research has created an overclass of successful research administrators who are today so busy consulting and giving speeches that they have no time to go into the laboratory and see what is happening. This overclass currently populates FDA advisory groups, national guideline panels, and similar entities to a disproportionate degree. If we eliminated this overclass by enforcing strict conflict of interest policies, and instead chose for our future panels the "underclass" of scientists who were conducting the hands-on research, we might find that we were getting better advice.[20]

But without a doubt, a university (for instance) pays a high price for its professionalism if it unilaterally puts a rigid policy in place, only to see all of its most productive scientists leave to go to less finicky schools. Regulations that create a level playing field are therefore a welcome addition to a resurgence in professional values. One strong reason to create the NIPD is that this becomes the only game in town; sleazy scientists cannot jump ship and go elsewhere to protect their sweetheart deals.

Professionalism and regulatory reform should reinforce each other. Ultimately, only professional values will "police" a university's (or the NIH's) conflict of interest policy. You cannot run an academic research institution like a police state, constantly snooping on everyone to make sure they follow the guidelines. But you can give real weight to professionalism with institutional policies that proclaim clearly the importance of these values at all levels, and that reassure the individual scientist that the next guy is not getting rich while I forego benefits.

American universities have developed a few promising models for conflict-of-interest policies for individual faculty members.[21] They have been much slower to find ways to police institutional-level conflicts of interest.[22] It is especially important that universities have strong institutional-level conflict of interest policies, to assure individual scientists that the institution as a whole is not acting in the same ways that it prohibits among its personnel. The lesson of the Olivieri case in this regard is clear. The outrageous behavior of the Hospital for Sick Children and the University of Toronto occurred not as a result solely of individual conflicts of interest among its faculty and administrators, though those conflicts played an undeniable role. In the end the University failed Dr. Nancy Olivieri, and the larger cause of scientific integrity, because the *University as a whole* imagined that its future well-being was tied to the financial success of a single company, and that it owed more allegiance to that company's bottom line than it owed to the health of patients under its care.[23]

The next time, for example, that the University of California at Berkeley decides to lease one of its research departments to a private firm, will there exist an institutional conflict-of-interest review process with the clout to call the deans, the president, and the board of regents on the carpet? The need for a national level of oversight seems apparent, even if precisely how to structure it is not. If, on the other hand, no one prevents the university from profiting from its name and reputation, while an individual faculty member is slapped if he owns a few shares of pharmaceutical stock, the hypocrisy condemns the entire arrangement.

Moreover, where standards exist, there is compelling evidence that universities today fail to monitor faculty relationships with industry to ensure that the relevant standards are met. One survey found that very few academic medical centers ensure that research contracts with industry meet the guidelines of the International Committee of Medical Journal Editors on matters such as access to data and control over publication.[24] This failure on the part of the academic medical center places all the onus on the shoulders of the individual investigator to go toe-to-toe with a giant pharmaceutical company to request that contract language be rewritten to meet standards of scientific integrity. Universities should both require their faculty to live up to standards of scientific integrity and actively support their faculty in pursuit of those goals.

Should something also be done about Bayh-Dole, since the academic stampede to secure patents appears to have triggered today's wave of undesirable commercial behavior among academic institutions? It is perhaps better to discuss that aspect of the problem when we address patents later.

THE FDA

The evidence seems overwhelming that at least since 1992, the FDA has veered too far in the direction of supporting the industry rather than protecting public interests. It did so because it was ordered to—first by Congress and later by the executive branch. The orders emerged from a free-market ideology and a desire to lower taxes. Now that we have seen some of the consequences of these actions, we can better judge both the ideology and what we have succeeded in purchasing in exchange for lower taxes.[25]

In the wake of the Vioxx recall, coming hard on the heels of the furor over suppression of antidepressant trial data, there were immediate calls for reforms at the FDA. Below are some proposals that seem the most compelling.

Repeal Industry User Fees

It seems to be no coincidence that the years when the FDA depended for a good part of its budget on user fees paid by the drug industry under PDUFA were also the years when quick approvals far overshadowed identifying safety risks. As Philip Hilts describes it in his FDA history, each time the FDA goes back to Congress to get more money, Congress is tempted to turn more to industry and less to taxpayer dollars. In turn, each time industry is asked to ante up more, it wrings out of Congress a few more concessions. Hilts believes that even the initial supporters of PDUFA would now have to admit its failure.[26]

The FDA needs a strong signal that however much it may need to collaborate with industry as a tactical matter, its primary client is not the industry but the American people. PDUFA is the wrong signal.

Independent Safety-Monitoring Wing

The model that has been proposed is the relationship between the Federal Aviation Administration and the National Transportation Safety Board. The former regulates the airlines and the latter investigates the cause of accidents. This seems to work well because we do not expect that those who were supposed to have prevented an airline crash in the first place to suddenly become objective in assigning the blame for what went wrong, and to take firm action for heading off future problems.

By analogy, it is dysfunctional to expect that the same people who approved a drug for use will now be unbiased in assessing whether that same drug is too risky to be allowed to remain on the market—that, in effect, they blew it the first time around. Yet that is how the FDA is currently structured, with the drug approval people, and the relatively small group of drug safety people like David Graham, all answering to the same boss.

In 1998, a group of experts on pharmaceutical issues called for the creation of an independent safety board, separate from the FDA.[27] This body would have two major functions. First, it would investigate drugs now on the market for safety, such as in the Vioxx case. Second, it would be much more proactive than the FDA is currently. It would no longer rely on a haphazard system of reporting, where all admit that at most 10 percent of all adverse drug reactions ever get sent in. The new agency would instead design and implement a modern surveillance system, based on up-to-date organization and technology—similar to what the Centers for Disease Control and Prevention use for monitoring infectious diseases and to contain any new outbreak of, say, influenza as soon as possible. As more and more hospitals and offices start to adopt computerized medical records, one could program these computers to notify the federal agency of all potential drug reactions, while still protecting patient confidentiality. On this model, instead of reacting after others had identified a possible drug risk, the drug safety agency itself would be the first to identify the danger.

After Vioxx, calls were renewed for a more independent drug safety monitoring agency.[28] I will not pass judgment on whether the ideal location for a drug safety monitoring agency is within the FDA but in a separate branch from the new drug approval process, or outside the FDA entirely. If other needed reforms were activated within the FDA, it might not be necessary to locate this function outside the agency. A critical reform will be for Congress to increase appropriations for this expanded, proactive safety monitoring function. We must as taxpayers accept the reality that ensuring the quality and safety of our drug supply is a public good and should be supported adequately from public funds. For-profit firms should pay their fair share of taxes but should not be expected to lift the burden from taxpayers' shoulders.

Graded Drug Approvals

In one particular way, Dr. Jerry Avorn thought that the FDA got it right in its final decision on Lotronex (chapter 13). Allowing a dangerous drug back on the market, but with additional special protections, angered a number of the agency's critics, but made excellent sense to Dr. Avorn. Drugs do not come in two types, safe and unsafe. Given that drug risks run along a continuum and cannot be assessed separately from benefits and costs, it seems silly that the FDA has only "yes" and "no" answers available to it when judging a new drug application. Avorn would favor the option for graded approvals.[29] For example, in hindsight, it would have made sense for the COX-2 drugs to receive a limited rather than a full approval when they first came on the market, before enough time had passed to see if they had any long-term side effects that early trials had not picked up.

Strictly Enforced Conflict-of-Interest Rules

The FDA frequently waives its own conflict-of-interest rules to allow paid consultants to industry to sit on its advisory panels, based on the rationalization that otherwise the FDA would be deprived of important expert opinion. As with NIH guidelines panels and other such expert conclaves, we need to be firm that good science and good ethics are not at odds with each other and that the true "expert" is one whose position is trustworthy. Strict enforcement of these rules should be standard FDA policy.[30]

The Revolving Door and Punitive Regulatory Action

Some of the FDA's harshest anti-industry critics—we must not forget that the FDA always has a claque of pro-industry critics who wish it would simply disappear and let the industry run its own affairs—judge the effectiveness and purity of spirit of the FDA by how many punitive actions it launches against firms, and by how effectively it shuts the revolving door that allows former FDA staffers to get lucrative jobs within the industry after they depart. Before we call for such "reforms," we ought to recall the warnings from John Braithwaite in his study of corporate crime in the pharmaceutical industry.[31]

Braithwaite was under no illusions as to how compliant the industry would be with high ethical standards if left to its own devices. He wrote his book, after all, to expose *crime*, not merely ethically suboptimal behavior—and he concluded that there was more corporate crime in the pharmaceutical industry internationally, at the time he wrote in the mid-1980s, than in any other comparable industry.[32] Nevertheless, Braithwaite was highly critical of those who urged the FDA to respond with the proverbial big stick, especially trying to use criminal prosecution as the answer to all serious problems. While "throw the bastards in the slammer" might be an emotionally satisfying response, especially when reading of egregious cases such as Chemie Grünenthal and thalidomide, Braithwaite's counterquestion is— should we aim to be emotionally satisfied or to make the supply of pharmaceuticals as safe as possible?

If our goal is product safety, Braithwaite argues that we have important allies within the industry itself. There are, for instance, scientists working in pharmaceutical plants whose job is quality control and who may be as concerned as any FDA inspector that no contaminants can enter the drug supply. Often a policy of trying to forge selective alliances with industry, to work collaboratively with forces on the inside who are in the best position to pursue safety and honest science, will work better than a punitive approach that will simply turn everyone in the company into an adversary. Having said that cooperation may yield more fruit, Braithwaite then goes on to say that the FDA must at least on occasion prosecute blatantly bad behavior vigorously, simply to show that it means what it says.[33]

Braithwaite has somewhat similar views on the problem of the "revolving door." In his view, the problem of the "door" is that it works only in one direction; it is not likely that the FDA will attract many people who previously worked for industry.[34] The ideal situation would be when people regularly move back and forth between the drug companies and the FDA. This increases the chance that an individual will identify a particular agenda as her major professional goal—such as doing good-quality scientific research—quite apart from who happens to be signing her paycheck at any given time. It also as a practical matter improves the FDA's ability to find out what is going on within the industry and what questions to ask company representatives when they testify.

Restrict Consumer Advertising According to Pre-1997 FDA Rules

We saw that when, in the fall of 2003, the FDA held open hearings on the regulation if DTC ads, the sessions were packed with those funded by the industry. Not surprisingly, the message that emerged was that DTC ads are a great source of information and a force for public good.

On January 6, 2005, the *Boston Globe* surveyed the scene in an editorial and saw a rather different landscape. In the wake of Vioxx having been taken off the market, the *Globe* saw the unbridled DTC advertising as a major reason that so many

Americans were unnecessarily exposed to significant risk of heart disease from COX-2 drugs.[35]

The *Globe* stopped short of calling for a total ban on DTC ads. However, by calling upon the FDA to require balanced presentation of drug risks and side effects, it indirectly suggested that a ban might be indicated. If the FDA were to implement such rules, it would come close, at least, to rolling back the clock to the pre-1997 days, when its regulations made it infeasible for most companies to advertise most prescription drugs on television particularly.[36] If the United States were to take this step, we would allow New Zealand to become the only developed nation in the world allowing widespread DTC advertising of pharmaceuticals. If, in a decade or so, we discovered that New Zealanders were markedly healthier than Americans, we might at that time have second thoughts. Today, however, it seems doubtful that anything of value would be lost if DTC ads were sharply curtailed. As Abramson has argued, we might be able to return to the day when "ask your doctor" suggested going to a professional for thoughtful advice, not going to a drive-up window to demand a particular consumer product.

CONTINUING MEDICAL EDUCATION

We ended our chapter on CME by quoting Derek Bok's grim prognosis—of all the horses in the academic-medical-center barn, the CME horse was farthest away over the hill when we began shutting all the gates, and so there's virtually no chance of ever getting that animal back into its noncommercial stall. Is it then impossible to apply the Divestment Strategy to CME?

We also saw that something unusual occurred in 2004. Impressed by threatened action from the inspector-general of DHHS, the industry appeared to be taking seriously the stringent new guidelines proposed by the ACCME.

If we adopt Bok's perspective, the only thing that would work at all for CME would have to be a very radical version of the Divestment Strategy. If, on the other hand, we take heart from what appears to have been true progress with the new ACCME guidelines, a case could be made at least temporarily for adopting the version of the Management Strategy that these guidelines represent. If there is an incentive to cooperate in creating strict firewalls to manage conflicts of interest in the design and administration of CME programs without totally eliminating commercial sponsorship, we might grant at least a trial period to see how well the current ACCME guidelines work. Only if those fail would we be justified in demanding a (complete) divestment alternative.

Current ACCME Guidelines: First Step

On its face, the new ACCME set of guidelines announced late in 2004 represent a serious effort to build firewalls. Commercial funders would be kept as far away as possible from the planning and content of the CME conference. Unlike previous guidelines, which relied mostly on disclosure of industry ties, the new guidelines would prohibit many speakers with direct ties to drug companies from appearing on CME programs at all.

These new guidelines, if effectively policed by the CME community, might amount to a de facto Divestment Strategy. That is, if industry influence were reduced as much as the guidelines promise, the industry might no longer find it worthwhile to fund CME programs. Alternatively, such funding would no longer come out of marketing budgets, as they apparently do today; companies would treat support of medical education as a charitable contribution, and not attempt to exert influence over program content. As charity, the industry would presumably fund CME much less generously. In either event, industry support for CME would plummet from its current level of more than half of total costs to perhaps less than 10 percent. At least some of the money saved by industry might be reinvested in non-CME programs such as dinner-lectures with selected pro-industry speakers—programs that would frankly be regarded as marketing. (Of course, I have argued that physicians of integrity would refuse to attend those dinners.)

Alternatively, companies might decide that CME helps to sell drugs, regardless of how much direct control they have over program content, and so it is still worth their while to fund CME generously even under the new guidelines. Presumably that would be the best-case scenario all around. The new guidelines, supposedly, would prevent the most egregious conflicts of interest. CME sponsors would continue to have levels of funding near their current levels with which to support programs. Physicians would continue to enjoy partially subsidized programs with lower registration fees, but would be better protected from commercially biased messages.

Explicit Divestment: Second Step

If in a few years it seems that even the current, more stringent guidelines are not working as intended, we would have yet one more bit of evidence that the Management Strategy simply won't work. The next step, then, would be to call for a more serious divestment of CME programs from industry support.[37] Either commercial support of CME programs would be banned entirely, or a limit would be placed at 10 to 20 percent maximum funding from commercial sources for any given CME program. Again, if this limit meant that industry effectively lost its influence over program content, that might amount to de facto total prohibition, as the industry would simply take its marketing money and go elsewhere.

Either through this second step, or through some of the scenarios possible with the first step, we could see a major reduction in funding available for CME programs in the United States. Organizers of CME programs would probably view this as a disaster. Such a dire assessment would not be accurate. First, if the programs eliminated were the programs that today contain the greatest amount of commercial bias, the medical profession has hardly lost a great educational resource. Second, if the loss of funds means that many of the special luxuries now routinely tacked onto CME programs are no longer affordable, a more spartan CME program might not be such a bad thing. Physicians who demand the accustomed luxuries—such as fancy receptions and dinners, and plush resort surroundings—might be willing to pay higher registration fees, and no one can complain if the professionals themselves pay a larger portion of the cost of their own education (plus added benefits).

In the end, we would probably see some combination of all three outcomes—some programs eliminated; some presented in a leaner fashion; and yet others supported with higher fees from attendees. As we noted, there is little evidence anyway that today's CME changes medical practice for the better. Even if it has little measurable impact on behavior, CME is a way for physicians occasionally to meet some other physicians in their field, and to be reminded of the importance the profession places on staying current. CME will for that reason probably never go away completely, no matter how lean the evidence that it has the desired outcomes.

Reduced Honoraria for CME Speakers

There is one practical way that all physicians involved in CME programs can strike a blow for professionalism and make it more likely that the current guidelines will be successful. This requires voluntary collective action to reduce the honoraria paid to physician presenters at CME programs.

I can put this suggestion into personal terms. When I began my career as an academic physician in 1980, I expected to do a certain number of CME presentations locally for free. For those that represented a special burden or that required out-of-town travel, it was a nice perk to be paid an honorarium of $100, $250, or (in extreme cases) $500. Today I receive honoraria for some of the CME programs that I would have imagined doing for free in my early days; and it is quite common to receive an honorarium of between $1,000 and $3,000. If I tried harder I could probably elevate my "going rate" to the $5,000 range.

Some of this rise represents inflation, and some (I would hope) my improved academic credibility and experience. But a certain amount of this inflation represents the general rise in the CME market caused by the heavy influx of pharmaceutical support. My apparent market value did not go up because I joined drug companies' speakers' bureaus. I primarily get invited to talk about medical ethics. For better or for worse, most drug companies are uninterested in that subject, which seldom prompts physicians to run home and prescribe more drugs. But as it became commonplace for drug companies to pay physicians on their speakers' bureaus fees of $3,000 to $5,000 per talk, the "expected" rate for *all* CME honoraria went up accordingly. The rest of us, without thinking about the cause, simply took for granted that we were worth that much, and that somewhere, printing presses were turning out enough new money for the CME system to pay all of us top dollar.

Of course the "printing presses" are mythical, and this inflation in speakers' fees is both a result and a cause of increased industry influence over CME programming. As industry cash flowed into CME coffers, programs could offer higher honoraria. As we speakers started to expect and demand these higher honoraria, as a matter of course (and even for topics far removed from pharmaceuticals), we made it that much harder for any CME program sponsor to put together a suitable panel of speakers without going, hat in hand, to the drug industry.

It may never have occurred to me that by coming to expect higher honoraria, I was advancing commercial interests. Ego being what it is, it would have been far more natural to assume that I was worth the extra money based on my merits. But now that we have confronted the entire system of commercial influence, with all its interconnections, I can no longer turn a blind eye to the role that I play. It will be necessary for me to moderate my expected CME honoraria if we are all to benefit from a CME system which is, overall, much less dependent on commercial funding. I call upon all my fellow CME presenters to do likewise.

PATENTS

The reforms already suggested would, if implemented, take some of the attention off the current patent system, because many of the most perverse financial incentives operating on the pharmaceutical industry would have been removed.[38] Still, some reforms aimed specifically at patents appear desirable.

Stop Evergreening and Restore Common Sense to the Patent Process

One set of interconnected reforms would not be necessary had the patent system, and the courts that rule on patent issues, kept firmly in mind the original principles—that to be worthy of a patent, a discovery or invention must be novel, useful, and nonobvious. The admittedly rare court ruling that allows a drug company to keep generic competition at bay because of a patent on some superficial feature of a drug, such as the color of the capsule or a particular coating, would seem to violate these simple precepts.

The problem will be difficult to rein in as long as the U.S. patent office continues to hand out patents wholesale on scientific discoveries for which a practical use might someday be found—such as most gene products and genetic testing procedures today—and on trivial modifications of existing products. But Marcia Angell makes the additional point that according to Hatch-Waxman, a brand-name company cannot block a generic drug based on just any patent. To be relevant to such actions, the patent must be listed in the FDA's Orange Book. If the FDA had adhered to its charge, irrelevant and superficial patents would never be listed there. The FDA, according to Angell, has abrogated its responsibility to police the patent wars. In the future, it could do better, without any changes in existing law.[39]

One set of reforms that addresses the problem directly would be a revision of the Hatch-Waxman Act to close many of the loopholes that have been most exploited by the industry—especially allowing the mere filing of a lawsuit, no matter how weak its merits, against a generic competitor, to automatically extend the patent by thirty months. Angell further argues for repeal of the amendment that provides for a six-month patent extension simply for testing the drug in children. This well-intentioned amendment was enacted due to concerns that the industry would make children "therapeutic orphans" by refusing to take on the expense of testing useful drugs in children to determine the ideal doses. In practice, Angell charges, the law has simply provided an incentive for companies to test many drugs in children even if there is no realistic chance that children would be prescribed the drug, merely to get the extra patent life. Angell reminds us that if the FDA were to develop the needed backbone, it could simply require appropriate pediatric testing as a condition of drug approval under existing law.[40]

Patents and Drugs for the Developing World

Activists often target drug patents as a barrier to making lifesaving drugs available in the developing world, especially in response to the AIDS epidemic.[41] Besides the question of making existing, patented drugs available is the question of whether new drugs for health problems in the developing world will be created at all. David Henry and Joel Lexchin summarize the larger system of economic incentives within which patents play a role: "The international pharmaceutical industry manufactures and distributes many drugs, displays generosity in its philanthropic activities, and has an important role in maintenance of manufacturing standards. However, evidence shows that companies have shifted their core activities from discovery and development of innovative drugs to marketing of products that keep profit to a maximum in high-income countries."[42]

As we have noted, the rhetorical shift that occurred when we stopped talking about "patents" and instead began talking about "intellectual property" appears to have been designed to elevate the status of patents as embodying a fundamental human right, and simultaneously to obscure the fact that economists view patents as government interference in a free market rather than as part of the operations of a free market. This rhetorical shift was rejected, however, by a United Kingdom commission studying the relationship between patents and policies toward developing countries: "The [intellectual property] right is best viewed as one of the means by which nations and societies can help promote the fulfillment of human economic and social rights. In particular, there are no circumstances in which the most fundamental human rights should be subordinated to the requirements of [intellectual property] protection."[43] The right to basic health care is, presumably, one of those "fundamental human rights" that should not be shoved aside in the name of the supposed sanctity of patents.

The document that shapes the relationship between patents and health needs in the developing world is the trade-related intellectual property agreement (TRIPS) of the World Trade Organization (WTO). Of particular concern was a statement from a ministerial meeting in November 2001 in Doha, Qatar (the "Doha Declaration"). Henry and Lexchin summarize the Doha declaration as affirming that TRIPS should not be interpreted so as to threaten basic public health and access to drugs. Nations can declare a public health emergency, in which case they can issue compulsory licenses for a patent-protected drug to be manufactured by the lowest generic bidder. Henry and Lexchin conclude by calling for "widespread voluntary licensing arrangements with the growing number of pharmaceutical companies in developing countries and freer trade between countries with varying amounts of manufacturing capacity."[44] Their call for voluntary approaches seems to be predicated on TRIPS allowing compulsory licensing in emergency cases.

Why would drug companies agree to voluntary licensing arrangements? The experience with AIDS drugs in South Africa, and with eflornithine for sleeping sickness, would suggest that a major factor is bad publicity. Companies do not wish to be portrayed as fat cats sitting on huge piles of profits while thousands of Africans die for want of their drugs—or, in the eflornithine case, that a company is willing to manufacture a drug to sell in rich countries to remove unsightly facial hair; but is unwilling to manufacture the same drug to save the lives of victims of African sleeping sickness.[45]

Fear of bad publicity may be sufficient to prompt companies to manufacture and distribute already existing drugs, but not to discover new, urgently needed drugs. There have been hardly any new drugs introduced for the treatment of such scourges as malaria and tuberculosis in the past three decades.[46] Our proposal for a National Institute of Pharmaceutical Development could address this problem as well. It might be a good deal cheaper to simply pay for this research with taxpayer funds than to try to design complicated incentives to prompt the industry to undertake this research on its own.[47] As Marcia Angell has noted, it is in large part because of various tax breaks showered upon the U.S. drug industry, in hopes of stimulating development of drugs for rare diseases ("orphan drugs") and other public needs, that the industry is taxed at a rate of about 60 percent of other comparable industries.[48] Recapturing even a small portion of the missing 40 percent of corporate taxes would fund a great deal of research into developing-world diseases and treatments.

Henry and Lexchin also mention the need for political action on the part of the major world powers. In recent years, under both Democratic and Republican administrations, the posture of the U.S. government in international trade talks has stressed protecting the financial interests of the pharmaceutical industry. If our government started wielding Teddy Roosevelt's fabled big stick in defense of the health and development needs of the poorer nations, we might see TRIPS in a somewhat different light.[49]

The best-case scenario for the United States, the pharmaceutical industry, and the developing nations is a combination of voluntary activities that provide needed existing drugs at affordable prices, whenever possible by increasing the local manufacturing capacity of generic medicine makers, and that also push the discovery of essential new drugs. The combination of better health of the local population, and increased economic growth through the support of essential local manufactures, would speed the emergence of real markets for U.S. exports in those nations and hasten the day when these countries could afford to pay higher prices for pharmaceuticals. If the pharmaceutical manufacturers are slow to realize that their interests lie in voluntary cooperation, it is essential that the U.S. government back the TRIPS option of mandatory licensing to meet public health emergency needs.

CONCLUSION

We have now reviewed a wide range of reforms, at the levels of both professionalism and public regulation. Skeptics will say that there is no way that all these reforms can be achieved. The skeptic is surely right, that without a great deal of will and energy, both within the medical profession and among the general public, little will be done. We have yet to see whether the "tipping" events of 2004 will galvanize all the parties to a higher level of commitment.

The preceding chapters, however, have explained why nothing less than this full plate of reforms will serve. First, the issues are larger, more serious, and more looming than most of us had realized. Second, the different levels of the problem are intricately interconnected, dooming to failure reforms that address only one level of activity.

We are left with one further criticism. Isn't the most basic problem the industry's reliance on a small number of "blockbuster" drugs to create the great bulk of profits? Isn't the real problem the drug companies' tendency to try to make average drugs into blockbusters? It's not quite, as Dr. Dale Console said decades ago, that the companies insist on marketing their failures. Rather, a successful drug is made into a failure by being promoted for tens of millions of patients when perhaps it really produces a net benefit for a few hundreds of thousands of patients. (Imagine, for instance, if the SSRI antidepressants had been promoted as somewhat safer drugs for patients unable to tolerate the side effects of the older antidepressants, but as generally not superior in their antidepressant properties.)[50]

Would real reform of the industry require that we eliminate the blockbuster system? We will address that intriguing question in a brief epilogue.

NOTES

1. J. Abramson, *Overdosed America: The Broken Promise of American Medicine* (New York: HarperCollins, 2004), 258.

2. D. Baker and N. Chatani, *Promoting Good Ideas on Drugs: Are Patents the Best Way? The Relative Efficiency of Patent and Public Support for Biomedical Research* (Washington, D.C.: Center for Economic and Policy Research, 2002), www.cepr.net/promoting_good_ideas_on_drugs.htm (accessed March 13, 2005).

3. Marcia Angell, despite her largely anti-industry position, agrees with this proposal for predictable patent life; M. Angell, *The Truth about the Drug Companies: How They Deceive Us and What to Do about It.* (New York: Random House, 2004), 247–48.

4. These qualifications, assuming maximal integrity on the part of universities and others, will result in the eventual publication of all trial results; so the real issue is control over the timing of publication, not whether or not it occurs at all.

5. Angell, *The Truth about the Drug Companies*, 240.

6. "For Truth in Drug Trial Reporting" [editorial], *New York Times*, June 20, 2004:12; "For Honest Reports of Drug Trials" [editorial], *New York Times*, September 11, 2004: A14.; B. Meier, "Democrats Take a Look at Drug Tests," *New York Times*, June 23, 2004:4.

7. L. Abboud, "Lilly Plans Broad Access to Results on Its Drug Trials," *Wall Street Journal*, August 3, 2004:B1; G. Harris, "Glaxo Agrees to Post Results of Drug Trials on Web Site," *New York Times*, August 27, 2004:C4.

8. S. Vedantam, "Journals Insist Drug Manufacturers Register All Trials: Editors Say That, Otherwise, Studies Will Not Be Published," *Washington Post*, September 9, 2004:A2; C. De Angelis, J. M. Drazen, F. A. Fizelle, et al., "Clinical Trial Registration: A Statement from the International Committee of Medical Journal Editors" [editorial], *N Engl J Med* 2004; 351:1250–51. See also K. Dickersin and D. Rennie, "Registering Clinical Trials," *JAMA* 2003; 290:516–23.

9. C. De Angelis, J. M. Drazen, F. A. Frizelle, et al., "Is This Clinical Trial Fully Regis-tered? A Statement from the International Committee of Medical Journal Editors" [edito-rial], *N Engl J Med* 2005; 352:2436–39. A few data, of solely administrative interest, are omitted from the list.

10. www.clinicaltrials.gov (accessed March 13, 2005). Others have recommended the World Health Organization as the ideal repository of such data; T. Evans, M. Gulmezoglu, and T. Pang, "Registering Clinical Trials: An Essential Role for WHO," *Lancet* 2004; 363:1413–14.

11. Angell, *The Truth about the Drug Companies*, 244–45, M. Goozner, *The $800 Mil-lion Pill: The Truth behind the Cost of New Drugs* (Berkeley: University of California Press, 2004), 251 (proposing an NIH agency to conduct head-to-head clinical trials); S. Krimsky, *Science in the Private Interest: Has the Lure of Profits Corrupted Biomedical Research?* (Lanham, MD: Rowman & Littlefield, 2003), 229; T. Lemmens, "Confronting the Conflict of Interest Crisis in Medical Research," *Monash Bioethics Review* 2004; 23:19–40.

12. Krimsky specifically envisions university-affiliated scientists applying for these grants. There would be no reason to exclude at the outset applications from the existing for-profit contract research organizations (CROs) and physicians affiliated with them. However, it would seem that the financial incentives that create the profit motive for these organizations would disappear under the new system.

13. Because of the sweeping reform called for by the effective decommercialization of so many clinical trials, I have not bothered to review many otherwise helpful reforms that as-sume less of a Divestment Strategy. For instance, the former editor of the *BMJ*, Richard Smith, has suggested that journals simply stop publishing clinical trials. The trials should all be posted on some neutral website, and the journals should compete with each other not to cap-ture the trial for its own pages, but rather to critique and comment on the trial; R. Smith, "Medical Journals Are an Extension of the Marketing Arm of Pharmaceutical Companies," *PLoS Med* 2005; 2:138. Smith also provides further reasons to consider either simply dispens-ing with journal supplements, or else requiring that the journals subject the supplement to the same editorial standards as the parent journal. Without the direct commercial pressure to "spin" research results, these otherwise admirable reforms would seem less necessary.

14. Reinhardt has estimated that an approximately one-half percent tax on pharmaceuti-cal revenues would be sufficient to fund a robust research program on the cost-effective-ness of drugs; U. E. Reinhardt, "An Information Infrastructure for the Pharmaceutical Market," *Health Aff (Millwood)* 2004; 23:107–12.

15. Fischer and Avorn estimate, for instance, that if all prescriptions written for antihy-pertensive drugs today were in concordance with evidence-based guidelines, the savings to government programs in the United States would be at least $1.2 billion; M. A. Fischer and J. Avorn, "Economic Implications of Evidence-based Prescribing for Hypertension: Can Better Care Cost Less?" *JAMA* 2004; 291:1850–56. This argues for physician compliance with existing guidelines rather than new drug trials to develop new guidelines; but hyper-tension is one of the relatively few areas where extensive head-to-head trials have already been conducted.

16. These figures are the result of an unpublished fiscal analysis of the interface between medicine and the pharmaceutical industry that I prepared along with John Goddeeris, An-drew Hogan, and Anders Kelto. More detailed analyses are provided in previous chapters on the specific topics.

17. For the $500 billion total, see A. Berenson, "Bad Medicine for Pillmakers: Pricey Drug Trials Turn Up Few New Blockbusters," *New York Times*, December 18, 2004:A1.

18. I am indebted to Dr. Peter Mansfield, of the Healthy Skepticism project in Australia, for even more optimistic projections—that the industry devotes about 10 percent of its

revenues to research and 30 percent to marketing, so that all these funds could be captured and reallocated to better ways of serving the health of the public independent of commercial bias. Imagining that only half of the relevant funds could effectively be reallocated, this would still amount to $100 billion in the United States—more than three times the current budget for the NIH.

19. D. Willman, "The National Institutes of Health: Public Servant or Private Marketer?" *Los Angeles Times*, December 22, 2004:A1, A26–A29; D. Willman, "Records of Payments to NIH Staff Sought," *Los Angeles Times*, December 9, 2003:12; R. Steinbrook, "Financial Conflicts of Interest and the NIH," *N Engl J Med* 2004; 350:327–30.

20. As a family physician I cannot help adding that we could replace these high-profile (as well as high-conflict-of-interest) scientific superstars with the Jerry Avorns of the world, primary care physicians with special training in clinical epidemiology and research methods, who often know more about the strengths and weaknesses of all the large-scale clinical trials conducted in a certain disease than do the principal investigators of trials. These nonsubspecialists are seldom asked today to serve on major panels.

21. H. Moses III, E. Braunwald, J. B. Martin, and S. O. Their, "Collaborating with Industry—Choices for the Academic Medical Center," *N Engl J Med* 2002; 347:1371–75; E. A. Boyd, M. K. Cho, and L. A. Bero, "Financial Conflict-of-Interest Policies in Clinical Research: Issues for Clinical Investigators," *Acad Med* 2003; 78:769–74; D. Blumenthal, "Academic-Industrial Relationships in the Life Sciences," *N Engl J Med* 2003; 349:2452–59; AAMC Task Force on Financial Conflicts of Interest in Clinical Research, *Protecting Subjects, Preserving Trust, Promoting Progress: Policy and Guidelines for the Oversight of Individual Financial Interests in Human Subjects Research* (Washington, D.C.: Association of American Medical Colleges, 2001), www.aamc.org/members/coitf/firstreport.pdf (accessed January 5, 2005).

22. F. A. Chervenak and L. B. McCullough, "An Ethical Framework for Identifying, Preventing, and Managing Conflicts Confronting Leaders of Academic Health Centers," *Acad Med* 2004; 79:1056–61; S. Lewis, P. Baird, R. G. Evans, et al., "Dancing with the Porcupine: Rules for Governing the University-Industry Relationship," *CMAJ* 2001; 165:783–85; M. J. Malinowski, "Institutional Conflicts and Responsibilities in an Age of Academic-industry Alliances," *Widener Law Symposium J* 2001; 8:47–73; AAMC Task Force on Financial Conflicts of Interest in Clinical Research, *Protecting Subjects, Preserving Trust, Promoting Progress II: Principles and Recommendations for Oversight of an Institution's Financial Interests in Human Subjects Research* (Washington, D.C.: Association of American Medical Colleges, 2002), www.aamc.org/members/coitf/2002coireport.pdf (accessed January 18, 2005).

23. Today the University of Toronto leadership claims that it has learned its lessons from the Olivieri case and has created a climate much more friendly toward scientific integrity; L. E. Ferris, P. A. Singer, and C. D. Naylor, "Better Governance in Academic Health Sciences Centres: Moving beyond the Olivieri/Apotex Affair in Toronto," *J Med Ethics* 2004; 30:25–29. Their account, however, ignores the fact that the University suffered *two* scandals in quick succession—first the Olivieri affair, and next the firing (or rather, unhiring) of David Healy to direct a psychiatric research institute. The Toronto defense never explains how, if the institution had learned its lessons the first time around, the second scandal was allowed to occur. On the other hand, Steinbrook credits the university with putting into place comprehensive standards for industry-sponsored research in 2001, claiming that the institution had learned from the Olivieri case; R. Steinbrook, "Gag Clauses in Clinical-Trial Agreements," *N Engl J Med* 2005; 352:2160–62.

24. K. A. Schulman, D. M. Seils, J. W. Timbie, et al., "A National Survey of Provisions in Clinical-Trial Agreements between Medical Schools and Industry Sponsors," *N Engl J Med*

2002; 347:1335–41. A later study, still showing considerable variation in contrast provisions among academic medical centers, is M. M. Mello, B. R. Clarridge, and D. M. Studdert, "Academic Medical Centers' Standards for Clinical-Trial Agreements with Industry," *N Engl J Med* 2005; 352:2202–10; see also Steinbrook, "Gag Clauses."

25. A. Marks, "How Drug-approval Woes Crept Up on FDA: Critics Charge Conflict of Interest in a System Where Pharmaceutical Giants Fund the Regulatory Process," *Christian Science Monitor*, November 26, 2004:2.

26. P. J. Hilts, *Protecting America's Health: The FDA, Business, and One Hundred Years of Regulation* (New York: Knopf, 2003), 280.

27. A. J. J. Wood, C. M. Stein, and R. Woosley, "Making Medicines Safer: The Need for an Independent Drug Safety Board," *N Engl J Med* 1998; 339:1851–54.

28. B. M. Psaty, C. D. Furberg, W. A. Ray, and N. S. Weiss, "Potential for Conflict of Interest in the Evaluation of Suspected Adverse Drug Reactions: Use of Cerivastatin and Risk of Rhabdomyolysis," *JAMA* 2004; 292:2622–31; D. Kohn, "FDA Critics Propose Key Changes for Drug Safety: Independent Review Board, Cutting Financial Ties Urged," *Baltimore Sun*, November 28, 2004:1A. The initial reaction of the FDA was both to defend its present structure and to call for an outside review by the Institute of Medicine; L. Crawford, "FDA's System Works," *USA Today*, November 22, 2004; A. W. Mathews, "FDA Plans Major Review of Procedures," *Wall Street Journal*, November 5, 2004:A3; M. Goozner, "Overdosed and Oversold," *New York Times*, December 21, 2004:A29.

29. J. Avorn, *Powerful Medicines: The Benefits, Risks and Costs of Prescription Drugs* (New York: Knopf, 2004), 179–80.

30. The double standard of the FDA in enforcing conflict-of-interest rules was made plain following the Vioxx debate when Dr. Curt Furberg, an unquestioned national expert on pharmaceutical clinical trials, was excluded from an FDA advisory panel because of an alleged conflict of interest. His sin, it appears, was having been outspoken previously on the need for the FDA to better monitor safety. That, presumably, constituted an unacceptable conflict of interest, whereas lining his pockets with drug-industry money would apparently have been all right; M. Kaufman, "FDA Bars Critic from Meeting," *Washington Post*, November 13, 2004:A5. Relman and Angell have suggested that FDA rules against financial conflicts of interest need to be further tightened; A. S. Relman and M. Angell, "America's Other Drug Problem," *New Republic* December 16, 2002, 27–41.

31. J. Braithwaite, *Corporate Crime in the Pharmaceutical Industry* (Boston: Routledge & Kegan Paul, 1984).

32. Braithwaite, *Corporate Crime*, 15. A great deal of the corporate crime that led Braithwaite to this conclusion involved bribery of foreign government officials, and so at least some might argue that his condemnation has relatively little to do with the state of affairs within the United States. Moreover, at least some of the countries in question have greatly improved their regulatory systems since Braithwaite's study twenty years ago.

33. Braithwaite, *Corporate Crime*, 291–98. Braithwaite also argued that passing tougher laws to regulate the industry usually gave highly paid industry lawyers more opportunities to figure out how to evade the laws; 314.

34. This might have been true when Braithwaite conducted his research in the 1980s; it is much less true today when the Bush administration has deliberately peopled the upper echelons of the FDA with industry-friendly staff.

35. "An Overdose of Ads" [editorial], *Boston Globe*, January 6, 2005:A10. In turn the *Globe* cited Abramson, *Overdosed America*.

36. Abramson, *Overdosed America*, 151–66; Angell, *The Truth about the Drug Companies*, 252; Avorn, *Powerful Medicines*, 288–91 (decrying bad consequences of ads without calling for ban); Goozner, "Overdosed and Oversold."

37. Angell, *The Truth about the Drug Companies*, 250–51; Goozner, "Overdosed and Oversold."

38. However, for the argument that eliminating patent protections for the pharmaceutical industry is pivotal to reform overall, see Baker and Chatani, *Promoting Good Ideas on Drugs*, www.cepr.net/promoting_good_ideas_on_drugs.htm (accessed January 18, 2005).

39. Angell, *The Truth about the Drug Companies*, 248–50. Angell generally provides one of the best overviews of the patent issues for a nonlawyer; see her chapter, 173–92. See also Relman and Angell, "America's Other Drug Problem."

40. Angell, *The Truth about the Drug Companies*, 248.

41. E. Goemaere, A.-V. Kaninda, L. Ciaffi, M. Mulemba, E. t Hoen, and B. Pecoul, "Do Patents Prevent Access to Drugs for HIV in Developing Countries?" [letter], *JAMA* 2002; 287:841–42.

42. D. Henry and J. Lexchin, "The Pharmaceutical Industry as a Medicines Provider," *Lancet* 2002; 360:1590–5; quote p. 1594.

43. Commission on Intellectual Property Rights (U.K.), *Integrating Intellectual Property Rights and Development Policy* (London: Commission on Intellectual Property Rights, 2002), www.iprcommission.org/papers/pdfs/final_report/CIPR_Exec_Sumfinal.pdf (accessed January 19, 2005); quote p. 10.

44. Henry and Lexchin, "Pharmaceutical Industry as a Medicines Provider," 1594.

45. S. Boseley, "Drug Firm Wakes Up to Sleeping Sickness," *The Guardian* (London), May 7, 2001:11.

46. G. Yamey and E. Torreele, "The World's Most Neglected Diseases," *BMJ* 2002; 325:176–77; S. Boseley, "Life: Dying of Neglect," *The Guardian* (London), December 11, 2003:6; T. W. Croghan and P. M. Pittman, "The Medicine Cabinet: What's in It, Why, and Can We Change the Contents?" *Health Aff (Millwood)* 2004; 23:23–33.

47. However, an interesting example of a private (but nonprofit) firm addressing the needs of the developing world is K. Ribbink, "To a Hale Champion," *Pharma Voice* 2004; 4:42–48.

48. M. Angell, "The Pharmaceutical Industry—To Whom Is It Accountable?" *N Engl J Med* 2000; 342:1902–4.

49. Henry and Lexchin, "Pharmaceutical Industry as a Medicines Provider."

50. This general principle that perhaps drug companies make successful drugs into failures by overextending their use will not justify the heavy promotion of Vioxx and the other COX-2 drugs. By all available evidence they were indeed failures at what they set out to do—substantially reduce the risk of gastrointestinal bleeding among patients requiring an anti-inflammatory drug—even though, in the test tube, they appeared to work wonderfully and to rely on an elegant molecular mechanism. It is hard to believe in retrospect that this degree of failure was not evident to the industry even at the time of FDA approval.

Epilogue

INDUSTRY WOES AND
PROFESSIONAL OPPORTUNITIES

This growing gap [between actual scientific evidence and widespread medical and public perceptions] is at the core of the crisis in American medicine. And why are we surprised? The drug companies have no more responsibility to oversee the public's health than the fast-food industry has to oversee the public's diet.

—Dr. John Abramson[1]

"The worldwide drug industry is ailing," reported Alex Berenson in the *New York Times* on December 18, 2004.[2]

The year 2004, as we saw in the introduction, had already seen plenty of bad news for the industry—most notably the SSRI scandal on suicide risk in children, followed by the withdrawal of Vioxx. But those were not the stories that Berenson focused on.

On December 17, three major companies all had bad news for Wall Street. Pfizer, after months of claims that its blockbuster, Celebrex, was safe for the heart (unlike its competitor Vioxx), was forced to admit that it too had found an increased incidence of heart problems. AstraZeneca disclosed that its lung cancer drug Iressa, introduced with great fanfare a year before, did not prolong lives in a new trial. Eli Lilly reported on two patients who had developed severe liver disease after taking its highly touted new drug for attention deficit disorder, Strattera.

Wall Street reacted in typical unforgiving fashion. Stocks of the three companies fell. According to Berenson, the combined market value of the three companies shrank by thirty billion dollars in a single day.

What did all this signify for the future? Berenson noted that for several years, analysts had been warning of problems in the industry pipeline. Older blockbuster drugs were going off patent and becoming available in generic form. Despite the escalating costs of trials to discover new drugs, fewer and fewer new drugs of real value were emerging. The industry doubled its annual spending on new drug development between 1996 and 2003, but the number of new drugs approved by the FDA dropped from fifty-three to twenty-one in those respective years.[3] And, as we have already seen, the vast majority of those "new" drug approvals were for me-too drugs, not true innovations.

The companies were reacting to this crisis by insisting that everything was really all right by marketing ever more heavily the drugs that it had on the market and by raising the prices of existing drugs. In short, they were protecting their profits at the cost of irritating consumers, payers, and well-informed physicians. And now the chickens were coming home to roost.

Worse, Berenson went on, the windfall expected from the biotechnology explosion had failed to materialize. Pharma had looked to Biotech for its next wave of blockbuster drugs. But Biotech had so far produced only sporadic and inconsistent breakthroughs—such as Iressa. The revolution spawned by the new genomic discoveries had turned out to be farther off down the road than most companies had bet on in the 1990s. (And if the Gleevec story was any indication, the results of the new genomic research might be drugs that did a wonderful job for ever-smaller numbers of patients—scientific breakthroughs but marketing nightmares.)

Berenson did not say so, but the situation looked very much as if the industry had simply spent the last several decades picking off the low-hanging fruit. It should come as no real surprise if, following such a large number of impressive drug advances, it cost a good deal more to reach up to pick the fewer and fewer pieces of fruit that were higher and higher up on the tree.[4] The idea that there were an infinite number of molecules out there, all of which were poised to fix some serious ill of the human body without causing dangerous toxicity, was, after all, a matter of faith rather than hard science.

Berenson quoted Dr. Jerry Avorn of Harvard, author of the recent book, *Powerful Medicines*.[5] Dr. Avorn suggested that there was a direct link between the scandals of 2004 and the drying up of the drug development pipeline. Produce fewer new drugs, and the only way to make a profit is to sell more and more of your existing drugs. The only way to sell more is to market ever more aggressively. And when you market aggressively, the last thing you could ever afford to do is admit that any of your drugs have serious risks. He might have added that we had perhaps arrived at the time when a company's leveling with the medical profession about the true risk-benefit profile of any of its drugs was tantamount to slitting its own throat on Wall Street—a terrible catch-22 for any industry executives who wanted to behave ethically.

By many outward signs, things were still in a state of bliss for the industry. Berenson noted that Pfizer stood to report an incredible fourteen billion dollars in profits for 2004 on fifty-one billion dollars in sales. Nevertheless, investors were getting skittish—pharmaceutical stocks as a whole had lost 7.9 percent in value during 2004 after many years as everyone's favorite. Perhaps most important, Berenson was not able to locate any scientists who thought they had any sure-fire advice for the industry, on where and how to look for the next set of blockbusters.

HOIST BY UNDULY HIGH EXPECTATIONS

Marcia Angell told PBS' *Frontline* that the industry today was caught in a trap of its own and Wall Street's making:

> The problem—and this is an interesting thing—the problem is not how profitable is the industry, in a sense. It's how much are the profits increasing, because that's what investors want. The investment market is an odd thing. It doesn't look at what the profits are making. It looks at, "Are they more than they were yesterday? Can I sell my stock for more than I just bought it for?" So in a sense, investors say to the drug companies, "What have you done for me today? Never mind that you pulled in last year 18.5 percent of your sales in net profits. Never mind that. What's it going to be this year?"
>
> Of course, no industry can keep climbing like that. They can't, and they haven't, in the last couple of years. They can't keep going up in these astonishing, stunning profits. It can't be done. But it shows how responding to their investors can, in a sense, put them between a rock and a hard place, and distort what they call innovation, so that it's the very opposite. It's less risky to make an empty "me too" drug than it is an innovative drug.[6]

Earlier, journalist Katharine Greider had written that the blockbuster system, as a way to structure the pharmaceutical industry, would sooner or later become unsustainable.[7] As 2005 dawned, however, it was not only the critics of the industry that were talking about the "dying blockbuster model."[8]

On Angell's view, the industry is in a no-win situation. It can continue its present course, and perhaps bully its way through the next few years—in the process, giving up almost any semblance of true scientific innovation in its in-house research—but will sooner or later run into the brick wall beyond which the public simply cannot afford to pay the ever-higher prices it will demand. Or industry leaders can tell the investment world frankly that the present course is unsustainable and that the large firms must restructure themselves to live in a world of fewer major breakthroughs, less reliance on a few blockbuster drugs, recapturing true innovation in research, and getting by on leaner profits. That way lies plummeting stock prices and hostile takeovers.[9]

One industry game that had traditionally won it fans on Wall Street was the merger game—or as an insider joke had it, "You know you work in the pharmaceutical industry when you've sat at the same desk for four years and worked for three different companies."[10] But when Gardiner Harris of the *New York Times* interviewed industry scientists in the fall of 2003, he was hard-pressed to find anyone who thought that these mergers had improved research productivity. The majority opinion was that the mergers were disruptive and distracting to research staff. Harris also quoted the former CEO of SmithKline Beecham, Jan Leschly, as saying that his company's successor, GlaxoSmithKline, needed five major new drugs each year to sustain appropriate growth, and that at present the company could manage only one per year.[11] If we multiply the number of major drug firms by five, we reach a number of novel drugs that, if they were truly to be therapeutic breakthroughs, far exceeds the number of new molecular entities that the present scientific establishment could conceivably produce; and we would probably exceed any conceivable learning curve of the medical profession to add these new drugs appropriately and with discrimination to its existing armamentarium. We would be back in the post–World War-II drug boom, in spades.

Even at a smaller scale, it is not clear that the industry currently has the capability to make choices that fit with its own long-term interests or sustainability. Pharmaceutical industry analyst Richard T. Evans told PBS *Frontline*:

> Assume that you run a drug company and prices are cut and what you would really like to do, quite honestly, is fire salespeople. . . . There're just way too many salespeople. We're spending as an industry far more on sales and marketing than needs to be done. . . .
>
> The best thing to do, for the industry model, is to pull back sales and marketing 5 percent and spend it on R&D. . . . So, let's say you go ahead and do that, but you move first. This is a marketplace, this market responds to sales promotions. So you cut back your sales promotion first.
>
> Your biggest problem is your competitors have more share voice in the market and more product demand than you do. So, you not only lost price, you lost market share. If you cut your sales force, the market reality is it's a pathway to putting yourself out of business. It is not that the industry loves having a lot of sales reps—I don't know a single CEO that wouldn't prefer to trade salespeople for research. You can't unilaterally disarm.[12]

Richard Schuerger of Campbell Alliance, a management consulting firm, agreed with the notion of a "salesforce arms race," noting that between 1998 and 2002 the average rep was able to complete 29 percent fewer details. But he immediately pointed out the irony that at the same time, companies had seen an 18 percent increase in revenues per rep. Finally he came to the bottom line: "There also is no motivation to reduce headcount in the absence of an alternative, proven selling model that ensures a company's ability to influence target customers as effectively as the current one."[13] No one has figured out a better way to market drugs to physicians.

Small wonder that when the industry magazine *Pharma Voice* tried to get beyond the stresses and scandals of 2004 by pointing out new directions for the year 2005, its commentators seemed equally divided between those who advised taking a hard look in the mirror and trying to get a fresh start, and those who urged continued "spin" by signing up even more celebrity spokespersons to give enthusiastic testimonials.[14]

So where do we go from here?

It is possible, but unlikely, that we will somehow turn the clock back to the 1930s. A large, successful drug company will no longer define itself by a handful of blockbuster drugs. Rather, it will manufacture virtually all drugs that physicians need to practice. It will attract market share based on several factors. It will offer the highest quality drugs—no longer much of a distinction, since the FDA has been quite successful at eliminating impure drugs from legitimate U.S. firms.[15] But the quality of its product will extend far beyond the chemicals it manufactures.

The reinvented pharmaceutical company will be as much an information system as a drug manufacturer. It will in many ways become a pharmacy benefit manager, but without the lack of transparency that currently plagues that institution.[16] From the physician's side, the company is both a source of drugs and a source of computer software that aids in patients' clinical management by matching the individual patient's needs to an evidence-based treatment selection process. From the side of those paying for health care, the company offers price for value. The payer no longer pays for insulin, metformin, or rosiglitazone; it pays for improved blood sugar control and a lower incidence of blindness, heart attacks, strokes, and limb amputations. The company helps the insurer to monitor treatments and patient outcomes so that the results are what both the insurer and the patients desire.[17]

Turning the clock back to the 1930s is unlikely; it is rather more likely that the industry will move in the direction of value-based pricing and integrated information management. Another scenario that appears unlikely is that a new technological breakthrough will appear in the next few years that suddenly increases the crop of low-hanging fruit and leads to another boom in novel drug identification and development. It is no doubt true that there may be some low-hanging fruit (to pursue that metaphor) that we have not yet picked, simply because we did not realize that it was edible; a new scientific discovery may reveal that an entire class of common molecules has therapeutic potential, because we come to understand a method of application that was previously unknown. The key discovery may come from the new genomic science, or it may come from quite another direction.

I don't doubt that eventually there will come one or more breakthrough discoveries that will radically change how we view pharmaceuticals and that will lead to a period of intense development similar to the boom at the end of World War II. My prediction, quite simply, is that no such breakthrough can be conveniently programmed to meet the demands or expectations of Wall Street.

Instead I will offer the prediction, based admittedly on slim grounds, that the industry is bound in the short term to go through a period of hardship and reorganization. This is bad news for investors and good news for the rest of us. A window of opportunity may be created in which the policy and professional reforms I have called for will be facilitated, simply because the status quo is no longer viable, and everyone knows it.

Finally, what about the proverbial six-hundred-pound gorilla—the high price of drugs, threatening to make lifesaving treatment unaffordable for a large segment of the population?

I explained early on my simplifying assumption, that the price of drugs was part of the relationship between the pharmaceutical industry and society, whereas the focus of this book is on the relationship between the industry and the medical profession.[18] I will, however, offer a few closing comments.

The industry informs us that high-priced drugs are actually a bargain. These drugs perform daily miracles in saving lives and promoting health. The drugs save money because they treat patients successfully who otherwise would have required even higher-priced procedures such as surgery or prolonged hospitalization. (These savings, the industry insists, are real, even if no insurance company is able to discern them.)[19] And, of course, the huge profits are all reinvested in research to discover tomorrow's new miracle drugs.

If all this were true, and if we believe that individuals in a rich country like the

United States deserve decent health care at an affordable price, then we would be providing for great public benefits by subsidizing the purchase of drugs for all needy citizens. The problem, then, would not be the industry, but the stinginess of society that refuses to ante up.

I believe that all of this is true only to a degree, and not to a degree that justifies the exorbitant prices of drugs in the United States. If the industry believed its own rhetoric, I would expect PhRMA to support some form of national health insurance. A scheme of that sort would be the most efficient and streamlined way to pay for a universal prescription drug benefit. According to industry arguments, the high price now paid for drugs counts as a great public good, by funding research and protecting the American public from shoddy-quality imported drugs. Since the public would in effect be running the insurance plan, we would expect that any reasonably sensible public would be happy to arrange for drug prices to remain high. How likely it is that this would happen is shown by the fact that the industry lobbies vigorously against any proposal to consolidate buying power within any governmental agency, even in the absence of a universal, national insurance system. The industry's heavy lobbying to prevent Medicare from using its bulk purchasing power to drive down drug costs, as part of the 2003 Medicare drug benefit legislation, is just one example.[20] The industry certainly does not act as if it trusted the American public to believe the truth of its assertions.

The question of how long we are going to be content paying these excessive prices for drugs, then, simply boils down to the question of how long the United States will continue to think that it is unique in the developed world, and that the solution to its health care woes lies with the so-called free market—when all the rest of the world has come to realize that a free market will never guarantee universal access to affordable and decent care, and that the only trustworthy and efficient guarantor is some sort of government coordinating system coupled with a variety of competitive, market-based elements.[21]

In 1961, Dr. Charles D. May warned the medical profession that a serious ethical problem was arising in its relationship with the so-called "ethical" drug industry.[22] In 1974, Milton Silverman and Dr. Philip Lee warned the profession and the general public that the problem was still there and was escalating.[23] We paid no attention.

As the year 2004 drew to a close, medical opinion leaders and journalists were climbing over each other like lemmings to tell us that this problem was serious and something needed to be done right away. Perhaps, it seemed, we were beginning to pay attention.

We do need to do something. "We" in part is the medical profession, which must shoulder the burden of taking back its system of education from commercial influence, and breaking its longstanding addiction to drug company largesse of all forms.[24] "We" is also the American taxpayer, who must accept the fact that if we want scientific, unbiased research and safe drugs, we cannot expect a for-profit industry to foot the bill for us and allow us to enjoy one tax cut after another. We will have to accept the need to fund a major investment in pharmaceutical research and drug safety monitoring, to be sure that it is done in the public interest.

The fact that we have to do something might also be good for the industry:

The pharmaceutical industry is facing the greatest period of opportunity in its history. I submit that . . . with leadership, courage, and a real willingness to implement mean- ingful changes in those practices that lie at the heart of current concerns, the industry can emerge revitalized with its public image restored to respectability. In doing so, the industry can position itself to better meet the challenges of the new millenium and possibly avoid another round of reactive regulatory zeal.[25]

If we pay attention and do what needs to be done, a powerful industry that has always striven toward expanded human health and greater scientific innovation will be freed to pursue those goals.[26] And a worthy profession will resume the place of trust that it must occupy if it is to serve the needs of the sick and vulnerable.

NOTES

1. J. Abramson, *Overdosed America: The Broken Promise of American Medicine* (New York: HarperCollins, 2004), 243.

2. A. Berenson, "Pricey Drug Trials Turn Up Few New Blockbusters," *New York Times*, December 18, 2004. For a somewhat similar assessment, see "Special Report: An Overdose of Bad News—the Drugs Industry," *The Economist* (London), March 19, 2005:89.

3. It is important to recall that this doubling was in the dollars spent on research and development, not on the percentage of company revenues devoted to that purpose. The latter figure, according to sources outside the industry, remained largely unchanged at less than both marketing expenditures and profits. Indeed, it was recently noted that the indus- try paid out more in dividends and stock buybacks than it spent on research; J. Appleby, "Drugmakers Spend More on Dividends Than Research; Payouts, Buybacks Rise," *USA Today*, October 11, 2004:1B.

4. "Research might necessarily be becoming more expensive because the 'low-hanging fruit' has already been picked: Current areas of unmet medical need are increasingly those in which diseases are more complex and more difficult to understand and control, and drug targets more difficult to attack"; I. M. Cockburn, "The Changing Structure of the Pharma- ceutical Industry," *Health Aff (Millwood)* 2004; 23:10–22, quote p. 12. Uwe Reinhardt has also used the metaphor "low-hanging fruit" to explain the decreased research productivity of the industry in recent years; Interview: Uwe Reinhardt. PBS *Frontline*, June 19, 2003, www.pbs.org/wgbh/pages/frontline/shows/other/interviews/oldreinhardt.html (accessed De- cember 12, 2003).

5. J. Avorn, *Powerful Medicines: The Benefits, Risks and Costs of Prescription Drugs* (New York: Knopf, 2004).

6. Interview: Marcia Angell. PBS *Frontline*, June 19, 2003. www.pbs.org/wgbh/pages/ frontline/ /other/interviews/angell.html (accessed December 31, 2004).

7. K. Greider, *The Big Fix: How the Pharmaceutical Industry Rips off American Con- sumers* (New York: PublicAffairs, 2003), 164–65.

8. "The dying blockbuster model" figures prominently in E. Pena, "Sea Change: Turn- ing the Tide: The Product-Life-Cycle Management Wave," *Pharma Voice* 2005; 5 (Febru- ary): 12–25, quote p. 12. See also T. Ginsberg, "Party May Be Over for Big Pharma," *Phila- delphia Inquirer*, February 16, 2005.

9. M. Angell, *The Truth about the Drug Companies: How They Deceive Us and What to Do about It* (New York: Random House, 2004), 234–36.

10. G. Harris, "Where Are All the New Drugs? GlaxoSmithKline's Laboratories' Productivity Appears to Be Getting Worse," *New York Times*, October 5, 2003:BU1.

11. Harris, "Where Are All the New Drugs?" See also S. Gottlieb, "Mergers Won't Cure Diseases," *Wall Street Journal*, July 17, 2002:16.

12. Interview: Richard T. Evans. PBS *Frontline*, June 19, 2003. www.pbs.org/wgbh/pages/frontline/shows/other/interviews/oldevans.html (accessed December 31, 2004).

13. R. Schuerger, "The Salesforce Arms Race," *Pharma Voice* 2004; 4 (December): 60–61, quote p. 61. For anecdotal evidence of a recent physician backlash, with more physicians cutting back or refusing to see reps based on the sheer competition for face time, see B. Japsen, "Drug Sales Calls Wear on Doctors: Surge Prompts Some to Limit, End Access; Skepticism Grows," *Chicago Tribune*, May 8, 2005. Japsen noted that both Pfizer and Merck, based on feedback from the field, were planning to reduce the number of reps' calls on physicians.

14. "Year in Preview: 2005," *Pharma Voice* 2004; 4 (December). At the time, Lance Armstrong was one of the most frequently seen celebrities, telling every TV viewer who would listen how he owed his life and health to the industry.

15. The FDA has not been quite so effective in keeping counterfeit drugs out of the U.S. wholesale supply; P. Jaret, "Fake Drugs, Real Threats: Seizure of Counterfeit Medicines and Arrests on the Rise, Causing New Concerns," *Los Angeles Times*, February 9, 2004:F1; J. MacDonald, "FDA Still Balking at 1988 Drug Law, Tool to Fight Counterfeiting of Medicine Still in Limbo," *Hartford Courant*, February 1, 2004:A1.

16. B. Martinez, "Two Hats: Firms Paid to Trim Drug Costs Also Toil for Drug Makers," *Wall Street Journal*, August 14, 2002:A1; C. T. Zaneski, "Drug Brokers Scrutinized Costs," *Baltimore Sun*, April 7, 2004:1A; E. Silverman, "Top Rx Benefits Manager Tied to $200M in Kickbacks," *Newark Star-Ledger*, December 2, 2004.

17. J. D. Kleinke, "Access versus Excess: Value-Based Cost Sharing for Prescription Drugs," *Health Aff (Millwood)* 2004; 23:34–47; A. Towse, "The Efficient Use of Pharmaceuticals: Does Europe Have Any Lessons for a Medicare Drug Benefit?" *Health Aff (Millwood)* 2003; 22:42–5.

18. For a thoughtful ethical analysis of the implications of drug pricing, and a call to view pharmaceuticals as a public good rather than solely as a market commodity, see M. Fisk, "Making Drugs a Public Good," *Pharmaceutical News* 2001; 8:45–52.

19. There are, of course, individual instances in which these savings occur. A $100 injection of sumatriptan for acute migraine headache is a bargain if it averts a $200 emergency room bill. The industry insists that this is true across the board, in which case it would appear that any money-savvy health insurer would be very pleased to pay today's prices for pharmaceuticals and to demand more of the same—which, of course, is hardly the case.

20. D. Gellene and N. R. Brooks, "Drug Industry Scores Gains in Medicare Bill; Pharmaceutical Firms Would Escape Price Controls While Getting New Customers," *Los Angeles Times*, November 26, 2003:20.

21. I cannot of course defend in depth here any proposal for national health insurance. Recent books defending universal coverage include R. Mueller, *As Sick as It Gets: The Shocking Reality of America's Health Care—a Diagnosis and Treatment Plan* (Dunkirk, NY: Olin Frederick, 2001); D. L. Bartlett and J. B. Steele, *Critical Condition: How Health Care in America Became Big Business and Bad Medicine* (New York: Doubleday, 2004). Excellent background materials can be found on the website of Physicians for a National Health Program, www.pnhp.org.

22. C. D. May, "Selling Drugs by 'Educating' Physicians," *J Med Educ* 1961; 36:1–23.

23. M. Silverman and P. R. Lee, *Pills, Profits and Politics* (Berkeley: University of California Press, 1974).

24. Roger Rosenblatt was perhaps one of the first to use the "addiction" metaphor to describe medicine and pharmaceutical freebies; S. Verma and R. A. Rosenblatt, "A Matter of Influence: Graduate Medical Education and Commercial Sponsorship" [letters], *N Engl J Med* 1988; 318:52–54. See also: "Drug-Company Influence on Medical Education in USA" [editorial], *Lancet* 2000; 356:781: "It starts slowly and insidiously, like an addiction."

25. E. G. Koski, "Renegotiating the Grand Bargain: Balancing Prices, Profits, People, and Principles," in *Ethics and the Pharmaceutical Industry*, ed. M. A. Santoro and T. M. Gorrie, 393–403; quote pp. 402–3 (New York: Cambridge University Press, 2005). This volume appeared only after work on this book had largely been completed.

26. In chapter 2, I cited Leonard Weber's book, *Business Ethics in Healthcare*. During the several years that I was working on this book, Professor Weber, my longtime ethicist colleague at University of Detroit-Mercy, was working on his own volume, *Profits Before People? Ethical Standards and the Marketing of Prescription Drugs* (Bloomington: Indiana University Press, 2006). I did not have the opportunity to read his manuscript until this book was essentially completed. The person who reads our two books in tandem, as I would recommend, will be struck by the fact that Dr. Weber and I approached the topic from nearly diametrically opposed positions. I started out as a physician worried about professionalism; Dr. Weber imagined himself a business ethics consultant called in by the pharmaceutical industry to help resolve its present crises. I think it important that we ended up reaching mostly the same conclusions about needed reforms, starting from these divergent places.

INDEX

60 Plus Association, 236

Aachen, Germany, 258
Abbott Laboratories, 69–72, 79, 164n55
abortion, 45n3
Abraham, John, 96n17, 118, 260
Abramson, John, 106,112, 116n38, 233–34, 240, 316, 328, 339
academic detailing. *See* counter-detailing
academic freedom, 101, 307
academic medical centers, 9n15, 14, 69, 74–83, 89, 96n12, 98–106, 119–20, 144, 152, 153, 156–57, 182, 186, 209, 214n40, 244n14, 289, 294, 295, 297n5, 300, 323–24, 328
Accreditation Council for Continuing Medical Education (ACCME), 203–11, 227n14, 227n18, 290, 328–29; guidelines. *See* codes of ethics, ACCME
acetaminophen, 185
acid reflux, 40–41, 62, 92, 202, 232
activated protein C. *See* Xigris
"act of profession" (Pellegrino), 24–26
Actos. *See* pioglitazone
ACT UP (AIDS Coalition to Unleash Power), 261–62
acyclovir, 261
Adams, Samuel, 160n5, 264n9
addiction, 129, 136n25, 184, 254; drug in-dustry influence compared to, 5, 192, 344, 347n24
Advantage trial, 89, 137n40
advertising, 29, 140, 143, 145, 146–47, 148, 149, 150, 151, 156, 157, 163n46, 174–75, 186, 202, 210, 215, 216, 219–20, *219*, 221–26, *224*, 226n5, 228n27, 229n37, 230, 231, 244n14, 249, 250, 252, 301, 311–12, 315n29; by celebrity spokespersons, 234–35, 237, 346n14; direct mail, 145, 146–47, 148, 162n32, 202; direct-to-consumer (DTC), 18, 20, 40, 41–42, 48n37, 107, 142, 189–90, 230–35, 240, 242, 243n2, 244n14, 244n17, 266n55; FDA rules for, 231, 327–28
Advertising Age, 146, 313n8
Africa, 28, 68n35, 333
AIDS. *See* HIV/AIDS
akathisia, 133–34
Albany Medical College, 148
Albert Einstein College of Medicine, 77
Alice in Wonderland, 103
allergies, 18–21
alosetron. *See* Lotronex
alprazolam, 240
Als-Nielsen, Bodil, 128–29
Altman, Lawrence, 225
Alving, Barbara, 33

Florida State University, 77
Floxin, 63
flu, 279
food as gift, 36–37, 44, 169–74, 177, 183,
    193, 200, 203, 290, 291, 292, 295, 307
Food, Drug and Cosmetic Act (1938), 251
Forest Laboratories, 92, 180n32
formularies, drug, 60–61, 62–64, 104, 185,
    189, 236
Fort Wayne, Indiana, 205
Fortune, 142
Fortune 500 companies, 57, 86
Frasier, 237
fraud, 2, 56, 61, 62–63, 115n28, 121–24,
    140, 145, 172, 206, 250
Frazier Healthcare Ventures, 115n22
free market, 45, 46n12, 53–68, 72, 83, 206,
    207, 302, 324, 344. *See also* patents
Freedom of Information Act, 223
Furberg, Curt, 337n30
gabapentin. *See* Neurontin

Galicia, 185
Galson, Steven, 283n32
Garai, Pierre, 163n49
Garattini, Silvio, 91
Garb, Solomon, 148
Garland, E. Jane, 299
gastroesophageal reflux. *See* acid reflux
gastrointestinal stromal tumor (GIST),
    16–18
Genentech, 236
General Electric, 75
General Motors, 65n7, 67n30
generic drugs, 20, 55, 57, 58, 64, 65, 65n6,
    67n30, 69–73, 77–78, 83, 87, 90, 92, 98,
    105, 123, 159, 260, 295, 298n13, 304,
    317, 322, 331, 333, 339
generic names, of drugs, 145, 150, 254, 259
genetics, 69, 73–74, 82, 90, 92, 331, 340,
    343
Geneva Pharmaceuticals, 70–72
George Mason University, 314n24
Georgetown, 251
Georgia, 122–24
Germany, 254–58
Gerstein, Joseph, 60–61, 62
Gestal-Otero, Juan Jesus, 185
ghostwriting of journal articles, 83n8,
    129–35, 136n30, 225, 236, 323

gifts, 29, 37–38, 39, 49n58, 56, 148, 153,
    162n33, 166–67, 169–77, 178, 191,
    192–95, 198n33, 200–201, 205, 216,
    226, 227n10, 288, 290, 291, 294, 295,
    300, 301, 304, 305–7, 308, 312; appro-
    priateness of, 43–45, 182–83, 187–89,
    188, 193, 198n35; compared to bribes,
    151, 187; perceived influence of, 183,
    191; prohibited by anti-kickback laws,
    210; psychology of gift relationship, 44,
    49n58, 174–75, 176, 191, 193, 305. *See
    also* codes of ethics, on gifts from drug
    industry; food as gift
Giles, Thomas, 226n4
Gladwell, Malcolm, 1–2, 8n2
Glassman, Peter, 226n5
Glaxo Wellcome, 206, 237
GlaxoSmithKline, 2, 3, 4, 237, 341
Gleevec, 6, 13–18, 21, 21n3, 22n7, 54, 83,
    90, 92, 94, 318, 340
Glenbrook Labs, 236
Glivic. *See* Gleevec
Global Alliance, 89
Goddard, James, 118, 159, 259–60
Goddeeris, John, 227n12, 315n31,
    335n16
Goldstein, Jared, 167
Goodman, Robert, 114n19
Goozner, Merrill, 21n3, 76, 89
Gore, Al, 75
Gøtzsche, Peter, 127–28
Government Accountability Project, 281,
    284n35
Government Accounting Office, 263
government spending, 292
Graham, David, 277, 280–81, 283n32,
    284n36, 325
Grammar, Kelsey, 237
Grand Canyon, 178
Grassley, Charles, 281
grassroots organizations. *See* Astroturf;
    patient advocacy groups;
Great Britain, 2, 101, 110, 129, 190, 242,
    244n17, 250, 255, 262, 276, 277, 332
Greene, Jeremy, 161n18
Greider, Katharine, 58, 341
Gribbin, August, 193
Griesman, Kenneth, 71
Group Health Cooperative, 109
Gueriguian, John, 276, 283n20

medical devices. *See* device industry
medical education, 143, 144, 181, 192, 202;
as scientific, 144. *See also* academic
medical centers; continuing medical
education; medical schools; medical
students; residents, medical
Medical Education Systems, 117
Medical Journal, 149
medical journals, 3, 4, 29, 40, 111, 118, 127,
129, 131, 132, 136n30, 139, 144–45,
150, 151, 154, 185, 202, 215, 216, 219–
20, *219*, 221–26, *224*, 226n5, 252, 255,
288, 289, 292, 295, 311–12, 315n29,
319, 323, 335n13; reprints of articles
from, 110, 183, 224, 225, 252–53; supplements to, 128, 130, 132, 224, 225,
242, 335n13
Medical Letter, 152, 163n49, 300
Medical Marketing and Media, 229n37
Medical Meetings, 208
medical organizations, 7, 23, 39, 42–45,
150, 151, 152, 204, 212n9, 215–21, 225–
26, 226n5, 270, 288, 297, 300, 310–12,
322–23; contrasted with trade unions,
220–21, 311; dues charged by, 43,
217–18, 227n11
Medical Research Council (Canada), 98
medical schools, 74, 150, 153, 156, 160n13,
203, 204–5, 211, 306
medical students, 148, 151, 187, 192–93,
198n35, 290, 291, 294, 295, 305, 307;
debt load of, 192, 198n31; idealism and
cynicism of, 192; tours of drug plants by,
198n32
medicalization, 42, 240–41, 247n49,
247n53
Medicare, 56, 61, 210, 317, 322; drug benefit (Part D), 236, 238–39, 344
medicine, 23, 139, 150, 159, 166, 333, 345;
business vs., 23–24, 25; demoralization
in, 306, 314n22; goals of, 24–26, *26*; internal morality of, 24–27, *26*; means of,
ethically appropriate, 26, *26*; on-stage
vs. backstage aspects, 5–6, 50n65; as
practice, 24. *See also* physician-patient
relationship; profession
MedVantx, 298n13
MER-29, 253–54, 255, 258, 259
MER-32. *See* thalidomide

Merck, 3, 4, 28, 61, 63, 89, 107, 110,
137n40, 143, 172, 281, 346n13
Merz, Jon, 82
metformin, 91, 343
me-too drugs, 21, 62, 69, 90–92, 151, 301,
318, 340, 341
Michigan Central Railroad, 198n32
Michigan State University, 227n12
migraine headaches, 346n19
milnacipran, 130
Ministry of Health (Canada), 108
Minnesota, 152
Mintzes, Barbara, 232
Misbin, Robert, 276–77
Missouri, 168
Moloo, Jamaluddin, 188
Moore, Joseph, 74
Mora, Marc, 109
Mothers Against Drunk Drivers, 309–10
Moulton, Barbara, 251, 253, 266n48
Moynihan, Ray, 237, 241, 287
muckraking, 140, 160n5, 250
Mundy, Alicia, 270, 273
Murray, E. Joseph, 257

Naprosyn. *See* naproxen
naproxen, 89, 106, 112, 118–19, 137n40
National Academy of Sciences, 259
National Cancer Institute, 76–78, 261,
314n24
National Cholesterol Education Project,
33–34
National Diabetes Study, 276, 277
National Heart, Lung, and Blood Institute,
33
National Institute of Drug Testing (Krim-
sky), 321, 322
National Institute of Pharmaceutical De-
velopment (proposed), 318, 321–24, 333
National Institutes of Health (NIH), 75–78,
79–80, *80*, 85n39, 93, 117, 261, 275–76,
277, 314n24, 320, 321, 322, 323. *See
also* conflicts of interest, NIH guidelines
on
National Library of Medicine, 3
National Pharmaceutical Council, 66n14
National Public Radio, 1
National Research Council, 158
National Transportation Safety Board, 325

ABOUT THE AUTHOR

Howard Brody holds the John P. McGovern Centennial Chair in Family Medicine and is Professor and Director at the Institute for the Medical Humanities, University of Texas Medical Branch at Galveston. Prior to this appointment, Dr. Brody was University Distinguished Professor of family practice and philosophy at Michigan State University, where he also sat on the faculty of the Center for Ethics and Humanities in the Life Sciences; he served as director of the Center from 1985–2000. Dr. Brody completed his residency in family practice at the University of Virginia Medical Center. He received his M.D. from the College of Human Medicine, Michigan State University, in 1976, and his Ph.D. in philosophy, also from Michigan State University, in 1977. He specializes in ethics and the doctor-patient relationship. He has authored five books, among them *The Placebo Response: How You Can Release the Body's Inner Pharmacy for Better Health* (2000), *Stories of Sickness* (2002), and *The Healer's Power* (1993). Originally a native of Chicago, Dr. Brody now lives with his wife in Galveston.